MW00629244

Plays Well in Groups

Plays Well in Groups

A Journey through the World of Group Sex

Katherine Frank

ROWMAN & LITTLEFIELD PUBLISHERS, INC.
Lanham • Boulder • New York • Toronto • Plymouth, UK

Published by Rowman & Littlefield Publishers, Inc.
A wholly owned subsidary of The Rowman & Littlefield Publishing Group, Inc.
4501 Forbes Boulevard, Suite 200, Lanham, Maryland 20706
www.rowman.com

10 Thornbury Road, Plymouth PL6 7PP, United Kingdom

British Library Cataloguing in Publication Information Available

Library of Congress Cataloging-in-Publication Data

Frank, Katherine, 1968-
Plays well in groups : a journey through the world of group sex / Katherine Frank.
p. cm.
Includes bibliographical references and index.
ISBN 978-1-4422-1868-0 (cloth : alk. paper) -- ISBN 978-1-4422-1870-3 (electronic)
1. Group sex--History. 2. Sex--History. I. Title.
HQ21.F766 2013
306.77--dc23

2013009897

The paper used in this publication meets the minimum requirements of American National
Standard for Information Sciences Permanence of Paper for Printed Library Materials,
ANSI/NISO Z39.48-1992.

Printed in the United States of America

Contents

Acknowledgements

Does one dedicate a book on group sex? If so, perhaps an appropriate dedication would be: To those who can't keep to the road less traveled, but veer off into dark alleyways marked "Do Not Enter."

To say that the path to get here has been winding would be an understatement. It was, however, a path with heart, and I am grateful to everyone who supported me along the way. This book would not exist at all if not for a memorable night spent at a pub in Canada with Paul Vasey, at a time when I was struggling with how to move forward with my research on nonmonogamy. Although I might not have been able to do justice to our original ideas here, our conversations were the catalyst for this project.

As this manuscript took shape, Mustafa Emirbayer provided insightful comments on nearly every chapter, helping me clarify my thoughts and contributing greatly to the book. He also reassured me during the writing process when I was overwhelmed, encouraging me to "leave it all on the field" (and then patiently explaining the sports metaphor). He is a versatile intellectual and his enthusiasm for knowledge is inspiring. Michael Bader also provided invaluable comments on the entire manuscript. I am thankful for his wisdom, friendship, willingness to debate, and the critical eye he brought to my work.

Al Gelbard was on-call for clarifications of legal issues in the United States regarding sexual expression and pornography. Pardis Mahdavi and Staci Newmahr responded readily to my questions, and our conversations were as valuable to me as their research. Many other individuals offered comments on sections of the manuscript, and I am grateful for their time and expertise: Paul Vasey, Thomas Foster, Keith McNeal, Dany Nobus, Philip Castle, Ken Haslam, David Ruecker, Tina Davis, Robert Phillips, Michael Bailey, Gary Wynn, Kevin Yelvington, Sir Ivan, and Clayton Barlow.

Because the literature on group sex is scattered across disciplines, I appreciated the many colleagues who responded to my queries—*Did you hear of any consensual group sex when you conducted research in Romania? Cuba? Trinidad? The Democratic Republic of Congo? Kenya?* Many individuals provided leads or answered other questions about their research, methods, or field sites: Christian Groes-Green, Meredith Chivers, Jack Friedman, Jeffrey Mantz, Jafari Allen, and Thomas Strong, among others. My thinking on the issues arising here—pleasure, power, sex, transgression—was also enhanced by conversations with Salvador Vidal-Ortiz, Michelle Newton-Francis, Michelle Carnes, Jane Ward, Susan Frohlick, Ken Zucker, other colleagues, and my feminist theory students at American University. Neil Whitehead was influential in my willingness to more intensely explore the complexities of human violence in sexuality, back when this manuscript was just handwritten notes; many times during the writing process, I missed him deeply.

Some of my interest in how witnessing and being witnessed in transgressive sexual activity became meaningful to people across time and place originated during my postdoctoral research at the University of Wisconsin, Madison. John DeLamater was supportive of my work on sexual exclusivity in relationships and of my quest to broaden my disciplinary and methodological scope. He was also an excellent mentor and role model. Although at that time I did not anticipate writing this book, what I learned about nonmonogamy during those years became the foundation for some of my later questions on the practice of group sex across identities. Our research on sexual exclusivity was funded by a postdoctoral fellowship from the SSRC Sexuality Research Fellowship Program. As the SRFP also funded my dissertation research, I was involved with the program for many years and thus had an opportunity to dialogue with dedicated sex researchers across disciplines. Diane di Mauro, the program head, was also an excellent mentor. Becoming involved with the International Academy for Sex Research (IASR), another interdisciplinary group of scholars, has been beneficial in continuing these conversations.

For the second time in my career, I've written a book where I cannot acknowledge everyone by name. When I wrote *G-Strings and Sympathy* in 2002, it was still relatively transgressive. Some colleagues thought I should not come out as having worked as a dancer until after tenure and some people who provided feedback on the manuscript were worried about being named in the acknowledgments. But by the time that Danielle Egan, Merri Lisa Johnson, and I published *Flesh for Fantasy* in 2006, the dancers who contributed chapters were publishing under their real names—then, it was the customers who used pseudonyms. Times had changed, at least for some. I hope that the same thing will happen again—that people eventually do not have to worry about the stigma attached to their sexual practices, or about the stigma of others haunting them even if they are simply commenting on a manuscript. For now, though, I certainly understand, and am thankful to everyone who agreed to share their narratives with me or provide feedback on sections of this book anonymously, including those on Facebook who responded to my posts and queries over the last three years (*Will you take this online quiz for sex addiction? What childhood "sexploration" games did you play? What makes you feel 'alive'?*)

At Rowman & Littlefield, Sarah Stanton, Kathryn Knigge, and Christopher Basso were instrumental in massaging the manuscript into its final form. If it were not for their attentions and deadlines, I might still be investigating *just one more* fascinating example that should be included here.

My family deserves thanks for supporting me at every twist and turn, even if none of us were exactly sure where I was heading. Of course, so does my husband, who not only offers me the freedom to indulge my curiosity but also eventually asks the questions I should have, but didn't ("What *is* a meat pie?").

Chapter One

The Elementary Forms of Group Sex

August 2010, Black Rock Desert, Nevada

It was a dark and stormy night.
Well, dusty, anyway.
I tightened my fur hood against the spraying wind. Wearing goggles, industrial-strength dust masks, fur bikinis, and yards of pulsating electroluminescent wire to make us visible in the darkness, my comrades and I blinked our way into the wheel of camps making up Black Rock City.

For one week a year during the Burning Man festival, Black Rock City becomes one of the largest cities in Nevada, an intentional experimental community built on utopian ideals and rebellious nihilism. Quite literally another world, the "playa" at Burning Man briefly becomes home to around fifty thousand people. The event engages all the senses: crazy, colorful outfits and gigantic art installations that contrast with the starkness of the desert landscape; smells of dust, ash, and gasoline; scorching hot days and freezing cold nights; incessant music. Groups of citizens explore on foot. Bikes whiz along the curved streets. Art cars, the only motorized vehicles allowed as transportation at Burning Man, inch through the city at five miles per hour— sea creatures, buses, cupcakes, boats. At night, green lasers cut across the sky and lights stretch along the horizon, punctuated by giant bursts of flame.

Like a mirage, the city disappears on Labor Day.

A "temporary zone of altered reality" is an ideal place to be an anthropologist, especially one who studies sexuality. People shed parts of their identities and many of their inhibitions when they step out of their everyday lives. New systems of order and meaning emerge just as readily, although the results are not always predictable.

Tonight, we were on an expedition.

"Not too much farther," I yelled.

The wind whipped at the shelters along our route, pulling tent flaps loose from their stakes. Even the RVs weren't impervious to the driving sand. A sunshade dangled from a silver Airstream. A screen door banged back and forth on a Tioga Ranger; its generator gurgled, faced with a torturous death from dust clogs.

An ancient double-decker bus, lit with orange lights, pumped music into the wind, waiting for visibility to improve.

We were searching for the infamous "Orgy Dome." It was my third pilgrimage to Burning Man and I still hadn't found it. Truthfully, I hadn't even seen much sex yet, though I'd heard the stories: "a bunch of hippies having sex orgies in the desert," "sex, drugs, and house music," "make sure you avoid the orgy tents." I'd happened upon a few BDSM demonstrations and a workshop on sexual technique. A campmate had enthusiastically tested both the Spank-O-Matic and the Orgasmatron—she was always good to have along in the field. I'd seen three people making out on an art car, clothes on, "orgy lite." But not much more. It was unconscionable not to follow up, given my profession.

I was also curious.

As always when one confronts stories of orgies happening somewhere but hasn't personally seen any, one starts to wonder why. Were we too "vanilla"-looking to get invited? Did we not know the "right" countercultural representatives on the playa? Maybe we're not orgy material out here, regardless of how we fare with invitations back in the real world?

Or maybe all the orgy stories were told by hopeful frat boys or paranoid critics?

After all, there's the reality of Burning Man to consider. Playa dust is fine and powdery, but sticky. It gets into every crevice of your camping gear, clothes, and body. No number of baby wipes can compensate for spending a week at a desert rave without running water. Good sex spots are hard to find. RVs and tents offer little space to maneuver for a couple, much less a group. If you crawl into a remote piece of artwork, hoping for a quickie, you'll likely get jumped either by rangers using night vision devices to scout for drug dealers or by a frazzled San Francisco sculptor guarding his creation. And while it might seem intriguing to stage an orgy underneath "the Man"—the giant, centralized effigy that symbolizes, in true postmodern fashion, whatever you want it to and that is ritually burned on Saturday night—doing so will get you a quick trip to jail in Reno.

Thus the legendary allure of the Orgy Dome: a temperature-controlled oasis, sheltered from the prying eyes of the authorities. Towels, fresh water, and double mattresses, trucked all the way from Los Angeles for our orgiastic pleasure—could it really be true?

We were determined to find out.

Why do some people have group sex?

Group sex was depicted in Paleolithic cave art. The ancient Romans are known as much for their orgies as for their aqueducts and bridges. The Egyptian queen Cleopatra supposedly had sex with more than one hundred men in a night—tell that to all the folks who boast of being her reincarnation. The sex parties at the Hollywood Playboy Mansion are legendary, as are the orgies in Hollywood film, from *Ben Hur* to *Caligula* to *Eyes Wide Shut*. The Kennedys are rumored to have hosted sex parties at the Hotel Carlyle in New York City. Contemporary sex parties take place in trailer parks, private mansions in the suburbs, converted warehouses, and luxury hotels from Las Vegas to Venice.

Stigma often befalls those who fail to lock the bedroom doors, yet some people have always defied norms of sexual privacy—fascinating or outraging others in doing so. Based on ethnographic observation, interviews with participants, memoirs, journalistic accounts, academic publications, and personal experiences, this book offers a cross-cultural look at some of the manifestations and meanings of group sex: who has it, how they do it, and *why*.

Such an inquiry requires abstaining from judgment while we journey through the fields of biology, anthropology, and psychology. Keeping an open mind might not be easy at first, as group sex incites responses ranging from fear and disgust to fascination and arousal—sometimes all at once.

Group sex, after all, is *transgressive* (yes, even for those college coeds seeking another girl on Craigslist for their boyfriend's birthday "threesome"). Although anthropologists have identified few, if any, true human universals, taboos are widespread against exposure of the genitals, public displays of sexual behavior, and multiple consecutive partners. Having sex willingly in the presence of observers or with multiple participants crosses a line of social propriety in many societies. Where these lines are drawn is, of course, highly variable. Take the fact that promiscuity for women is fairly predictably discouraged, though not universally forbidden: when former French first lady Carla Bruni admitted to having fifteen lovers before marrying Nicolas Sarkozy, some labeled her a slut. Some found her count remarkably behind the times for a woman of her age. *Only fifteen*? Others—like myself—wondered how impressive her list of conquests might have been if she'd been a bit *more* adventurous, given rumors that she'd already ticked off Mick Jagger, Eric Clapton, Kevin Costner, Vincent Perez, Donald Trump, and former French prime minister Laurent Fabius, along with philosophers, other musicians, and eventually the French president. But in the same country where Bruni was quoted as saying, "Monogamy bores me terribly," poor women from a growing immigrant Muslim population still face threats of beatings, gang rape, and even murder if suspected of impropriety, which might mean simply talking in public to a nonrelative who is male. Regardless of the relative nature of promiscuity, however, having group sex is likely to get one labeled as promiscuous quickly. Group sex also transgresses expectations of monogamy in relationships and prohibitions against public nudity. Group sex participants are more maligned than either the plain old promiscuous or good old-fashioned cheaters because they break so many rules at once and do so in the presence of witnesses.

Of course, in a few times and places, group sex had loftier associations. Links between ritual sex and spirituality have been found throughout history, and words such as "bliss," "passion," and "ecstasy" can describe both spiritual and sexual highs. Ritual group sex, some scholars believe, marked natural cycles and transitions in certain tribal societies, such as when crops were planted or harvested or when couples were married. It was also purportedly used to attract the attention of the gods for favors. Whether these ancient rites were primarily sexual or primarily religious is still debated. Some of these rites must have been more religious than erotic—for example, sprinkling goat blood on the crowd was supposedly customary before orgies at Dionysian festivals. But does ritual animal dismemberment sit well with *your* libido? Some rites sound amusing—imagine dancing drunk around a giant wooden phallus as it is paraded through town on the way to a sex party. If that doesn't make you snicker, well, perhaps your ancestors hailed from Tyrnavos. Some rites seem cruel, even if arguably symbolic as well—as when a young virgin couple in a South Seas community was supposedly chosen to copulate publicly during a giant feast and then ceremoniously crushed under a pile of logs.

Christian authorities eventually clamped down on bawdy European pagan rites—canceling Greek phallic celebrations, banning the creative use of sausages in Lupercalia festivities, and doing away with the ritual sex, crossdressing, and other impieties of Bacchanalia. By the time the church began burning witches at the stake for, among other crimes, dancing "naked, lasciviously," and holding orgies "where incest and homosexuality prevailed,"[1] sex was firmly associated with sin and shame in mainstream religion. Group sex, as we shall see, was thought even worse. Christian missionaries spread these ideas far and wide, so although the older anthropological literature describes a sprinkling of ritual sex practices in places such as the South Pacific, Asia, and South America, contemporary enactments are rare. Sex, and occasionally group sex, remains sacred for some pagans and neo-pagans, and some Western Tantra practitioners believe sexual practices can amplify spiritual experience. Overall, however, sex has lost its connection to the divine in most contemporary organized religions.

One shouldn't forget, of course, that before they immolated suspected witches for their "sinful" and depraved ceremonies, some early Christians had themselves been accused of similar crimes by the Romans, crimes such as holding secret drunken orgies, "involving the most reckless incestuous sex between men and women of all ages" in addition to slaughtering children, drinking blood, and worshipping the genitals of their priests.[2] Groups that challenge mainstream beliefs, whether they are religious or not, may find themselves associated with orgies regardless of the accuracy of such claims. Even today, Wiccans have difficulty dispelling myths that their initiations involve secret midnight sex rites. In fact, charges of orgy hosting go along with all kinds of fearmongering, sometimes used to justify violence or oppression against particular groups. During the genocide in Rwanda, for example, Hutu extremist propaganda featured cartoons of Tutsi women having orgies with Belgian paratroopers and UN peacekeepers.[3] Stories about the customs of the Yanomami Indians of Brazil—including allegations of crazed orgies and bizarre or violent sexual practices—were used to provoke interventions against them. Is it surprising that such stories accompanied the discovery of gold on their lands? Before quite literally losing her head in the French Revolution, Marie Antoinette was charged with losing her marbles in orgiastic excesses. Accusing an enemy of sexual depravity is a long-standing political tactic.

Unless we're talking about children (or teens). The corruption of this particular group often signals the collective failures of a nation. In 2003, a guest on *The Oprah Winfrey Show* described "rainbow parties" to a horrified audience—oral sex parties where girls wore different shades of lipstick and boys collected rings of color around their penises. Commentators jumped on the story: What did this mean about American society? How could the youth of the nation go so wrong? By 2005, however, although admitting that oral sex was growing among teens, sex researchers remained dubious about how many actually participated in such parties. Rainbow parties are now dismissed as an "urban legend" rather than an "epidemic," though the media attention may have given some teens (and adults) ideas. Also in 2005, reports of teens engaging in after-school "daisy chains" caused panic among parents in London. Though the term "daisy chain" often refers to a circle of people performing oral sex on each other, in this context public health professionals used it to denote a wider variety of group sex activities by teens that was supposedly leading to higher incidences of STDs. According to some French parents, British perversity infected their teenagers through a cult television series called *Skins*. The show inspired a series of parties—*le Skins* parties—where the youth "cavort in little more than their underwear" or masks, hold "adolescent orgies," and "lose themselves in sex and drugs." Defenders suggest that *le Skins* parties are "tame compared with what goes on at the *clubs echangistes*," or the swingers' clubs popular with the older generation, and that the teens kiss but rarely go further.[4] Sadly, reports of gang rapes at high schools—such as the 2009 gang rape and beating of a teenage girl outside a California high school while other students watched or videotaped with cell phones—make rainbow parties, daisy chains, and *le Skins* seem downright quaint.

Group sex is often illegal as well as taboo, though restrictions vary. Throughout history and around the world, venues used for group sex are targeted in sex panics. Fears of sexually transmitted disease and crime, such as prostitution or illegal drug use, lead to sex clubs or parties besieged with "cleanups." Such fears—often unfounded—also impact legislation, arrests, and prosecutions. In an infamous raid in May 2001, fifty-two men were arrested on the "Queen Boat" in Egypt, a floating gay nightclub, for "habitual debauchery" and "obscene behavior." In 2010, Ma Yaohai, a college professor from Nanjing, China, was sentenced to three and one-half years in prison for "group licentiousness." His actual crime? Organizing swingers' parties for consulting adults. Of the twenty-one people arrested and charged with Ma, eighteen received jail sentences. Although such punishment seems harsh, Chinese commentators note that Ma Yaohai might have been sentenced to death twenty years ago, when attitudes toward sex were more conservative.[5] In April 2012, eighteen men were arrested in Manhattan Beach, California, in a sting at a public restroom. After police were alerted about "unusual activity" in the restroom, they began monitoring online conversations about the facility, eventually arresting the men on a variety of charges: "soliciting and engaging in lewd conduct in a public place, loitering, utilizing a peephole in a restroom, invasion of privacy and indecent exposure." The men's photos were posted online.

Despite potential stigma and legal penalties, consensual group sex occurs around the world and among people of varying sexualities, ages, ethnicities, and other social distinctions. Some libertines, accomplished at the art of the orgy, have been wealthy, famous, or powerful: Caligula, Hugh Hefner, Silvio Berlusconi. *Bunga bunga, anyone*? Most, however, are not. Some participants are gay, lesbian, or bisexual; many are straight. Though group sex participants may self-segregate based on sexuality, age, race, attractiveness, or other considerations, the link between practices and identities is rarely straightforward. Group sex is something that some people *do*, regardless of what they call themselves. Men who advertise on Craigslist and then meet for late-night sex in a hotel room may identify as gay or straight; some couples at a sex club might identify as "swingers," other people as "open" or "polyamorous," and still others as "just willing to party." Some individuals prefer group sex but rarely have it. Some alternative sexual communities involve group sex more than others. What starts as practice—men having anonymous group sex with men in public parks, for example—can become vital to identity formation. Or not. Precisely *how* identity becomes important in different scenarios and in relation to participants' erotics should be explored rather than assumed.

Sex isn't just sex; group sex isn't just "sex + 1 + 1 + 1."

Bathhouses, sex clubs, and erotic parties catering to gay men thrive in urban areas worldwide, as do those drawing heterosexual couples. "Dogging," the most notorious British sex fad of the millennium thus far, is a form of heterosexual cruising in public parks or large parking lots. Doggers also arrange group sex encounters involving multiple voyeurs and participants through e-mail or text messages; such technologies are well suited to participants' needs for both anonymity and speed, as encounters must be completed before police are alerted.[6] (If you have an Android phone, there's an app for that. . .) One researcher suggested that 60 percent of UK country parks were affected by dogging in 2003,[7] with its popularity growing. American "wife swappers" and revolutionary free lovers of the 1970s have given way to diverse groups of "swingers" around the world. Also termed "the lifestyle," recreational nonmonogamy among couples has seen a resurgence due to the use of the Internet to meet partners and the growth of erotic couples' tourism to places like Hedonism in Jamaica or Desire in Mexico. Not all swingers have group sex—some swap partners and "play" in separate rooms—but many do. "Hotwife" enthusiasts, or men who are turned on by watching their wives having sex with other men, trade stories online and arrange gang bangs at hotels.

Looks like orgies aren't just for the Romans anymore!

Men claim more voyeuristic fantasies than women across cultures; not surprisingly, they are more avid pornography consumers. Studies conducted around the globe also find men fantasizing more about group sex than women and expressing more interest in actually participating in it.[8] Reputable studies of sexual fantasy are lacking in most non-Western locales, however, and comparing sex differences in the desire for group sex is difficult. People sometimes respond to surveys in socially appropriate ways and may be ashamed to even discuss sex, much less admit to transgressive fantasies. A US study found that only 1 percent of women found the idea of group sex appealing compared with 13 percent of men.[9] But when *Marie Claire*, a popular women's magazine, features articles on threesomes, dogging, and swinging, one could say that group sex has an increasing presence in American culture.[10] (Across the pond, the French daily *Le Figaro* similarly reported on the regularity of threesomes among youth and quoted an eighteen-year-old woman as suggesting that threesomes were "a good way of spicing up your love life.")[11] In Pensacola, Florida, a savvy defense team wanted to argue that their client's adult website hadn't violated community standards of obscenity. Using Google Trends, software that analyzes the popularity of search terms, they found that "orgy" was more prevalent as a search term in Pensacola than "apple pie," "ethanol," or "boating"; "group sex" beat almost all nonsexual search terms it was compared with as well.[12]

"Gang bang" porn is a thriving niche in a worldwide industry. In 1995, Grace Quek, otherwise known as Annabel Chong, achieved infamy with the film *The World's Biggest Gang Bang*: she set a world record by engaging in 251 sex acts with 70 men. The competition has gotten stiff (and probably sore), however: Lisa Sparxxx currently holds the world record at 919 men in a single day, a title she claimed at the Third Annual World Gangbang Championship and Eroticon 2004, and Sabrina Johnson engaged in two thousand sex acts during a two-day event in honor of the new millennium. Records are held for the largest transsexual gang bang, gay orgy, all-female gang bang, and "reverse" gang bang (one man with numerous women). Porn waxes creative as well as competitive when it comes to group sex, however. Bukkake porn, originating in Japan but since spreading around the world, showcases group scenarios where multiple men ejaculate on a woman's face or body. Japanese porn directors also bring us "fucking contests," "dildo races," and other orgy-themed game shows. Japan also boasts the record for the largest orgy, a choreographed production of 250 couples copulating in synchrony. The video, *500 Person Sex*, is available online.

Take that, Cleopatra.

Not all group sex, unfortunately, is consensual. Gang rape has been used to control and punish for centuries. Although the last reported incident in the group occurred in 1940, the Mehinaku Indians of the Amazon used the threat of gang rape to prevent women from entering sacred male space.[13] Similar threats, direct or indirect, have been used in the United States to keep women from competing in male-dominated sports, covering news stories in war zones, and attending military academies such as the Citadel. Gang rape is prevalent in prisons around the world. In the United States, a 2010 report suggests that more than one hundred thousand people a year are sexually assaulted in prison; many of these are group attacks.[14] Transgendered prisoners are at an increased risk for gang rape, especially if they are housed according to their birth sex rather than other factors, such as a feminine appearance. Victims may even be punished when they turn to the courts. In some Muslim countries, rape victims can be charged with "fornication" or "adultery" if they are unlucky enough to become pregnant from the assault; male victims can be arrested for homosexuality. In 2007, a nineteen-year-old woman was gang raped in Saudi Arabia for meeting with a man who was not her relative. Though her seven rapists were given prison time, the victim was also sent to jail and given up to two hundred lashes. After the violence of the 1990s in the former Yugoslavia, mass rape was successfully prosecuted as an act of genocide, although gang rape has occurred in warfare for centuries.

At the same time as violent group sex can maintain order by establishing hierarchies or enforcing the status quo, out-of-control group sex—the stereotypical, excessive *orgy* depicted in Western literature and film—is associated with both individual and social breakdown. Aldous Huxley's *Brave New World* ends with a scene of frenzied sex and violence while the crowd chants, "Orgy-porgy, orgy-porgy." One of the most scrutinized scenes of Stanley

Kubrick's 1999 film, *Eyes Wide Shut*, is the orgy scene of masked participants, which ends in the murder of one of the prostitutes involved. It is impossible to forget the literary (and real) orgies of the Marquis de Sade, which he explicitly invests with revolutionary—and cautionary—meaning. Orgies, it seems, rarely end well. Losing control sexually is believed to have a domino effect on one's individual morality and sense of self as well as on society as a whole.

Something far more significant than "boot knocking" is going on here.

Still, there isn't a lot of information to be found about group sex if you want more than titillation or advice on where to find it. *Gang Bangs and Group Sex* is a collection of "true submitted tales of orgies, gang bangs, groups, public sex, incestuous parties, and many other taboo and exotic erotic events." (It comes in a Kindle version, better for those reading on airplanes.) If you don't know the "ten commandments of orgies," you can pick up *Sex Parties 101* or *Nina Hartley's Guide to the Perfect Orgy*. Don't forget, you probably need a date if you've managed to score an invitation: you might want to buy *Getting Your Wife or Girlfriend to Become a Swinger*. If you're a gay guy looking for group action, there are dozens of books and websites to help you find it: check out the *Spartacus International Sauna Guide & Bathhouses*, which has a multilingual edition.

Yet academics have barely touched the subject of consensual group sex since the 1970s publication of a book called—you guessed it—*Group Sex*, which was actually about swingers. Searching for "orgy" in the academic literature will find it used metaphorically as an example of out-of-control excess or in reference to a scene in a film or work of literature; only rarely will it refer to sexual activity. Group sex is sometimes brought up as a form of risky sexual behavior in the context of the HIV crisis, particularly for gay men. Research on contemporary heterosexual "swingers" focuses more often on the cerebral aspects of the topic—jealousy in couples or negotiations between participants, for example—than on what people are doing with their bodies.

But what *are* people doing?

Let's take a tour—quick, before someone shuts us down.

The journey begins with the symbolism of "orgies," looking at historical accounts, art, and literature, from the ruins of Pompeii to the beaches of Tahiti, and then moves on to examine group sex practices around the globe. Violent group sex is explored: "jackrolling" in South Africa, mass wartime rape in Bosnia, and group assaults on college campuses. Recreational group sex participants appear as well, from individuals who use Craigslist Casual Encounters to lifestyle couples looking for a "rock star" experience. You'll peek inside businesses catering to group sex participants: BDSM clubs, swingers' conventions, and gay bathhouses. You'll hear from people who have group sex and people who wish no one would have group sex. The quest for altered states of consciousness through group sex is investigated, from "sex addiction" to "cosmic ecstasy." Along the way, a series of questions is posed about how group sex dramatizes relationships between individuals and between the individual and society: What can we learn about human sexuality more generally by exploring a form of behavior that is not only taboo but relatively widespread across geographic locales and time periods? How does the human propensity to experience disgust, shame, or guilt affect the meaning of group sex, either as violence or as union? What do our tendencies to both regulate sexual activity and repeatedly break the rules teach us about desire? And why is group sex so emotionally and symbolically powerful?

ANTHROPOLOGY IN THE BEDROOM (AND ELSEWHERE)

I never set out to write a book on group sex.

My original research questions about sexual desire and fantasy first sent me into strip clubs—while working as a stripper—to study the motivations and experiences of the other dancers. But after working in the clubs for a few months, I became much more interested in the regular male customers. Why were these men willing to spend so much money for an interaction ending with a hefty credit card bill instead of an orgasm?

While my approach to gathering data seemed unconventional to some, it was in many ways quite traditional. As an anthropologist, I was committed to participant observation. *Do as the natives do*, the famous anthropologist Bronislaw Malinowski suggested, to truly understand how other people live. His research on Kula exchange among Pacific Islanders, at first glance, appears worlds away from my exploration of why so many married, middle-class men enjoy folding dollars into the G-strings of young women. Yet, at some level, both practices are about establishing identity, forming relationships, displaying status, and acting in ways that feel deeply personal to the individuals involved but are embedded in cultural systems of meaning. How better to understand what people thought they were doing in strip clubs as well as what they were doing without realizing it than to actually participate in those interactions? My questions thus first emerged as I observed strip club "culture" as an outsider, but they were answered only as I immersed myself in that world.

While working as both a stripper and an anthropologist, I learned that many of the committed customers were struggling with monogamy. They loved their partner and wanted to remain faithful; at the same time, their desires for *more*—more sex, more connections with people, more freedom, more understanding—sent them questing into the clubs. This search for more became the basis of my next research project. In it, I explored how people

thought about sexual and emotional exclusivity in different relationships—
monogamous relationships, those where one spouse or the other was secretly
cheating, and open relationships. How did people define "cheating"? Why do
people ask their partners to "forsake all others" physically, socially, or emotionally? In addition to surveying and interviewing couples for this research,
since the mid-1990s I have attended swinger (or "lifestyle") events, parties,
and conventions in the United States, Canada, Mexico, and Europe. Again, I
took on multiple roles: as a single woman, as part of a couple, as a hired
stripper, as a researcher, and as part of a convention crowd. And after a time,
I again "went native" and began negotiating monogamy rather than expecting
it in my own relationships. Sometimes my personal questions aligned perfectly with my intellectual inquiries. Other times, as when I unpacked my
suitcase after an anthropology conference and repacked it for a lifestyle party
in Miami, trading slacks and blouses for shimmering bikinis and Lucite
heels, I was aware of inhabiting two different worlds. Once again, my questions developed out of multiple perspectives: outsider, insider, anthropologist, participant.

My interest in writing this book on group sex was to broaden my analysis
of human behavior. After years of focusing intently on specific communities
and field sites, I wanted to think about sexual practices more generally. I also
realized that because of my experiences as a stripper, in the lifestyle community, and as a sex researcher who rarely passes up opportunities to explore
erotic nightlife, I had developed another unique combination of insider/out-
sider perspectives on a form of human sexual behavior that is not necessarily
rare but that remains a mystery for many: group sex.

So—have I been to a real *live* orgy?

I knew you'd ask.

Yes. I've been to orgies where the rules were strictly enforced, right down
to when one's clothes were removed. I've been to sex parties where nervous
couples huddled together until the wee hours, gulping drinks and wondering
who would make the first move. (Sometimes no one does.) I've been to
week-long events, where parties were interspersed with zip-lining adventures, visits to Mayan ruins, or a group excursion to Cirque du Soleil. Occasionally the participants were famous; sometimes they were stay-at-home
moms, contractors, or schoolteachers. I've gone to house parties, BDSM sex
clubs, swingers' clubs, orgies hosted by movie stars and musicians, and
lavish invitation-only events where potential participants are screened by
existing club members. I've been to parties where the rules of engagement
became more nebulous with each line of cocaine disappearing from the
nightstand, and where group erotics became a way to fight for attention
rather than express desire. (And yes, there were catfights, tears, and girls sent
home in taxis—all the dramatic elements that make you suddenly wonder, at
4 a.m., whether you're being filmed for a reality show.) So I've seen a lot of

group sex. In fact, I've seen so much group sex that I can discuss the weather or the irritations of rush-hour traffic as the action unfolds around me. Nude bodies—even copulating nude bodies—have lost any impact they once had.

But perhaps I am a different sort of person in this regard anyway, as walking into an orgy always sent my thoughts spinning more toward Freud, Durkheim, or Bataille than to sexual pleasure. My curiosity, not my sex drive, stimulated my explorations of human sexuality in the first place. In fact, part of my intellectual fascination with sex stems from the fact that sex is *not* itself very significant to me: I enjoy it but I don't crave it, feel guilty having it, or worry much about whether my fantasies and desires are "normal." I am, however, captivated by transgression. People from all walks of life regularly risk *everything* for sexual experiences—their relationships, jobs, health, and even their lives—and endlessly seek ways to push the boundaries of acceptability. Others never find the courage to explore the things they secretly or shamefully fantasize about and spend their lives struggling to control their sexual desires. Still others choose to explore but live complicated "double lives." I am interested in why sex means so much to so many people and the underlying reasons for cultural and personal struggles over sexuality. And I am also interested in why we are so often told "no" when it comes to sexual exploration.

In some settings discussed in this book, I had firsthand, participant, observer,[15] or research experience. Although I did not anticipate writing this book, my interest in sexuality, disciplinary training in cultural anthropology, and previous use of participant observation as a research tool meant that I paid close attention to details and social dynamics in these settings. My informal observations became important as this project took shape, as did my tendency to analyze my experiences through an academic lens. Thinking about group sex from such an insider's perspective presents an intriguing opportunity. Because sex is generally private, researchers studying sexual behavior rarely observe people in the act. Instead, they rely on reports of what people *say* they do in the bedroom, and as we all know, people don't always tell the whole truth about what they do and why (nor could they if they wanted to, as some motivations are unconscious). But I had the chance to watch and, at least in some settings, ask questions. I developed ongoing relationships with participants involved in different sexual enclaves. My own experiences became a source of questions and information.

As contemporary researchers increasingly study in, or write about, their own communities, questions arise: Where does research begin and end? Which identity—participant or researcher—is most salient in a given situation? How does one write about people, places, and experiences without jeopardizing confidentiality or violating one's personal boundaries? Both to protect the confidentiality of others and direct attention toward a bigger picture, this book is not a "tell-all" or confessional memoir. If an experience is recounted in the regular body of the text or the name of a person, place, or event is presented there, it has been rendered as accurately as possible. Interview material is identified as such, and while these sections are edited for clarity and confidentiality, substantial changes have not been made here, either. These interviewees were men and women of different sexualities, ages, races, social classes, and nationalities, although they cannot be said to be representative of any particular population. The italicized sections are composite narratives drawn from both my experiences and those of people I interviewed over the years. These sections provide sensory details, illustrate themes emerging in the discussions, or hint at the diverse meanings of group sex experience.

Places where group sex occurs are not universally accessible. Women, both lesbian and straight, are usually turned away from bathhouses for gay men, for example, except on special occasions. Single men are not welcome at many sex clubs catering to couples. And despite popular misunderstandings about the inclusiveness of "orgies," invitations to sex parties are not extended to everyone wishing to attend. The interpretations and observations given here thus reflect the privileges and disadvantages of my sex, age, appearance, race, social class, and nationality. Whether or not I had firsthand knowledge of a particular setting, I sought interviews with experts and drew on published scholarly work, which is admittedly sparse. Sometimes I invited people to send their recollections of group sex experiences or drew from published memoirs. Journalistic accounts and blogs also provided information about how group sex is conceptualized, practiced, and policed, although I was limited to material produced in English or that could be translated. These sources allowed me to include relatively recent or obscure events that had not appeared in the peer-reviewed literature, although it is important to remember that journalistic pieces are written with a particular audience in mind; many newspapers, websites, and news blogs recirculate the same stories.

Examples of group sex from multiple countries appear here, although a lack of reliable cross-cultural data makes it impossible to systematically canvass the globe. If a BDSM club in Germany is discussed, the information should not be taken as generalizable data about *all* Germans, *all* people involved in BDSM, or even all Germans involved in BDSM. Further, although many of the group sex participants discussed here are relatively privileged and have access to the Internet as a means of seeking partners or information, this does not mean that consensual or recreational group sex is unique to these populations. Global and local power dynamics affect the stories that can be told about various places and the aspects of sexuality deemed possible and worthy of study. Are there sex parties in Khartoum, for example, that might have been described to balance the discussion of gang rape in Darfur? Just because I have not found accounts of swingers' clubs, bathhouses, or erotic parties in Sudan in the mainstream press or the academic literature does not mean that some people there do not pursue pleasure, adventure, and escape through sex. But in some countries, the legal and religious climate, along with the politics of gender, sexuality, and ethnicity, make it both risky and difficult to conduct research on sexuality. Journalists and scholars may focus on sexual violence, sexually transmitted diseases, or the perils of reproduction because these are serious issues faced by populations around the world, but also for practical reasons—people are understandably reluctant to share their experiences when sex is considered shameful or if they risk criminal penalties. Scholars may also fear being stigmatized at home or in the field. Even anthropologists who have observed, heard about, or partaken in consensual group sex rarely write about their experiences. Because the research on consensual group sex is heavily biased toward the United States, Western Europe, and Australia, I have included examples of violence from these places as well. Such a strategy is an imperfect solution to the problem.

Historical data is also challenging to evaluate. Some accounts of sexual customs in tribal cultures, for example, were produced by missionaries or colonial officers. Although some of these individuals were also excellent observers and ethnographers, others were untrained or primarily interested in controlling the populations or managing public opinion back home. Sometimes, our knowledge of a supposedly customary practice is based on a single description or on retrospective accounts given by community members who may not have even participated (and probably had good reasons for including or leaving out certain details). Thus, while we cannot expect multiple observers to have reported on tribal customs in the 1700s, we do need to contextualize existing accounts and be aware of how they are retold over the years. When it was impossible to verify particular descriptions of group sex using reasonable or contemporary academic standards, or even to trace them back to an identifiable source or ongoing debate, these accounts are usually explored as myth or discourse, as there is still much to be learned from how people talk about group sex.

These are limitations faced in every chapter. Nevertheless, this book offers privileged descriptions of some of the ways people have group sex. Beyond that, I also hope to shed light on some of the *whys*, on the personal and cultural meanings with which group sex is endowed.

MAKING SENSE OF SEX

Why do people have group sex? And what does it mean when they do?

Scientists distinguish between proximate and ultimate causes for behavior. Proximate causes are the closest explanations of a phenomenon; ultimate causes are its underlying reasons. The existence of both kinds of explanation, importantly, invalidates neither of them. Many of us are not aware of the underlying reasons for our behavior, though it is still meaningful to us and to others. Parental investment theory, for example, predicts that women will be more selective than men in their mating practices because their costs of reproduction are greater and the obvious benefits of having multiple partners are reduced. Even if a female mates with one hundred males in a year—or in a day, like Cleopatra or Annabel Chong—she can still only bear one child in nine months. Parental investment theory thus suggests an ultimate explanation for why women around the world generally report fewer sexual partners than men in surveys as well as less interest in group sex. More information is necessary, however, to explain why *some* American women still have more sexual partners than some men, enthusiastically participate in college "hook-up" culture, or refuse to count anal or oral sex as "sex." More information is necessary to explain sexual practices among the Mosou in China, who once celebrated sexual freedom for women but have been harassed by the government into adopting more conservative attitudes.

My perspective on sexual behavior here is multifaceted and interdisciplinary. Human sexuality involves more than a universal drive to reproduce, although it has important biological and physiological components. Patterns of sexual behavior and meaning are shaped by historical, political, legal, and economic factors, cultural values, religious beliefs, distributions of power, gender norms and expectations, parenting styles, and ideas about love, sex, reproduction, and marriage. Parents, consciously and unconsciously, transmit their own beliefs and feelings about sex and those of their culture to their children. Sometimes these beliefs and feelings are contradictory, triggering anxieties and stimulating desires in both unique and patterned ways. Prohibitions against certain desires or acts are generated through individual histories and cultural norms; these prohibitions, in turn, can become exciting—and shameful—to transgress.

Group sex, as defined here, is *erotic*[16] *or sexual activity that implicates more than two people and consists of various possible configurations of participants and observers.* Including erotic activity allows us to sidestep the numerous difficulties with defining sex: Do blow jobs count as sex? What do we call it if a married couple has sex while another couple watches them? Is a public demonstration of a violet wand on a "slave" at a kink venue considered sex? What if onlookers are allowed to participate? All of these activities might be considered erotic—although to different degrees—for at least some of the participants. Because my discussion ranges across place and time, however, I also discuss activities that may not be considered erotic by some or all participants but that still involve witnessing or being witnessed in sexual practices or situations—gang rape, defloration and initiation ceremonies, fraternity hazing, or bachelor parties, for example. Part of the difficulty in studying across boundaries is that setting definitions beforehand forecloses some of our ability to discover what is going on and what any of it means to participants. On the other hand, without an idea of the territory we are interested in exploring, it is tough to come up with even a rudimentary map (or decide when it is time to turn around).

In any given encounter, participants may witness or engage in a variety of activities—kissing, masturbation, mutual masturbation, oral sex, vaginal sex, anal sex, and so on—with multiple or sequential partners. This definition covers orgies, "daisy chains," bukkake, "horseshoes," "circle jerks," and the ménage-à-trois. Some group sex encounters are distinguished by the sexual activities that occur, as when swingers differentiate between "soft-swap" (no intercourse) and "full-swap" encounters or when gay men attend a "jack off" party where intercourse is forbidden. Such distinctions are important to participants who use them to state preferences or maintain boundaries. Such distinctions may also be important to public health researchers or others concerned with counting "risky" behaviors or changing practices. Here, however, it is the "group" aspect that is key to my inquiry.

Cross-cultural research demonstrates that desires for sexual privacy of some sort are widespread among humans.[17] Only rarely is copulation allowed in public with any degree of social approval, for example, during rituals or "moral holidays," such as a fertility rites or festivals, or during aggressive and sometimes punitive displays, such as a collective rape.[18] Defloration ceremonies were occasionally performed publicly before marriage by the bride's relatives or future husband. Some societies require public proof of consummation (and prior virginity) upon marriage, as when a blood-stained bedsheet is presented to family members or religious authorities. Fewer societies require, or allow, witnesses to intercourse itself, however. Some tribal groups purportedly held wedding orgies, where a husband's friends or relatives publicly had sex with the bride. Other societies supposedly had such liberal attitudes toward sex that privacy was an afterthought. Unfortunately, because such examples are relatively infrequent, the same few accounts have been extracted and retold for decades, often becoming both decontextualized and politicized in the process. Sorting out truth from fantasy—or political spin—in such descriptions can be like a game of Chinese whispers.

Privacy is relative, of course. For groups such as the Siriono of Bolivia, for example, privacy was unavailable at night because family members shared tight quarters; appropriate intercourse thus took place in the late afternoons in the forest.[19] Most societies also have norms of discretion, or "social rules against noticing or even discussing specific human actions" that serve as a substitute for, or supplement to, privacy.[20] Young people around the world have sex in cars out of necessity; sometimes the couple in the front seat pretend the couple in the back aren't there. An American teen walking in on his parents having sex would undoubtedly act as if it hadn't happened, although he might tell a busload of friends if he had interrupted two school-mates instead. Specific notions of privacy are also cultural and historical. Modern American ideas about privacy, for example, have their roots in complex legal and political discourses, some of which recognizably emerged during the Victorian era.[21] Discourses of public health and medicine add another layer of meaning: people who seek privacy for acts like urination, defecation, and copulation are considered more civilized, dignified, intelligent, or healthy than those who do not. Even bodily attentions of less consequence, such as bathing, shaving, or dressing, are considered private matters in the United States. A homeless person washing in a public restroom is more likely to arouse disdain than sympathy. The United States fosters a confessional culture with regard to inner feelings, thoughts, and desires, however; many disclosures that Americans readily make—sometimes even on television—violate norms of privacy elsewhere in the world. Still, desire for some level of "protection or escape from other human beings" is panhuman—that is, existing in every human society where conditions permit.[22]

In 2008, Max Mosley, chief of Formula One racing, was caught on video-tape engaging in kinky BDSM with five prostitutes wearing "Nazi" uniforms. The video caused a media frenzy. Mosley sued *News of the World*, the tabloid that broke the story, for breaching his privacy. He had a point. Group sex is not the same thing as "public sex." Although group sex cannot truly be "private," it *can* occur in private spaces such as homes or hotel rooms. The court agreed, and Mosley was awarded $120,000 in damages (although he has not been successful at compelling Google to prevent discussions of the incident from appearing in searches). Public sex, on the other hand, is sex occurring in public places such as parks or nightclubs. Sometimes the presence of witnesses is important to the participants. But other times public sex is dyadic in intention, for example, when homeless individuals have sex in a crowded shelter or a couple have sex in an alley because they find it erotic. In these situations, norms of discretion are usually maintained; that is, unintentional observers avert their gaze rather than watch, masturbate, or attempt to join in.

Some psychoanalysts argue that even dyadic sex comprises more than two people at the level of fantasy. In addition to the couple, for example, sexual encounters could be said to involve each person's unconscious Oedipal rivals and Oedipal ideals—basically, the psychological remnants and elaborations of their parental relationships (or other significant emotional relationships, if we prefer to put Oedipus to rest). And if that doesn't make the bed crowded enough, we could invite the other fantasy figures that consciously, but often secretly, animate any given encounter—past lovers, the partner's past lovers, hoped-for future lovers, and any number of porn stars or celebrities. Some couples fantasize together openly about including others.

But although such complexities are fascinating, the focus here will be on situations where we could actually call for a head count.

My definition of group sex extends far beyond "orgies," as is probably clear. The meaning of the word *orgia*, from which orgy is derived, is "secret worship." Not that historical orgiastic practices were all that secret—Dionysian ceremonies in ancient Greece, for example, reportedly involved public drunkenness and "every aberration of sex, the one leading up to the other,"[23] which sounds more like a scene from MTV's *Spring Break* than a clandestine woodland prayer circle. The word "orgy" implies that sexual partners are taken on indiscriminately, perhaps because participants have lost their inhibitions due to the power of ritual, the use of mind-altering substances (drugs or alcohol), social breakdown, or insanity. It also suggests that participants are all seeking pleasure, which is certainly not the case with violent group sex. Over time, the word "orgy" has expanded to denote unrestrained excess in a variety of forms—gluttony, drunkenness, and even murder ("blood orgy"). Because of these dense historical associations, the phrases "group sex," "multiperson sex," or "plural copulation" are often more accurate.

The term "monogamous" is used here to mean sexual exclusivity in a relationship, rather than referring to a form of marriage where individuals have only one spouse at a time. Group sex is by definition nonmonogamous in this colloquial sense if couples are involved, although not all kinds of nonmonogamy involve group sex. Religious polygamists, for example, may have sex privately with each spouse. Similarly, contemporary polyamorists, who have multiple romantic and sexual partners, do not necessarily have sex with more than one at a time—except on late-night television. Inuit "wife swapping," where male guests were offered a night with an Eskimo's wife in the name of hospitality, or suburban American "key parties" like the one depicted in the film *The Ice Storm* (1997), where the women pull a set of car keys out of a bowl and leave with someone else's husband, are other examples of nonmonogamy that do not involve group sex.

This book does not address the question of whether monogamy is or should be the sexual ideal for humans, nor does it consider whether "swinging," BDSM, or any other practice discussed is good or bad for individuals, relationships, or society as a whole. The focus here is on what people actually *do*. And some people have group sex. Some have a lot of it.

Some social scientists will see an attempt to theorize across practices, places, and identities as being invested with intellectual hubris, doomed to failure. Every concept we attempt to deploy across settings—culture, individual, ritual, and so on—can ultimately be deconstructed. Strict relativists might argue that the meaning of group sex is so different in Tehran that we can't even begin to compare it with group sex in Atlanta. And if we are comparing heterosexual teens in contemporary Tehran and adult gay men visiting bathhouses in Atlanta during the 1970s? Forget it. Certainly, in some ways, this is true. Developing the richest understanding of group sex in either setting requires much excavation, perhaps even years of study. Still, as anthropologists Robert Edgerton, I. M. Lewis, and others point out, a statement of incommensurability is already a comparison. From another perspective, then, it is interesting to explore patterns arising despite the variation. Some of the meanings of group sex overlap from time to time. People have group sex because it *does* things in human societies, and some of those things are similar across historical, geographic, and cultural boundaries. Some of those things are examined here, although I make no claims to have exhausted the possibilities.

Realistically, I am merely shouting out the tip of an iceberg. But, as those on the *Titanic* could attest, sometimes that can be a good start.

Chapter Two

What We Talk about When We Talk about "Orgies"

The orgy breaks all the rules. It transgresses notions of monogamy, the distinction between public and private space, and the idea that sex should be aiming towards reproduction rather than pleasure. It promises multiple thrills. Voyeurism mixes with the opportunity to have every appetite satisfied. There is always more at an orgy. More bodies, more orifices, more positions. [1]

"ORGY" IS NOT JUST ANOTHER WORD FOR GROUP SEX

Sandwiched between pubs, restaurants, and the infamous strip clubs that line Bourbon Street in New Orleans is *Marie Laveau's House of Voodoo*. Tourists buy "spell kits," "mojo bags," and "voodoo dolls," hoping to hex their exes or vex their enemies. The salespeople insist that Vodou is about fostering love and protection, not seeking power or revenge, but the popular conception of Vodou as a source of dark magic and ritual remains entrenched.

And Marie Laveau remains its Louisiana figurehead.

Born in the French Quarter of New Orleans in 1794, Laveau was the daughter of a white man and a free Creole woman of color. She was a Roman Catholic who attended mass regularly, nursed yellow fever and cholera victims, visited condemned prisoners, and worked with orphans. [2] This part of her spiritual life, however, was overshadowed by her decision to become a Vodou priestess.

Blacks around New Orleans had long practiced Vodou secretly. In the early 1800s, however, an influx of Creole planters and their slaves from the Caribbean led to an increase in both practitioners of the religion and its visibility. Laveau held weekly Friday night meetings for followers in her home, drawing on Catholic rituals, prayers, and symbols but also incorporat-

21

ing African dancing and chanting. Vodou rituals, followers believed, allowed spirits to enter the bodies of congregation members, offering advice and granting favors. Laveau gained her powerful reputation, in part, by cultivating a multiracial following, something transgressive for the times. Most of her followers were black, but whites occasionally paid a fee to attend her ceremonies, hoping to succeed in business, politics, or seduction.

In descriptions of her rituals and ceremonies—and their effects—fact and fiction blur. Laveau and one of her daughters, who resembled her so much that they were often mistaken for each other, became known as the "Vodou Queen of New Orleans." Many believed in Laveau's "psychic powers" (though some historians believe that her work as a hairdresser, her networks in both black and white communities, and her observation skills were the real source of her information). Laveau was said to possess supernatural healing powers, use a snake named "Zombi" in ceremonies, and "organize secret orgies for wealthy white men seeking beautiful black, mulatto, and quadroon women for mistresses."[3] According to folklore, Laveau also ran a brothel, influenced court cases, caused the deaths of several politicians, and haunted the community as a ghost.

To the general public, Vodou was both frightening and fascinating. An early account of a Vodou service presented by Creole colonist Medric Louis Moreau de Saint-Mery in 1797 set the tone of descriptions to follow:

> The delirium keeps rising. . . . Faintings and raptures take over some of them and a sort of fury [takes] . . . the others, but for all there is a nervous trembling which they cannot master. They spin around ceaselessly. And there are some in this species of bacchanal who tear their clothing and even bite their flesh. Others, who are deprived of their senses and fall in their tracks, are taken . . . into the darkness of a neighboring room, where a disgusting prostitution exercises a most hideous empire.[4]

Police frequently raided Vodou places of worship during the 1850s and 1860s. Newspaper accounts of the time condemned the "revolting rites" and "unrestrained orgies" of followers. An article in the *Daily Picayune* warned that such mixed-race rituals and the deviant behaviors they fostered were on the rise:

> Carried on in secret, they bring the slaves into contact with disorderly free negroes and mischievous whites, and the effect cannot be otherwise than to promote discontent, inflame passions, teach them vicious practices, and indispose them to the performance of their duty to their masters. . . . The public may have learned . . . what takes place at such meetings—the mystic ceremonies, wild orgies, dancing, singing, etc.[5]

Journalists capitalized on public interest in the "Vodou Queen" and her well-known celebration of the summer solstice at Lake Pontchartrain on St. John's Eve. News stories told of "bonfires, bloody animal sacrifice, savage drumming, chanting, dancing, drunkenness, nude bathing, and interracial fornication,"[6] along with—surprise, surprise—orgies. After her death, the *New Orleans Democrat* described Laveau as "the prime mover and soul of the indecent orgies of the ignoble Voudous." The *New Orleans Times* predicted that her death would be followed by "midnight orgies on the Bayou."[7]

What do Marie Laveau's nineteenth-century Vodou worshippers have in common with Roman Bacchus cult members, accused witches in medieval Europe, and 1960s San Francisco hippies?

They all threw some crazy sex parties.

No—supposedly, they had *orgies*.

They weren't the only ones accused of such antics. Whether Martin Luther King Jr., Marie Antoinette, Grigory Rasputin, Alfred Kinsey, or the sons of Saddam Hussein, accusations of orgy hosting have been raised against certain politicians and public figures. Similar accusations have been leveled at scientists, religious leaders, entertainers, and criminals. Social groups, even whole countries or cultures, have been accused of holding orgies. From the hippies and ravers at Burning Man to the tech-savvy Pokémones of Chile, contemporary youth cultures come under suspicion of encouraging orgies as rebellion or—even more terrifying to some—as an antidote to adolescent boredom. Halloween is still condemned as a pagan ritual by some fundamentalist Christians in the United States, said to involve "sex with demons" and "orgies between animals and humans."[8]

This chapter looks at a few of the many stories about orgies to explore what precisely is at stake in such accusations. What do orgy stories mean? Who tells them, and why?

Certainly, some people who are called out for it *really do* partake in orgies. Some of them even admit it. The Beatles, for example. Charlie Sheen. Dennis Rodman. Dominique Strauss-Kahn.[9] For some celebrities, orgies are a way to display status. For others, that's just the way things are. Vince Neil, lead vocalist for the rock band Mötley Crüe, admits to having lined up "half a dozen naked girls on my hotel room floor or facing the wall," then "run[ning] a sexual obstacle course"—but only when he "really needed a distraction."[10] Like rock stars, politicians seem to have a special weakness for orgies—or, perhaps more accurately, orgies are a weakness easily exploited by political rivals. In 2004, Illinois Republican Jack Ryan was pressured to withdraw from the US Senate race, despite leading in many polls, after his divorce custody proceedings indicated that he had visited swingers' clubs and pressured his ex-wife to have sex in public. (This incident had long-term political implications—Alan Keyes, Ryan's replacement, lost the election in a landslide to Illinois state senator Barack Obama. By 2008, Obama was leaving the US Senate for the presidency. As a friend of mine jokes, "We've had swinging presidents in the past, but Obama may be the first president *brought to us by swinging*.") Members of the German parliament were caught attending sex parties organized by Volkswagen, one of which was described as an "all night champagne and prostitute-filled romp" at a nightclub called Sexworld.[11] Japanese former pro wrestler Atsushi Onita took major hits to his political career after group sex with "a female bureaucrat, a hostess, and a porn actress."[12] (One wonders how they got along.) Even Arnold Schwarzenegger has been rumored to have been to an orgy or two, although during his California gubernatorial campaign he claimed he hadn't done anything so deviant since the 1970s, back when everyone was doing it, and then only while traveling in Brazil and smoking lots of weed, or something like that. We'll get to such real scenes of group sex soon enough. This chapter is less concerned with the truth or falsity of orgy claims than with the underlying symbolism and meaning of orgies.

This chapter, then, really *is* talking about orgies.

So what makes an orgy different from group sex?

Try this: close your eyes and imagine walking into an orgy. What does it look like? Who is there? What are they wearing, if anything? (This exercise works best if you haven't gone to many orgies. If you're an experienced orgiast, you already know the answer to the question.)

People who have group sex know there are differences between what they do and the orgies of literature, film, and the popular imagination. In fact, many will go out of their way to point this out, as "orgy" can be a bad word, used by newbies, gawkers, journalists, and lawyers. What we're talking about in this chapter when we talk about orgies, then, are the layers of history, images, beliefs, and fantasies that color our understanding of group sex whether or not we have actually participated in or witnessed it. After all, the details of the orgy you just imagined may or may not have a basis in reality. They might come from film and literature, history books or an anthropology course, the media, or whispers about what "some people" do. Hearsay. Speculation. Imagination.

What does the orgy symbolize when you peel apart the layers?

Let's start with the Romans—even though they'd probably blame it all on the Greeks.

ROME: LAND OF THE ORGY

Ancient Romans contributed greatly to the development of Western civilization. They accomplished feats in civil and military engineering: well-designed bridges, paved roads, and underground aqueducts, to name just a few. Leaving aside the question of whether lead from the pipes used in the aqueducts leached into the drinking water, causing rampant insanity among the upper classes, we can also certainly credit the Romans with influencing European legal systems, developing those fancy Roman numerals, and bequeathing Latin to the world, a form of torture still inflicted on high-school students today.

So, how about those orgies?

You'd know a Roman orgy if you saw (or imagined) one: jovial, toga-clad guests; banquet tables piled with fruit and delicacies such as peacock brains or sow udders; a magnificent roasted pig, apple in mouth, at the center of the feast; jugs of wine; golden loaves of bread. Guests drying their hands on the long hair of the slave boys, who are offered as party favors at the end of the night. Beautiful entertainers who might be executed at the whim of the emperor. As guests become increasingly intoxicated, they shed their inhibitions like their togas in anticipation of the main course: an evening of decadent, indiscriminate, kinky sex among slaves, dancers, soldiers and their wives, and the sovereigns.

Roman orgies have had as much of a stranglehold on the Western imagination as Middle Eastern harems. Slaves, prostitutes, gluttony, and a thirst for cruelty and blood in the nation's rulers and gods—these elements make for lascivious plotlines. And such tales we certainly have about the debauched exploits of Tiberius, Caligula, Nero, and Carinus. It wasn't only the men, though, who overindulged their carnal desires. The Roman empress Messalina, third wife of the emperor Claudius, was said to have hosted orgies for upper-class women, engaged in numerous affairs, and competed with a local prostitute for the highest number of sex partners in a day. (She purportedly won the contest after taking on twenty-five men, though this paltry number would have her laughed out of the World Gangbang Championship today.)

Roman orgies are not often depicted as religious, despite the influence of Greek mythology on their system of deities and practices of worship. The Greeks are known for some of the first recorded orgies, which were associated with cults and festivals dedicated to the worship of Dionysus, the wine god (who later, in Rome, became Bacchus; occasionally, both are entwined with Pan, the god of fertility). The Dionysian mysteries were secret rituals supposedly meant to return individuals to a more natural state of being and involved drinking, dancing, parades, and sexualized festivities. Volumes have been written on the many celebrations and secret cults associated with Dionysus that spread from Greece to Rome—and further, into Egypt and Asia—before the time of Christianity.

The Romans did not universally embrace Bacchanalia, and in fact, many leaders considered the ceremonies a threat to the empire. Bacchanalia were suppressed by restricting the number of people who could be present at ceremonies and through other formal and informal measures, including propaganda. Livy's *History of Rome*, written sometime between 27 and 25 BC, contributes to the archive of Roman orgy lore. Livy describes secret Bacchic ceremonies involving not only orgies but also torture and murder:

> The pleasures of drinking and feasting were added to the religious rites, to attract a larger number of followers. When the wine had inflamed their feelings, and night and the mingling of the sexes and of different ages had extinguished all power of moral judgment, all sorts of corruption began to be practiced, since each person had ready to hand the chance of gratifying the particular desire to which he was naturally inclined. The corruption was not confined to one kind of evil, the promiscuous violation of free men and of women; the cult was also a source of supply of false witnesses, forged documents and wills, and perjured evidence, dealing also in poisons and in wholesale murders. . . . The violence was concealed because no cries for help could be heard against the shriekings, the banging of drums . . . in the scene of debauchery and bloodshed. [13]

The portrayal of orgies that remains, after many similar accounts, is tilted toward decadence and violence rather than spiritual communion.

The Roman orgy, however, may be as much myth as reality. "There have been more orgies in Hollywood films," classical scholar Alastair Blanshard claims, "than there ever were in Rome." The orgy's "promise of indiscriminate sex," accompanied by images of "elaborate feasting and decadent luxury," has "proven irresistible to countless moralists looking to be appalled and libertines looking for inspiration," although accurate and trustworthy historical references to orgies are lacking. In fact, Blanshard believes the Romans would have been appalled at our image of them. [14]

Blanshard's point is well taken. There are very real limits to what we can infer about the group sex experiences of people living in ancient times. Historical records are incomplete and decontextualized. Because the Dionysian mysteries were part of a secret religion, the uninitiated had little access to details, especially about ritual behaviors. As the Dionysian mysteries spread across the Mediterranean, other cults and practices were sometimes absorbed and confused with one another. With the rise of Christianity, already secretive rites were further driven underground; information about them is thus scarce and of debatable accuracy. So what *do* we have? We can examine artifacts such as erotic art found during excavations of Pompeii. Some erotic scenes painted on urns or mosaic tiles depicted threesomes or larger groups, and others featured heterosexual or homosexual couples having sex. "Gigantic free-standing phalluses" and other "bizarrely erotic objects" such as lamps and furniture resembling genitals or sex toys were also unearthed. To eighteenth-century European scholars, tourists, and art dealers, these items implied that the lost citizens of Pompeii were comfortable with sex, even with "perversions." [15] Still, understanding what such images actually meant is complicated, filtered through the beliefs, fantasies, and expectations of the person making the interpretation. When facts fail, emotion and imagination take up the slack. What might seem pornographic to a contemporary observer could have been fertility imagery, appearing as banal, non-sexualized, or religious to a native. Were these items used daily, displayed in homes like family photos? Or did such pieces signal a departure from accepted social interactions, like the flashing neon nude figures advertising adult entertainment venues today? The giant phalluses depicted on urns and mosaic tiles might have been as unremarkable as Barbie's giant breasts are to legions of children. Perhaps people even responded with humor when confronted with such disproportionate male members. *Hey, you know that if his penis was really that big he wouldn't be able to stand up?* In fact, when archaeologists working in Pompeii unearthed a phallus "eighteen inches long and jutting from a building wall," with an inscription underneath that read "'*Hic habitat felicitas* (here dwells happiness)," they first assumed that the building they were restoring was a brothel. The building turned out to be a bakery, however, and many more phalluses were found in shops around the city, serving as signs of good luck.[16]

One thing seems certain: Whenever humans invent a new communicative or artistic technology, they'll inevitably use it for sharing erotic imagery, whether that means drawing with mammoth blood on cave walls, working with clay, or "sexting" at work.

We can also look to myths, fables, or written texts for clues to what life—and sex—was like for ancient Romans. The *Satyricon*, written by a courtier to Nero named Petronius, is one such relic. (Of course, some will be more familiar with Fellini's scandalous film adaptation of the same name.) Scholars debate whether *Satyricon* was meant as a moral satire or as a critique of particular rulers; either way, it is not an unbiased account of everyday life. So which sections should be considered fact, and which are fiction? Did Petronius really observe an aristocrat serving a pastry fashioned like a roast pig and stuffed with live birds? Did the birds fly madly around the banquet table after the fake pig was carved? Or are these fictional details? Do we trust that his accounts of the orgies are accurate? How do we even know he was invited to any?

Even scholarly texts produced by intellectuals of the time cannot be elevated too far beyond the fictional. Even though Livy was a known scholar whose chronicle of Roman history is believed accurate by many, for example, critics allege that he embellished certain sections to promote his own political beliefs and to please his superiors. Given that historians were executed if the emperor disliked their accounts, this was a shrewd move—but not one that makes for the most reliable work. Similarly, though some nineteenth-century anthropologists described Roman customs and beliefs, many accounts they drew on were collected second- or thirdhand and are as difficult to substantiate as the existence of Pegasus. Sir James George Frazer, for example, whose famous comparative study of religious myth and ritual *The Golden Bough* (1890) is regularly cited as a source of information on ancient Rome and elsewhere, never conducted his own fieldwork. He relied on letters, reports, and journals by missionaries, explorers, or colonizers. His citation practices are sketchy by modern standards. Even in his day, Frazer was challenged in the press for his lack of firsthand knowledge—"An authority on savages. But he has never seen one."[17] Yet the book remains a classic.[18]

Speculating about everyday sexual behavior in the Roman empire from a few provocative etchings or texts is admittedly disingenuous—a method akin to watching a few Evil Angel videos and deducing that American housewives are as lusty and acrobatic as the porn star Belladonna. This doesn't mean, however, that the Romans were "vanilla" in their sexual practices. Some of them probably had orgies. Group sex has most likely occurred in every culture and time period whether such events ended up in the historical record or not. Whether Blanshard is correct about the prevalence of orgies in ancient Roman society is thus a matter for historians to debate.

But what do such scenes of human licentiousness mean to modern individuals? After all, Roman orgies ended up not only in history books but also in the public imagination. Edward Bulwer-Lytton's *The Last Days of Pompeii*, published in 1834, alludes to the "magnificent debauches" of the priests of Isis; while the novel is a warning against decadence, its popularity was in part related to its salaciousness (at least in Victorian terms). The story has been retold numerous times over the years. Fellini recognized this fantasy element to orgies, calling *Fellini Satyricon* (1969) a work of "science-fiction" where we "journey to the past" instead of the future. Roman-style orgies have graced the big screen in numerous other films—*Caligula*, *Titus*, *Eyes Wide Shut*—and more recently have even found their way to television with Bravo's miniseries *Spartacus*. Roman orgies also occupy a vital spot in Western erotic life. Many swingers' clubs host "toga"-themed sex parties, celebrating the legacy of these ancient easy-access garments. In 2002, an invitation-only event in New York City made the mainstream news. Called "Caligula's Ball," the event featured on-premises opportunities for sexual activities and Roman-themed performances—men dressed as legionnaires, choreographed intercourse between "Caligula" and "Drusilla," and the toga-clad hostess riding on a bench representing Incitatus, the horse that Caligula appointed to the Senate.[19] And where would porn be without the Roman orgy? The set of *The World's Biggest Gang Bang* was decidedly Roman, featuring white columns and sculpted urns. Annabel Chong, initially clad in a long, white gown, reclined on a raised settee while dozens of men queued up before her like slaves. Chong, in fact, admits to being inspired by the tale of Messalina.

THE ORGY AS A SYMBOL OF SOCIAL DECAY AND SUBVERSION

Since the eighteenth century, when Edward Gibbon's *The History of the Decline and Fall of the Roman Empire* became an overnight classic, scholars concerned with the stability of civilizations have pondered the lessons of ancient Rome. As one commentator notes: "We have been obsessed with the fall: it has been valued as an archetype for every perceived decline, and hence, as a symbol for our own fears."[20] Theories about what caused the demise of Roman civilization abound: Christian officials wresting power from the emperors, barbarian attacks, heavy metals poisoning the drinking water, uncontrollable economic decline and political corruption, or cultural and geographical divisions across the empire growing unmanageable. Contemporary scholars believe a combination of factors was most likely responsible for changes in Roman power structure, which may or may not be accurately termed a "fall" politically. Perhaps the most colorful explanation for the decline of Roman civilization, however, and one that illustrates how contemporary fears are expressed through fantasies of the past, is that Roman citizens brought ruin upon themselves by embracing an immoral, excessive lifestyle. Tolerance of decadence in any realm, according to this perspective, can spur widespread social degeneration, eventually leading to sexual depravity, insanity, and homicide. Fellini's *Satyricon*, for example, depicts far more than group sex occurring in Rome: prostitution, bondage, flagellation, coprophilia, homosexuality, and sexual slavery. The "fall," here, is a moral one. Regardless of the veracity of such depictions, Rome has become symbolic of the dangers to any society that fails to control the urges of its people.

Worries about outbreaks of orgies among a population can accompany liberalizing social change, from gay men serving in the US military to Bedouin women watching Western soap operas. The archaic Chinese crime of "group licentiousness," rarely invoked in recent decades, became the focus of debate twice in 2010, when it was used to charge individuals allegedly participating in orgies. The first accusation was against Nanjing professor Ma Yaohai, caught organizing swingers' parties; the second was against a seventeen-year old girl videotaped having sex with three men in Guangzhou. Her father claimed his daughter was drugged and raped and that she was arrested when the crime was reported to police. (Incidentally, the men appearing in the video were also tried for the same crime, although most press coverage appears focused on the girl). An eighty-four-year-old legal professor and special consultant with the Supreme People's Court of China, however, defended the charges in both Nanjing and Guangzhou, stating that group sex, consensual or not, "disrupted the social order." Regardless of the circumstances, he argued that such actions caused irreparable damage: "If everyone just does whatever they want, then how should we maintain the normal social order of things?" Concern about the spread of consumer values and other

outside influences on the population has grown as China has undergone a
social revolution over the past few decades. Though many attitudes toward
sexuality remain traditional, a generation gap is widening as younger, urban
Chinese adopt more "Western" ideas about love and sex.[21] The eighty-four-
year-old professor is the proverbial Dutch boy sticking his finger in a leaky
dyke, hoping that cracking down on sex parties (or rape victims, depending
on the facts) can prevent a torrential flood of immoral behavior.

Questionable accounts detailing certain groups' dangerous sexual practices have been used as propaganda throughout history, deflecting attention
from underlying political, social, or economic agendas and from the racism,
classism, and sexism of the day. In this way, orgy stories reveal the fears of
powerful elites, especially fears of "political subversion, resistance and dissent."[22] Religion scholar Hugh Urban argues that many demonized groups,
from ancient Greece to the Middle Ages through the eighteenth century, such
as the Gnostics, Bogomils, and Cathars, were seeking liberation from the
existing social order. Thus, even though many were ascetic or even antisexu-
al, "they were attacked as dangerously subversive, not because of what they
were actually doing—namely, challenging the dominant systems of marriage
and religious authority—but instead for the imaginary crimes of sexual license and black magic."[23] It is also worth noting that the Bacchanalia ceremonies Livy described in Rome were suppressed at that time for political
reasons. Though scholars differ on whether Livy's account is fabricated or
merely exaggerated, some believe the Roman Senate wished to control Bacchanalian cult members not because they actually participated in mass orgies
and ritual murders (if so, how could they have been kept so secret anyway?)
but because of the political challenges posed by their acceptance of women
in leadership positions and the fact that many members were poor or were
slaves.

Similarly, men's fear of women's segregated religious rituals throughout
history led to fantasies of female infidelity, sexual licentiousness, cruelty,
and murder. According to Blanshard, subsequent commentators took these
stories as truth rather than "as the scandalous comic exaggerations or the
paranoid fantasies that they so clearly are."[24] While orgy scenes were un-
common in early European treatises against witchcraft, where witches of
both sexes were figured primarily as sorcerers, later writings homed in on the
"perverse sexuality" of witches. Women joined forces with the devil through
witchcraft, in part, because of their sexual insatiability. Pierre de Lancre, a
medieval European prosecutor under King Henry IV who burned more than
eighty women at the stake, described the witches' sabbat as a ritual where
witches rode on broomsticks, communed with Satan, murdered infants, paro-
died the Catholic Mass, and then socialized in a very particular manner:

Naked witches danced lasciviously, back to back, until the dancing turned into a sexual orgy that continued to the dawn. Incest and homosexual intercourse were encouraged. Often the devil would climax the proceedings by copulating—painfully, it was generally reported—with every man, woman, and child in attendance, as mothers yielded to Satan before their daughters' eyes and initiated them into sexual service to the diabolical master.[25]

During the last two-thirds of the fifteenth century, a huge increase in the number of witch trials leads some scholars to suggest that this later picture of the female witch as a sexual deviant was more disturbing to elites than earlier versions.[26] The threat supposedly posed by witches to the existing social order was then used to incite prejudice and expand state control over certain segments of the population. Beliefs that their form of worship involves secret midnight orgies continue to haunt contemporary Wiccans.

There are more recent examples as well. In Germany during the 1940s, Nazis fought against the "decadence and orgies" of young people who had taken up swing dancing—not swinging, just swing *dancing*—even sending some organizers of swing events to concentration camps.[27] The Mau Mau rebellion of the 1950s in Kenya has been called a "civil war between the rich and the poor." Under Jomo Kenyatta, who eventually became the first prime minister, Kikuyu peasants attempted to overthrow British rule. Instead of viewing the Mau Mau as a political movement, British colonialists termed the uprising a "crime wave," casting the poorly armed rebels as "gangsters who indulged in primitive oath-taking ceremonies, cannibalism, witchcraft, devil worship and sexual orgies."[28] In the United States, revolutionary groups and their leaders have also been accused of hosting orgies. The Black Panthers, a radical African American organization, found their San Diego offices raided in the late 1960s after local police were told they were "having sex orgies on almost a nightly basis." Dr. Martin Luther King Jr. was accused both of being a communist sympathizer and of having orgies with white women. In Turkey, Sunni Muslims have long accused Alevi Muslims of holding orgies as part of their worship, a belief that has fueled prejudice and violence against them. Some rumors about Alevis also throw in incest, pederasty, and murder. Allegations of satanic ritual abuse, including forced participation in brutal orgies, have caused panics around day-care centers worldwide, though the McMartin trial during the 1980s in the United States remains exemplary. Allegations of forcing children and others into orgies have also plagued gay men across the globe.

When youth are viewed as willing participants—using orgies to cure boredom or rebel against tradition—blame is hurled at working moms, HBO, illegal immigrants, or anywhere else it might stick at that point in history. Concern over a younger generation's sexual activity can result when the older generation forgets its own transgressions—or remembers them—and from anxieties surrounding social, political, and technological change. In the United States in the 1950s, particularly in the South and the Midwest, stories circulated about "non-virgin clubs," which supposedly required the performance of certain sexual activities for membership. A non-virgin club in Memphis, for example, was said to mandate that each girl have thirteen sexual encounters; another required male recruits to perform oral sex on every female member. An April 1, 1954, article in *Jet Magazine* warned that sex parties were becoming a "fad" among teens "in virtually every US city." In Danville, Virginia, a group of young white girls were caught "dancing nude and drinking liquor" in a "dirty ramshackle shanty owned by a Negro called 'Sneaky Pete,'" who reportedly held "wild sex parties" for girls in their early teens on a regular basis. The explosion of teen sex was blamed on "the 'smut' trade (lewd pictures)" and "the seeking of new thrills."[29]

Each of these examples is infinitely more complex than can be addressed here. And for every social conflict where accusations of orgy hosting circulate, other instances could be found where orgies do not make even a cameo appearance in propaganda on either side. There are other ways, of course, to denigrate an opposing group and stir fears about social change. The point is that the orgy is a powerful symbol frequently used to express anxieties regarding the development and stability of societies, which are seen as vulnerable to the weaknesses and failings of their citizens and the destabilizing influence of both marginalized internal groups and "dangerous" outside forces.

To understand the symbolic persistence of the Roman orgy, we must explore another type of orgy that persists as a dark fantasy in Western culture—the tribal orgy.

THE SEXUAL RITES OF SAVAGES: THE ORGY AS A SYMBOL OF THE PRIMITIVE

The "tribal orgy" is almost as recognizable as the Roman one: just substitute coconuts for the golden loaves, drums for lutes, and strategically placed palm leaves for togas. Replace the drunken laughter with ominous chanting. And don't forget the gigantic pot, encircled by spear-carrying, stomping revelers, used for boiling any hapless explorers who wander into the ceremony at the wrong time. (Roasting a sacrificial victim for post-orgy refreshment is perhaps the ancestral equivalent of a modern swingers' midnight buffet.)

Like the Romans, "savages" got pretty wild when they had group sex.

Archaeologist Robert Suggs describes ancient Polynesian ceremonies combining feasting, drinking, drumming, singers, "troops of naked girls," and "the fast pounding staccato of broad, brown dancing feet." These occasions lasted several days, culminating in an orgy that would have compared favorably with the best that pagan Rome would offer at the nadir of its decadence. With passions aroused by several days of erotic songs and dances and public ritual intercourse, the population could scarcely be restrained from joining in the festive mood. As a result, most ceremonies ended in a fury of drunkenness, overeating, and pro-digious sexuality in every form known to mankind, so shocking and outraging the tender sensibilities of the early missionaries that they could bring them-selves to refer to them only in the vaguest terms.[30]

Suggs stomachs a bit more description:

> Much of the really heavy drinking done by the adults was done in the spirit of a contest to see who could manage to drink under the table the husbands of the most accessible females and still remain conscious enough to possess the victor's prize. Many such contests soon became sexual orgies, with discretion and custom thrown completely to the winds; wives took lovers right beside their dead-drunk husbands; young boys lured women of their mothers' genera-tion into the bush.[31]

Anthropologist Bronislaw Malinowski writes of Melanesian and Polynesian native ceremonies called *kamali kayasa*, which involved a similar relaxation of customary social rules around sex:

> Sexual acts would be carried out in public on the central place; married people would participate in the orgy, man or wife behaving without restraint, even though within hail of each other. The license would be carried so far that copulation would take place within sight of the *luleta* (sister, man speaking; brother, woman speaking): the person with whom the strictest sexual taboos are always observed.[32]

As in tales of Roman orgies, customary sexual partners were supposedly passed over for those who were normally forbidden or rejected.

The breaking of multiple cultural taboos in quick succession is a recurring theme in writing about "primitive" or "tribal" orgies. In his work on sex and religion, Ben Zion Goldberg spins a story that "man" was born free but ended up in the chains of sexual restraint as social life grew increasingly complex: "sex worship came to break the fetters and, if only for a brief space of time, to bring back to man the freedom that had been his."[33] "Pagan religious rites generally ended in open sex orgies," he writes: "Whatever behavior bonds on the sex impulse existed within the tribe were lifted for the moment. Sex indulgence that was so taboo as to be punishable by death was permitted in religious worship and was entered into with a vengeance."[34] The more strict a society was in regulating sex, he argues, the more likely it was that relig-ious rites could lead to an orgy; once uninhibited sex broke out, violence could follow. The Oraons of Bengal, Goldberg writes, performed a ritual remarriage of the village priest and his wife, after which they indulged in the "wildest orgies with the sole object of making mother earth fruitful." The Tarahumare of Southwest Mexico and Nicaragua, a group he describes as "peaceful, orderly and reserved," drank "testivo" during religious ceremonies: "as the intoxicant was becoming effective, men and women entered into open promiscuous sexual relationship in which they engaged until well nigh dawn." (They still observed incest taboos, he notes, despite the "debauch").[35] He describes Mayday celebrations in England; one "credible" source from 1553 reports "of forty, three score, or a hundred maidens going to the wood overnight there have scarcely the third part of them returned home again undefiled."[36] Early worshippers of Cybele, Aphrodite, Baal, and Dionysus, Goldberg claims, reached such peaks of excitement during their orgies that they lost a sense of reality, becoming impervious to pain, wounding themselves, purposely or accidentally, and even murdering their fellow celebrants.

For the religious historian Mircea Eliade, in "primitive societies" the orgy was a form of "'magico-religious ritual' aimed at enhancing the fertility of crops and restoring humankind to the primordial, unformed chaos from which all life proceeds: 'the orgy sets flowing the sacred energy of life.'"[37] "Unbounded sexual frenzy on earth," he suggests, "corresponds to the union of the divine couple." Ritual orgies were used to avert social or cosmological crises or as part of initiation ceremonies. He invokes many of the same examples as Goldberg but also mentions that the Baganda in Africa and the Fiji Islanders used orgies to mark weddings and the birth of twins.[38] Orgies could produce a regressive state of "biocosmic unity": "Like seeds that lose their shape in the great underground merging, disintegrating and becoming something different (germination), so men lose their individuality in the orgy, combining into a single living unity."[39] By "abolishing norm, limit, and individuality," a complete breakdown and regeneration is possible. The ritual orgy is a means by which to move from order to chaos to order.

The breaking of sexual taboos was once again linked to the transgression of other cultural taboos. On occasion, orgiastic rituals allegedly ended with purposeful human sacrifice. Joseph Campbell, for example, discusses a ritual of the men's societies in New Guinea that "enacts the planting society myth of death, resurrection and cannibalistic consumption":

> There is a sacred field with drums going, and chants going and then pauses. This goes on for four or five days, on and on. Rituals are boring you know, they just wear you out, and then you break through to something else.
> At last comes the great moment. There has been a celebration of real sexual orgy, the breaking of all rules. The young boys who are being initiated into manhood are now to have their first sexual experience. There is a great shed of enormous logs supported by two uprights. A young woman comes in ornamented as a deity, and she is brought to lie down in this place beneath the great roof. The boys, six or so, with the drums going and chanting going, one

after another, have their first experience of intercourse with the girl. And when the last boy is with her in full embrace, the supports are withdrawn, the logs drop and the couple is killed. There is the union of male and female again, as they were in the beginning, before the separation took place. There is the union of begetting and death. They are both the same thing.

Then the little couple is pulled out and roasted and eaten that very evening. The ritual is the repetition of the original act of the killing of a god, followed by the coming of food from the dead savior. [40]

Granted, Campbell is interested in the myth being enacted through the above ritual, and he is careful to stress that being sacrificed in such societies is "not what we think." Interpreting such rituals through our own moral lens or cultural beliefs would be a mistake. To prove this point, he uses the example of an ancient Mayan Indian game—somewhat like basketball, but not really—where the captain of the losing team cut off the head of the captain of the winning team on the field. [41]

Perhaps the "little couple" and their families were deeply honored by being chosen.

Still, it is difficult for even seasoned ethnographers to retain a position of cultural relativism in the face of what looks—at least to many of us—more like gang rape, double murder, and cannibalism than Catholic Communion. The historical information that we have is thus often filtered through ethnocentric biases. Eliade, for example, relied heavily on the assumption that "primitives" thought about and experienced the world more simplistically than his contemporaries—a problematic supposition. Western notions of "the savage" are also filtered through fantasies about the sexual lives of different cultural groups. Even without human sacrifice or incest, orgy sex is transgressive from the standpoint of Western morality (and many other belief systems around the world). After all, it involves sex not necessarily tied to reproduction, marriage, intimacy, or even pleasure. Descriptions of orgies in these early texts tend toward the melodramatic: the orgies are "indescribable," "appalling," and "unspeakable."

Suggs, for example, drew on missionary accounts, military reports, and anthropological studies to reconstruct his picture of Marquesan culture before European contact. While he paints himself as a scientific observer and suggests that readers refrain from judgment, his prose occasionally seems equivalent to what you would find in *Star Magazine*. Yet we cannot simplistically assume that such ceremonies—even if they unfolded exactly as Suggs describes—were significant to Marquesans in the same way they would be to his readers. In fact, Suggs admits that sexuality among the Marquesans was much less restricted than in Western cultures. During childhood, Marquesans were likely to witness adults having sex, for example. Young boys and girls engaged in premarital sexual play, occasionally in groups. "Promiscuous girls" who sometimes left their families and moved into vacant houses so that they might more easily have sex were stigmatized but not ostracized. Again, Suggs explains, young men occasionally visited them in groups. Extramarital sex was also common, increasing in frequency toward middle age. Men sought sexual partners "mainly among the wives of friends (many of whom may have been former lovers), promiscuous girls in the community, and younger virginal girls," with whom they took on "the role of sexual initiator." Women, occasionally into old age, also sought lovers "among married males and the young boys of the community." So were they really being "lured into the bush" or was it a less sinister, more playful encounter? The age differences between the "young boys" and women of "their mother's generation" might not have even been great enough to inspire "cougar" jokes today, given that women began having babies shortly after puberty. Extramarital encounters were usually concealed—evoking jealousy from spouses when discovered—but occurred within a tight social network where sexual relations were frequent.[42] Hence, while the "ritual orgies" Suggs described may indeed have diverged from Marquesan behavior as usual, this break with the everyday was likely incremental rather than cavernous. The individuals involved may have already been intimate with each other, possibly already had group sex experience, did not necessarily experience shame around "nudity"—itself a relative state—or sexual behavior, and did not expect strict monogamy of either men or women.

Some reports of orgiastic sexual customs had a basis in reality—the repetition of themes across numerous cultures is indicative of at least a mythological importance to ritual group sex. Some people of every era and nation have also probably had group sex regardless of whether it held any cosmological meaning. As with the ancient Romans, however, we cannot truly know how Polynesians or Melanesians practiced group sex before contact with the Europeans who wrote about them. The European missionaries and colonial agents producing the accounts of tribal customs relied on by "armchair" anthropologists like Frazier were often unfamiliar with native languages. One can imagine the confusion resulting from attempts to understand native kinship systems, which were sometimes based on affinity rather than consanguinity (think "brother from another mother" but with more significance). Certain areas of Polynesia, for example, used a simple classificatory system of kinship that distinguished by generation and gender but not by parental lineage—thus, all females of a parent's generation might be called by the term for "mother" and all males by the term for "father." Some African societies used naming patterns to extend kin relations, so females bearing the same name as one's sister—even from a faraway tribe—would also be called "sisters." Could this be part of the reason that so many horrified European witnesses reported that the "savages" engaged in blatant incest or copulated within view of close family members?

The descriptions of incest, violence, and human sacrifice often accompanying accounts of tribal orgies have undoubtedly contributed to both perceptions of the authenticity of the reports and to their persistent reappearance in art and popular culture—you just can't make that stuff up. Or maybe you *can*: Goldberg conspicuously lacks citations; he is also accused of inventing many of the descriptive passages that made his book so appealing to readers over the years. Similarly, the men's house ritual described by Campbell, which can be traced to a 1928 text on the Marind-anim, was termed a "cock and bull" story in 1966 by Dutch cultural anthopologist Jan Van Baal. The Marind-anim practiced ritual group sex, according to Van Baal, but stories of accompanying murder and cannibalism were likely due to misunderstandings or deliberate embellishment on the part of either the missionaries or Marind-anim.

Unfortunately, some missionary and colonial reports about native customs were fabricated or exaggerated to justify interventions and even violence against native populations. (Even distinctions between cultural groups were occasionally artifacts of such colonial interests.) Appealing to offenses against morality to stir public sentiment against a particular group was as effective then as it is now, perhaps even more so because there were few possibilities for the targeted people to set the record straight, if they were even aware their traditions were being discussed in French cafés or British tearooms. Accusations against individuals, groups, or societies of having orgies can be disparagements of their social and moral development. Carolyn Long, a scholar who researched Marie Laveau's life and legend, sees a political element to the accusations that Laveau and her Vodou followers held orgies. Whites needed a reason to justify slavery in nineteenth-century Louisiana, Long argues, and the supposed superiority of "civilized" whites over "savage" Africans provided one. Instead of being represented as a religion, Vodou became caught up in the politics of the time, associated with immorality, devil worship, interracial fraternization, and, unsurprisingly, sexual deviance.[43] In fact, Moreau's description of the "hideous" orgies of Vodou worshippers—often "accepted as the classic New Orleans Voodoo ceremony"— was actually taken from a history of colonial Saint-Domingue published in 1797. This account reappeared in 1883 in a travel journal published by a New Orleans resident and was then paraphrased and repeated for decades as a true account, even though the details are unsubstantiated and the origin was forgotten.[44]

Further, native peoples were increasingly pressured to adopt the moral systems of their colonizers and penalized if they did not. The sexualized rituals and practices that did exist were driven underground, denied, or attributed to other groups, making it difficult for later researchers to substantiate the details. Unlike Frazer, Malinowski spent extended amounts of time living in the communities he studied. Still, he admitted to never witnessing a *kaya-*

sa or even confirming that one had occurred within the twenty years prior to his arrival, a methodological problem he attributed to the impact of missionaries.[45] Malinowski also found that his informants denied engaging in such behavior themselves; those from the north, for example, pointed to the southern districts as most likely to indulge in such transgressions. *Yausa* was another custom involving ritualized group sex, a violent encounter between insiders and outsiders. If a male stranger passed through a southern district during the "communal weeding" period, he was open to attack by women working in the fields: "first they pull off and tear up his pubic leaf," then "try to produce an erection." If the women were successful in arousing him, they would have intercourse with him, "use his fingers and toes, in fact, any projecting part of his body, for lascivious purposes," and "pollute" him by urinating and defecating on his face and torso. Malinowski was unable to find people with personal experiences of *yausa* and even refers to it as "hearsay." He suspected that *yausa* tales were used by northerners to amuse themselves at the expense of southerners (or vice versa) but nonetheless heeded warnings that "no stranger . . . would dream of going there at that season." He did not follow up.[46]

Who can blame him, really?

Sexuality also plays a key role in the portrayal of the "noble savage," the flipside of the "dangerous primitive" and an idealized image rather than a denigrated one. Early eighteenth-century European explorers initially reported on the "natural," "shameless," and permissive sexuality of the Tahitians, for example. The island gained a reputation as an earthly paradise where nearly naked women swam out to ships to greet explorers and enthusiastically traded sex for nails (one captain reportedly had to take drastic measures to keep his sailors from completely dismantling the boat). Frequent casual sex and even public copulation arises in accounts of traditional Tahitian sexuality, as natives were said to have "gratified every appetite and passion before witnesses."

Yet in addition to the problems of decontextualization, ethnocentrism, and misinterpretation, and as with stories of Roman orgies, accounts of native sexuality can become entangled with political debates—and sometimes those of multiple eras. In his journals, for example, Captain Cook recounts an event that occurred at Point Venus, Tahiti, in 1769, where his team was recording the transit of Venus across the sun. In a passage that has reverberated far more widely than his astronomical observations, Cook described an "odd scene" at the gate of the British fort where a "young fellow above 6 feet high lay with a little Girl about 10 or 12 years of age publickly before several of our people and a number of the Natives." Cook writes that "it appear'd to be done more from Custom than Lewdness" and notes that several observers "instructed the girl how she should act her part, who young as she was, did not seem to want it." After the expedition, Dr. John Hawkesworth was commissioned by the British Royal Navy to transform Cook's journals into an official narrative of the journey. Hawkesworth's description in *Voyages*, which was widely read, differs from the original. The "odd scene" now became a "Divine Service" and an "extraordinary spectacle": "A young man, near 6 feet high, performed the Rites of Venus with a little girl about 11 or 12 years of age, before several of our people, and a great number of the natives, without the least sense of its being indecent or improper, but, as appeared, in perfect conformity to the custom of the place." Hawkesworth also altered Cook's wording slightly, but significantly, around the interaction with witnesses: women of "superior rank . . . gave instructions to the girl how to perform her part, which, young as she was, she did not seem much to stand in need of."[47] Hawkesworth further added a paragraph suggesting that the incident raised a philosophical question: "Whether the shame attending certain actions, which are allowed on all sides to be in themselves innocent, is implanted in Nature or superinduced by Custom?"[48] Some scholars believe that Hawkesworth's changes—increasing the girl's age, mentioning the "superior rank" and "great" number of natives in attendance, and naming the "Rites of Venus" as a "Divine Service," for example—were meant to make Cook's observations more palatable for readers. Nevertheless, Hawkesworth was harassed after the publication of *Voyages* for his scandalous rendering of island life and the questions he raised about morality.

The scene clearly hit a nerve.

Voyages contains hundreds of pages of observations, but the paragraph now known as the "scene at Point Venus" has continued provoking emotional responses for hundreds of years. The passage inspired writers from Diderot to Voltaire, not to mention an eighteenth-century brothel owner named Charlotte Hayes, who sponsored a performance of the "Rites of Venus" for her high-end clients.[49]

Yet although Tahitians certainly had more liberal attitudes toward sexuality than Europeans, painting their culture as a childlike utopia requires overlooking the inequalities and complicated social relationships that existed, both internally and in their interactions with explorers. A divergent historical perspective of the maidens "greeting" the European boats, for example, suggests that Tahitian women offered themselves to French soldiers as a survival strategy rather than out of native "hospitality,"[50] *after* the community had been fired on by explorers. The Point Venus scene, rather than an example of uninhibited, unselfconscious native sexuality, has been alternately posited as an act of obedience to *Ariori* religious leaders who wished to use sex to acquire the "mana" of Europeans or even a satirical dramatization of the first sexual contact between a sailor and a Tahitian woman (which somewhat accidentally took place "completely in the open, the young Irishman concerned being in great haste to have the 'Honour' of inaugurating such relations"[51]). For scholars who return to the original texts, the ambiguity in wording adds to the cryptic nature of the event. Did the young girl not seem to "want" the instruction because she did not desire the sex or because although "young as she was," she already knew what to do? Was this an "odd" scene where "Custom" should be read against "Lewdness" to mean "perfunctory" (without real desire between the lovers), or was it a "Custom" in the sense of being an essential or regular part of Tahitian life? Such quibbles over wording might seem like "nit-picking" if public sex had indeed been routine in Tahiti, anthropologist Nicholas Thomas points out. "But the behavior that Cook described is mysterious," Thomas writes, "and nothing quite like it is ever reported again."[52]

As one historian queries, "What was in that young girl's mind so far away and long ago? What did she really want at Point Venus on 14 May 1769? How can we ever know?"[53] Well, we *can't*. We can, however, inquire as to why the story has been so frequently told.

A complete analysis of the symbolism underlying contemporary Western understandings of tribal orgies is beyond the scope of this book, as it would require delving into the history of European colonization—a time when stories about "natives" began to fascinate "polite society"—as well as the rise of social Darwinism and the development of ideas about race. But what is important here is that orgy stories told over the past several centuries draw some of their meaning from powerful historical distinctions made between "primitive" and "civilized" cultures. Early tales of orgiastic ritual were bolstered by the belief that cultures "evolved" or progressed through the same stages until they finally reached an apex of civilization. That apex, incidentally, looked a lot like Western Europe at the time—although not everyone was equally pleased with it. Other cultures became emblematic of what had been gained, or lost, in this process. "The European view of the non-Western world," according to archaeologist Brian Fagan, "fluctuated throughout the centuries." Sometimes, non-Western peoples were portrayed as "brutish and violent," while other times they were romanticized as uncorrupted, in harmony with nature, and "still living in a more or less paradisal state."[54] Similarly, native sexuality was sometimes characterized as spiraling into "unbounded sexual frenzy" and "unspeakable orgies," and other times as communal and pleasure oriented, a throwback to the innocence of the Garden of Eden. Although one view or the other might predominate, neither completely supplanted the other, providing evidence of the ambivalence with which Europeans viewed their own society. The story of public copulation at Point Venus thus hints at the "paradise" (or degeneracy) that supposedly existed in Tahiti before the Europeans came, "with their civilization and their shame"[55] —regardless of whether it was a genuine description of a cultural tradition that was later repressed or an exaggerated account of an unusual incident.

Much has changed since the eighteenth and nineteenth centuries, but Hawkesworth's rendering of the scene at Point Venus continues to circulate, used to denounce the sexual inhibitions of westerners, challenge gender inequality and the double standard, or illustrate the cultural construction of monogamous marriage. A 1958 book by Bruno Partridge, *The History of Orgies*, presents public sex as commonplace in Tahiti, an educational activity rather than a ritual occurrence: "Young men and girls often copulate publicly before the people, receiving good advice from the bystanders, usually women, amongst whom the most important inhabitants are to be found. Thus the girls (of 11 years) receive their information at an early age."[56] Fifty years later, in *Sex at Dawn: The Prehistoric Origins of Modern Sexuality*, the scene is offered as an example of "shamelessly libidinous behavior."[57] The many times and places the "scene" crops up in the interceding years would be difficult to count.

The association of orgies with "primitive" cultures, rituals, and moralities remains strong. Italian prime minister Silvio Berlusconi became embroiled in a sex scandal in 2010 when a young prostitute claimed she'd been paid to attend "bunga bunga" parties at his mansion near Milan. The phrase "bunga bunga," which has now become everyday lingo in Italy, supposedly dates back to 1910, when it appeared in a joke about African tribal rituals.[58] Some news agencies reported that Berlusconi was referring to a rite participated in by Colonel Qaddafi's "harem," where the women stripped and "pleasured him."[59] Sources close to Qaddafi, however, claimed that the women surrounding him were bodyguards, not playthings.[60] Although properly referred to as "the Revolutionary Nuns," the women were termed "the Amazonian Guard" in the Western media. Despite being trained at a special military academy and appearing in uniforms, the women could not sidestep sexualization: the Amazons, after all, are a mythological all-female warrior tribe, themselves no strangers to orgies, often with a bit of self-mutilation and male sacrifice thrown in for good measure.

MARCO VASSI: THE ACID-LADEN ORGYMASTER

"Are you . . . searching?"

It is the opening line to Marco Vassi's autobiography, *The Stoned Apocalypse*, a question to which he replies, "Yes, you might say I am searching."

Thus begins a journey that takes the young man from coast to coast, questing after a higher level of existence. Marco Ferdinand William Vasquez-d'Acugno was born in New York City in 1937. Although known in his younger days as Fred Vasquez, he changed his name to Marco Vassi, invoking the voyager Marco Polo. From his early readings of Gurdjieff (a spiritual teacher who believed that humans needed to transcend their state of "waking sleep" to achieve full potential) to LSD trips, from Scientology to communism, and from hippie encounter groups to gay bathhouses, Vassi was a tireless explorer. He was also a prolific writer, publishing more than a dozen books, along with essays and short erotic stories.

Over the course of his spiritual and intellectual travels, Vassi focused more and more on sex as a source of enlightenment and human potential. As his friend David Steinberg writes: "Sex for Marco wasn't just about getting laid (except sometimes), not just a question of neurons and orgasms. For Marco sex was a lens on life itself, a magnifying glass through which the dynamics and foibles of being human become intensified, and so his pursuit of sexual knowledge and experience took on the color of a philosophical quest. He saw himself at once as the Avatar of Eros and an eager student of Zen enlightenment." Vassi's ambition was to "exhaust all the subjective aspects of the sexual act" so that he might transcend male-female dualism and the limitations of human culture and finally achieve true liberation. He explored sex with men and women, along with any kink he could imagine— fetishes, BDSM, loving intimacy, casual encounters. "Sex is a key to door-ways of knowing," he wrote. He claimed to have been with more than five hundred women and "twice that many men."[61]

Shortly after relocating to California from New York in the 1960s, Vassi began experimenting with group sexuality at the Experimental College, a student organization at San Francisco State University. Guided by the "twin threads of sexuality and mysticism," Vassi led classes that moved from relax-ation, massage, and suggestive imagery to spontaneous movement, where students pretended to be puppets on a string. His classes became more sensu-al as Vassi asked students to remove their clothing and gaze at each other, attempting a spiritual communion made flesh. But the sexual energy of the class built to an uncontrollable level, and Vassi found he could not keep himself from "sinking under the sheer sensuality of the scene."[62]

The sessions, of course, were facilitated with pot and LSD.

Vassi began to develop a following. As word of his teachings spread, Vassi had a realization: "Without doing a single thing but following the inner logic of my madness to its most baroque extension, I was becoming a guru to an entire generation."[63] He took the role to heart: "He shaved his head and went barefoot, wore a leopard-skin coat, and carried a wooden staff. Instead of talking, he played the harmonica. If he wanted to dance in the street, he danced in the street. If he wanted a particular girl, he had only to smile at her."[64]

Vassi continued wandering the West Coast, visiting an estate called Olompali, where horses frolicked and hundreds of people tripped on pure THC. He spent time at Harbinger Springs, a commune led by a physicist who believed he'd journeyed in a flying saucer (and managed to tell a believable story about it). During a weekend in a "haunted chalet" with eighty "young acid graduates," Vassi found that their religious fervor for producing "posi-tive vibes" as a form of salvation easily erupted into an orgy: "It was the single most happy sexual time I experienced, and more taboos came ringing down in an hour than Ellis was able to catalogue in a lifetime."[65]

Group sex, he believed, was a means of both connecting with others and challenging the status quo, which many of his contemporaries believed was ready to crumble. He started teaching classes again in Haight-Ashbury, reveling in the power he was gaining among the throngs of hippies:

> I was high on my own potency and on acid; I was high on the continual flow of energies coursing through the commune; I was high on the potential of the human species when it begins to really swing in a beautiful way. And I was high on the sight of a dozen naked women who looked to me as a guru and were ready to experience the ALL under my supervision.[66]

During a particularly memorable encounter session, while tripping on acid, Vassi hallucinated that he was an Aztec priest. In the vision, he saw himself baking in the jungle heat before thousands of screaming worshippers, wearing a plumed helmet and a cape, and wielding an obsidian knife. After asking the crowd for a virgin volunteer, he quickly realized "it was an absurd request" and settled for a Virgo, a young co-ed named Adrienne. Lying her facedown on the floor, he invited the group to join in his fantasy:

> Just relax, and get the sense of a very hot sun burning into your shoulders. See if you can feel the sweat trickling down your arms, and the way the light makes your eyes hurt. You are staring up at a very high altar where the priest of the tribe is going to sacrifice a young virgin for the health and prosperity of the people. Picture the girl, much like Adrienne here. She is lovely, heavy-limbed. She has never known the touch of a man's lips, the ecstasy of a caress. She has never had the moment of sheer bliss when two human beings interpenetrate and become one body, one consciousness. She has never known love.[67]

Sensing the crowd had become animated with a communal "blood lust," he continued: "She is frightened and excited. She is going to experience brutal, painful, swift death, before she has even begun to taste the juices of life . . ." Vassi turned the young woman over, noticing that her breathing had become heavier as the tension in the room had risen to "sublime heights." Gazing at an LSD-induced Peruvian sky, he offered a "silent prayer to the deities who hovered overhead, waiting for the soul of the girl."

Without further ado, he let out a "savage cry" and plunged the heavy stone knife into her gut.

What happened next, Vassi recalls, was terrifying: Adrienne let out a hair-curling wail. Screams emerged from the crowd. Someone fainted. Other people rose, striving to see whether their guru was tearing out the young Virgo's still-beating heart. Vassi himself, noticing how Adrienne "folded in half," worried he had somehow materialized an actual knife through the power of suggestion. Had he killed her?

When Adrienne then rolled over onto her stomach again, shaking, Vassi looked at her with relief—and desire. Realizing "that there was a delicious naked woman" in front of him, "so flipped-out she was ready to relive being a human sacrifice," he did what any self-respecting "acid-laden Aztec priest" would do: "I lifted my robe, lowered myself on her quivering form, and fucked her with rapid, mounting pleasure."

Within minutes, Vassi noticed the others had followed suit. As he observed the naked bodies copulating around him, he realized his "career as an orgymaster was beginning to assume a distinct direction."[68]

THE ORGY AS A SYMBOL OF LIBERATION

As we saw in the symbolism of the Roman orgy, orgies can serve as a sign of the crumbling of civilization due to a loss of traditional morality structures. One might expect orgiastic behavior among "savages," but in a supposedly civilized population, orgies were a symptom of greater trouble ahead. On the other hand, for those critical of an existing social order, such collapse was potentially revolutionary; myths of the tribal orgy bolstered aspirations that humans might return to a more natural state through sexual transgression, whether "savage" or "innocent."

Orgies are thus dangerous to the status quo, imbued with the power to shatter social structures (along with the boundaries of the individual, as we shall see). The Marquis de Sade (1740–1814) was a French aristocrat and writer living at the turn of the nineteenth century who was preoccupied with orgies. There are so many orgies in his books that it would be difficult to count them. Not surprisingly, a few of his fictional orgies were set in Roman temples, further strengthening popular associations of the orgy with decadence and depravity. Sexual transgression was of the utmost importance for Sade—personally, politically, artistically, and philosophically—and he viewed sexuality as inherently violent. His fictional orgies involve copious forms of torture and forbidden sexuality, from the violation or corruption of nuns, priests, and children to the sexual use of religious objects. In his personal life as well, Sade was believed to regularly participate in orgies, occasionally with his wife, that is, except during his years in jail, which he spent writing about orgies instead. All told, he spent about thirty-two years in prison for various sexual and political crimes, including poisoning a group of prostitutes with "Spanish fly" during one of his debauches. Although rumors thrived that the Marquis de Sade was also involved with torture, sexual perversion, and even murder like the characters in his novels, he denied such claims: "Yes, I am a libertine, I admit it freely. I have dreamed of doing everything that it is possible to dream of in that line. But I have certainly not done all the things I have dreamt of and never shall. Libertine I may be, but I am not a criminal, I am not a murderer."[69] Yet even if just a libertine, he was too much for society. In 1801, Napoleon Bonaparte called for his arrest after the publication of *Justine* and *Juliette*, and Sade was again imprisoned. He was later transferred to an insane asylum, where he continued to write scandalously until he died.

Some commentators on the Marquis de Sade focus on the conservative aspects of his writing—the violence against women and children, for example. Still others are intrigued by the ambiguities arising in his texts: victims become torturers, women become as powerful as men through imaginative cruelty, and morality repeatedly loses to "human nature," which is violent yet authentic. Other commentators highlight his obsession with freedom from social norms and institutions and see his literary works as offering a philosophy of liberation through purposeful and systematic sexual transgression. For Sade, violating social norms around sexuality, especially moral and religious prohibitions, becomes a path to one's true self.

Aleister Crowley (1875–1947), known for the phrase "Do what thou wilt," was another libertine who believed in sexual transgression as political rebellion and personal liberation. Sexual excitement, he believed, was a "degraded form of divine ecstasy"; the bonds of social convention caused the sexual instincts to "assume monstrous shapes."[70] Crowley had an appetite for adventure, traveling widely and courting both mystical and sexual experiences, including encounters with prostitutes and men. After he decided to dedicate himself to occultism, he founded a magical order, the Argenteum Astrum, or A.˙. A.˙., and despite his misogynistic views on women, he attracted many female followers. His rituals were said to include "unspeakable orgies," a belief he augmented through his own writing, which included publishing a journal and producing both philosophy and fiction. *Diary of a Drug Fiend* described his drug use, sexual proclivities, and obsession with sin and transgression: "Pleasure as such has never attracted me. It must be spiced by moral satisfaction." His "ultimate goal" was "to explode the boundaries of all morality and conventional models of sexuality in order to achieve an intense experience of superhuman liberation."[71] Absolute personal freedom was not in the cards, however, as Crowley became addicted to heroin later in his life, using increasingly large doses. Instead of attaining magical rebirth for himself, his followers, and the world, he ended up physically debilitated, impoverished, and depressed.[72]

For other movements and individuals critical of the inequality or violence of modernity or capitalism, authentic sexuality is conceptualized as loving rather than sadistic; the potential of the orgy is to aid in the recovery of a natural connectedness to the world and its peoples severed by industrialization and other forms of cultural "progress." The belief that small-scale tribal societies are more harmonious than modern ones, internally and in relation to "nature," is sometimes referred to as the "myth of primitive harmony" (and linked, of course, to the idealized noble savage). Problems in tribal societies could be traced to colonialism, and like those in Western culture, to the spread of unhealthful sexual repression accompanying modernization. Suggs, for example, argues that group sex once played an important role in Marquesan society as a religious ritual cementing social solidarity. But when the Marquesans' "elaborate and colorful pagan religion" was swept aside by Christianity and their social and political organization destroyed by colonialism, their ceremonies were also corrupted, becoming scenes of "endless debauchery," disruptive, meaningless, and of no value to their society.[73] Likewise, although some missionaries saw Tahiti as an example of uncivilized debauchery—"no portion of the human race was ever perhaps sunk lower in brutal licentiousness and moral degradation"[74] —other writers argued that Tahiti had been "contaminated" through contact with the West. That explorers also spread venereal disease among the island inhabitants was, for some, further symbolic of the destructiveness of Western cultures.

When authentic or "natural" sexuality is conceptualized as unproblematic, peaceful, and egalitarian, vanquishing sexual repression can become seen as a route not only to individual liberation but to creation of a better civilization as well. Wilhelm Reich, an Austrian American psychoanalyst sometimes credited with coining the phrase "sexual revolution," began working with Freud in the 1920s. Later, he became a controversial figure in psychiatry because of his radical ideas about sexuality's revolutionary potential. Much of his later career focused on attempts to isolate and harness "orgone energy," the universal life force he believed was released at orgasm. Reich was eventually jailed for making "misleading claims" about his "orgone accumulators," and the Food and Drug Administration destroyed much of his research. Still, other thinkers, from philosophers such as Herbert Marcuse to contemporary queer theorists to activist sex workers such as Annie Sprinkle, have endorsed ideas that society can be improved by challenging negative attitudes toward sexuality and the restrictive bodily and sexual practices those attitudes engender. In Western culture, overcoming shame about sexuality and liberating oneself from cultural inhibitions—as in "gay pride" movements, for example—became an ideal in the past century as a means of exercising personal freedom and fighting political oppression.

Group sex can serve as an affirmation of such ideals and appear as a powerful antidote to repression. The orgy as a symbol of "free love" and peaceful revolution is perhaps not as deeply entrenched as that of the orgy as a symbol of animalistic degeneracy, but is still widely recognizable. The first "summer of love" of 1967, beginning with a gathering in San Francisco's Golden Gate Park, was an outgrowth of 1960s youth movements championing individualistic rebellion against mainstream beliefs and norms: "Do your own thing, wherever you have to do it and whenever you want. Drop out. Leave society as you have known it. . . . Blow the mind of every straight person you can reach. Turn them on, if not to drugs, then to beauty, love, honesty, fun."[75] The goal of dismantling the "death machine" of the state was linked to the release of sexuality from social conventions. Overcoming shame about the human body and experimenting with alternative sexual life-styles became important as links were made "between sexual liberation and the larger goals of social, political, or psychological liberation." In addition to the creation of a new "tribe" of people outside of "the destructive system of the nations," underground political groups also aimed at bringing a "sense of festivity into public life whereby people could fuck freely and guiltlessly, dance wildly, and wear fancy dress all the time."[76] The musical *Hair*, which debuted in 1967, presented many of these controversial ideas to the broader public. The musical drew on tribal themes: it was subtitled *The American Tribal Love-Rock Musical Smash*, the youth called themselves a "tribe" and wore loincloths, and appearances were made by African witch doctors, "Indians," and a woman referred to as Margaret Mead, the cultural anthropologist whose controversial research on sexuality in the South Seas was used to exemplify the social benefits of sexual freedom. One of the songs suggested, "Join the holy orgy / Kama Sutra / Everyone!" The production included profanity, scenes of drug use, and onstage nudity.

As monogamy was criticized as part of the establishment, group sex became a political statement. Sam Sloan, president of Berkeley's Sexual Freedom League in 1966 and 1967, organized forty-two weekly sex parties on campus. These meetings were also ostensibly to discuss free speech and other political issues (though he admits his motivation was as much to gain access to attractive women as to effect social change).[77] The underground Weatherman group held a "national orgy" in Cleveland, Ohio, in 1969, in an effort to integrate politics and pleasure and to promote the organization's belief that abandoning monogamy would lead to revolutionary progress. Swinging gained popularity, from Sandstone Retreat in California to Plato's Retreat in New York, practiced by some couples as a utopian politics. Allen Ginsberg, a leading "Beat" poet, suggested that the orgy could become "an acceptable community sacrament—one that brings all people closer together." He wrote:

> America's political need is orgies in the parks, on Boston Common and in the Public Gardens, with naked bacchantes in our national forests. . . . I am not proposing idealistic fancies, I am acknowledging what is already happening among the young in fact and fantasy, and proposing official blessing for these breakthroughs of community spirit. . . . What satisfaction is now possible for the young? Only the satisfaction of their Desire—love, the body, the orgy.[78]

Although there were many other important social developments during the 1960s and 1970s in the United States, the image of long-haired, androgynous merrymakers chucking aside their sexual inhibitions along with their flowered bell-bottoms remains pervasive.

Yet freedom is not easily won. Sexual liberation, Urban notes, has a tendency "to become mingled with less admirable sorts of things, such as misogyny, drug abuse, or simple commercialization."[79] While there is no doubt that hippies had an impact on sexuality in the United States and that their ethos spread around the world, many of their grander hopes were not realized. Disillusionment accompanied realizations that "freedom" is limited by preexisting inequalities. Liberation was not as simple as abandoning bras, "smashing monogamy," or tossing aside derogatory terms like "faggot" or "slut." Despite the introduction of "the Pill," an active feminist movement, and the relaxation of social norms around sexual practices, for example, the double standard of sexual behavior for women remained. Some feminists even decried calls for nonmonogamy as simply allowing men greater sexual access to women's bodies. Symbols of revolution were as easily swallowed and regurgitated by consumer culture then as they are now. Although my daughter's Skechers are decorated with rainbow-colored peace signs, we are still far from making love instead of war.

Sometimes sexual revolutions change more than patterns of sexual behavior and produce the intended effects—at least initially. But pervasive social change remains more elusive. As queer writer and activist Pat Califia remarks, "I do not believe that we can fuck our way to freedom."[80]

Perhaps we are asking too much of sex.

Or perhaps true freedom is illusory.

THE ORGY AS TRANSGRESSION

Many societies allow for sanctioned forms of rule breaking during certain holidays or festivals, in some altered states of consciousness, or in everyday practices such as humor. For example, Carnival festivities in Brazil, the Caribbean, and other Roman Catholic countries are public celebrations where people wear masks or costumes and otherwise step outside of everyday expectations by partying in the streets, staying up all night, and engaging in behaviors usually forbidden or discouraged. Some holidays or ceremonies allow men and women in societies with strict gender roles to swap positions for a given period of time, a night or a week. People may be allowed to publicly ridicule their leaders, expressing discontent or hostilities that are usually controlled. During Roman Saturnalias, masters and slaves might dine or gamble together, or otherwise overlook typical distinctions in status. A contemporary American "roast" involves joking about and even insulting the guest of honor. Such carnivalesque inversions are a form of circumscribed resistance that staves off rebellions and preserves exploitative power structures. Societies sanction certain forms of rule breaking in other ways as well, such as assigning "ineligibility" to persons assumed unable to follow rules (small children or those with mental disabilities), or allowing for "time-outs" (periods of time where customary social rules and the penalties for breaking them are temporarily relaxed, as in drunkenness).[81] Some theorists speak of "cultural safety valves," or controlled opportunities for people to relieve tensions caused by the process of socialization—which is never complete—or pressure to conform. Many types of behavior arguably function as safety valves: adultery, political demonstrations, criminal activity, witchcraft, sports, and creative expression (music, art, or literature), to name just a few. Carnivalesque inversion, "time-outs," and "safety valves" are all concepts addressing how human societies attempt to maintain stability over time despite the existence of conflict, some of which is endemic to human societies—such as intergenerational conflict—and some of which is related to specific power structures.

In *The History of Orgies*, Partridge analyzes the orgy as carnivalesque: "an organized blowing-off of steam; the expulsion of hysteria accumulated by abstinence and restraint." As such, he believes, the orgy is often cathartic, releasing tensions as well as "rearousing by contrast an appetite for the humdrum temperances which are an inevitable part of everyday life."[82] Carnivalesque orgies offer only a temporary rebellion: after the party is over, people go back to their everyday roles and lives, leaving the power structure unchanged.

Transgression, then, is ultimately conservative in its social effects.

The writer Georges Bataille (1897–1962) also saw the orgy as an organized transgression, although he took a more psychological approach. Like Sade, Bataille saw "violence as an inherent aspect of the erotic." He was intrigued by human sacrifice. However, while Sade focused on violence turned outward toward victims, Bataille was interested in erotic violence as jeopardizing one's sense of self. Eroticism, he believed, is the way that humans manage the fact that we desire to experience "continuity" with others—the state of being both before birth and after death—but while alive, we have only our individual body and consciousness, our "discontinuity." We repetitively and impossibly seek both experiences: the obliteration of the boundaries of the self *and* the preservation of our individual existences. Sex, he wrote, becomes the "half-way house between life and death," as during erotic activity we ideally experience some fusion with others. We may also experience continuity in religious activities. But such experiences are only momentary, as we are either thrust back into discontinuity (our own body and consciousness) or the self is dissolved, which means death. Religions thus turn sex and death into sacred matters, surrounding them with taboos. Transgression of those taboos, for Bataille, is important because it allows us access to this realm of the sacred: "The sacred and the forbidden are one."[83] Transgression may suspend a taboo but cannot destroy it. In fact, transgression— and this essential area of human experience—cannot exist without taboos. Bataille put his ideas into practice through his writing, which spans essays to fiction, featuring urination and defecation, orgies, insanity, enucleation, blood, necrophilia, and death. He has been called both a philosopher and a pornographer.

Reading Bataille, Crowley, the Marquis de Sade, or other writers of transgressive literature (a category including writers from Petronius to Hubert Selby to Bret Easton Ellis) can initially be an intense experience. Artists and filmmakers have similarly pursued the politics and aesthetics of transgression. Pushing the boundaries of the body—through "deviant sex," the ingestion or eroticization of body fluids, mutilation, torture, or murder—becomes a way to explode moral, social, and psychological boundaries believed to be restrictive of personal freedom. Yet after a while, the shock wears off. The stories or images become repetitive. Oh, we're doing something with urine or poop again? *Yawn.* Semen? *Bor-ing.* Maybe mix the body fluids together in a glass and force a girl to drink them after some rough sex? (That is, in fact, the premise of the porn series *Gag Factor*, although the political effects are less calculable than the profits; the series boasts at least eighteen DVDs, indicating that the repetition is working for some viewers.)

Maybe keep transgression alive by desecrating religious artifacts with bodily fluids—who could forget artist Andres Serrano's *Piss Christ*?

But that was so 1987.

What about involving religious figures in orgies?

Enough to earn Salman Rushdie a fatwa, but they won't bat an eye over at www.dirtypriest.com.

Libertines may hope for the complete destruction of rules, norms, and boundaries rather than a temporary suspension of them. Some people, in some societies, do resist the return to the "humdrum" or expected after their moral holidays. Thus, while a society can set up "safety valve" rituals, "time-outs" where individuals are temporarily excused for their behaviors, or other opportunities for sanctioned rule breaking, sometimes those strategies fail to reintroduce an individual to the fold. There are times as well when personal experiences of transgression indeed produce lasting changes in one's worldview, perhaps leading to political action. Yet while one might always be able to shock *someone*—perhaps even or only oneself—a politics of transgression eventually dead-ends. Rules can change over time; after all, the bikini was once transgressive. But if liberation is tied to violating taboos, one *needs* taboos, regardless of whether any particular limit shifts, mutates, or dissolves. One may even become increasingly dependent on the very elements one wishes to challenge. Reflecting on Aleister Crowley's eventual heroin addiction and emotional despair, Urban suggests disillusionment might be the risk of transgression as a strategy: "What is there left to do after every forbidden desire has been indulged and every taboo has been trans-gressed?"[84] Invoking postmodern philosopher Jean Baudrillard, he argues that

> the problem for our generation is not so much that we are still in need of sexual liberations or freedom from the prudish taboos of our Victorian forefathers; rather, the dilemma today is perhaps that we have passed through too many sexual revolutions, that we have violated so many sexual, moral, and social taboos that we don't really know what sex *is* anymore. We are thus left in the strange, ambiguous state of a "post-orgy" world, wondering what sex is even supposed to be about in a postmodern, late capitalist world.[85]

As Baudrillard's fictional orgiast proposes to his partner: "What are you doing *after* the orgy?"

THE ORGY AS THE BEGINNING—AND END—OF THE INDIVIDUAL

What *do* people do after the orgy?

Do they smoke a cigarette and *go home*?

In many Western myths and stories, orgiasts meet an unpleasant end. At best, in these warning stories, participating in an orgy places the self in serious jeopardy, potentially prompting a descent into an animal nature and the basest of sensual desires, whether temporary or permanent. At worst, such descriptions serve as warnings that surrendering to the carnality of the orgy can lead to a loss of one's sense of morality, purpose, self, sanity, and life. In sensationalist descriptions of the orgies of Bacchus, for example, Grecian women were described as coming close to this edge:

> The gravest matrons and proudest princesses suddenly laid aside their decency and their dignity, and ran screaming among the woods and mountains, fantasti-cally dressed or half-naked, with their hair disheveled and interwoven with ivy or vine, and sometimes with living serpents. In this manner they frequently worked themselves up to such a pitch of savage ferocity, as not only to feed upon raw flesh, but even to tear living animals with their teeth, and eat them warm and palpitating.[86]

Despite—and *because of*—these dangers, there is another perspective on the loss of individuality associated with the orgy: the possibility for feelings of intense communal belonging. As Allyn writes:

> In an orgy, the gulf between self and other—the source of psychological alienation and spiritual loneliness which has troubled philosophers throughout the ages—momentarily disappears. Collective fervor and communal pleasure erase the typical boundaries between individuals. An orgy allows participants the opportunity to explore every aspect of human sexuality, to translate fantasy into reality. Orgies satisfy both our voyeuristic and exhibitionistic desires, and at an orgy, the lines between heterosexuality and homosexuality inevitably blur. An orgy reflects human beings' social nature—it engages them in communal activity for their collective gratification—and their animalistic past.[87]

This effect links orgies to religious rituals as an "expression of the ecstatic." For Bataille, these moments of altered consciousness arising out of the collective violation of taboos produce a "momentary ecstasy,"[88] or sense of continuity. At the subjective level, transgression can be experienced as transcendence. Experiencing desire, pleasure, and connection beyond the boundaries of identity, then, is seen as a potential promise of group sex—yet, still, one that puts the self at risk. Outside of the work of a few philosophers, however, this view has been marginalized in Western culture.

Aldous Huxley's *Brave New World* is a novel using the fictional dystopia of World State to criticize American culture of the 1930s. In the name of happiness and stability, the masses of World State are drugged with a substance called soma, individuality is discouraged, and novelty and consumption are privileged over intrinsic value. The state has also taken over reproduction, child rearing, and other social relations, believing that stability is jeopardized by the strong emotion inherent in such relationships. Because intense emotion is also triggered by sexual repression, the orgy becomes a sanctioned form of release—anonymous, instantaneous promiscuity that is believed safer than monogamous, dyadic sex because emotional bonds are less likely to form. "John the Savage" is brought to World State after growing up on an isolated reservation. Seeing through the eyes of an outsider, he is critical of the state vision of emotional stability and instant gratification. At the end of the novel, John engages in public self-flagellation, desperately trying to resist the pressure to conform to World State ideals, and attacks a woman with whom he has developed a relationship. His violence spurs an orgy among the people gathered to watch him, who begin chanting a popular folk verse: "Orgy-porgy gives release." Instead of continuing to strive for freedom, John loses control and joins the masses.

The next day, realizing what he has done, he commits suicide.

Huxley worried about the loosening of sexual mores, which he saw as tied to the growth of consumer society. Despite the reversal of the terms "savage" and "citizen" in Huxley's novel—the savage being the one who aims for decency and depth—his orgy serves as an example of the defeat of the individual by the horde, a warning against allowing desires for sensual and immediate pleasure to overtake loftier goals. Much could be written (and most likely has been) about the influence of Freud's ideas on Huxley's novel, as the "happiness" and "stability" of World State citizens is achieved in part by eradicating sexual repression and the anxiety and dissatisfaction it supposedly caused. The elevation of the orgy to a semireligious ritual, an emotional safety valve offering instant gratification, holds participants captive to the state and to their bodily pleasures as they are unable to self-actualize or form deep attachments to others.

In *Last Exit to Brooklyn* (1965), another fictional account warning against the devastation—both personal and cultural—wrought by the failure to curb human impulses toward sex and violence, Hubert Selby spins the story of Tralala, a young urban prostitute. Tralala is immersed in a world of violence, hustling and robbing her customers. The disturbing tale culminates with Tralala offering to have sex with an entire bar of drunken men. The men drag her to a wrecked car, push her into the backseat, and strip off her clothes. A rowdy line forms, beer is passed out, and the crowd grows. Tralala drinks beer with the men and yells, among other things, that she has the "biggest goddamn pair of tits in the world." Though the men grow increasingly sadistic toward her, Tralala seemingly cooperates. When a beer can is shoved into her mouth, she curses and spits out a piece of tooth, laughing and continuing to drink along with the crowd. She eventually loses consciousness, although it is unclear as to whether it is from the abuse or intoxication. Her sudden lack of response angers the young men who are still in line. They continue to assault her. When it is clear that Tralala is dead, the men grow "bored" and wander away, leaving her body in the abandoned lot with a broomstick "jammed up her snatch" and blood leaking from between her legs.

Sexual licentiousness sometimes *does* either precede or accompany other cruelties and breakdowns in the social order. What happened to Tralala—the escalation of sex into gang rape and then into murder—has happened to women around the world in situations of criminality, conflict, or warfare. What differs in Tralala's story is her supposed willing participation in her own degradation, at least until she loses consciousness. She turns against her own body and life, becoming part of the mob and escalating their aggression. The self becomes other, not in ecstatic communion but in destruction.

Sex promises pleasure, and group sex promises even more. Yet, such tales warn, this pleasure comes with a price. The dangerous forces of sexuality are contagious, and when unleashed *en masse*, the risk to one's individuality and humanity is multiplied. Emotional attachments to others, if they existed, are severed. Individual preferences, choices, and purposes are drowned in the desires of the crowd; an indiscriminate attitude regarding one's sexual partners is taken as a step toward the loss of individuality. Once the taboo against group sex is broken, other remaining taboos, such as those against incest, suicide, or murder, lose their hold on what is left of the human conscience.

The tragic end result for the individual can be degeneration into undifferentiated madness.

John the Savage and Tralala are not the only fictional orgiasts to lose control of their impulses and become complicit in scenes of violence and death as a result. Examples could have been chosen from other time periods or media forms. From classic works of literature to pulp novels, we find orgy participants overwhelmed by the force of the primal horde: crazed men castrating themselves in a libidinal frenzy or women who mount gigantic carved phalluses in fits of desire, splitting themselves open in the process. Tales of Messalina's sexual exploits, especially her offers to take all comers like a prostitute, are invoked to suggest her descent into madness; promiscuity in women is still often linked with insanity. These two examples, however, draw explicitly on the layers of oppositional meaning explored in this chapter thus far—between the primitive and the civilized, cultural progress and decay, social control and freedom, power and resistance, and the troubled relationship between the individual and the group, or self and other.

GROUP SEX, SOCIETY, AND THE SELF

The idea that sexuality and society are ultimately in conflict runs through the history of Western thought, explored by philosophers, sociologists, anthropologists, psychologists, novelists, artists, and others. This notion is not only or primarily Western, although the ways it manifests differ around the world. In *Civilization and Its Discontents*, Sigmund Freud posits a fundamental tension between civilization and the individual. Each individual, he argues, has conflicting drives for fusion and destruction: Eros, the life drive, and the death drive (later termed Thanatos). These primitive human instincts, expressed through the desire to kill and the desire for sexual gratification, must be repressed, or sublimated, in the name of cultural progress. The price of progress is usually guilt and neurosis instead of happiness; unfortunately, in Freud's model, such a price must be paid for civilization. Societies, if they wish to survive, must somehow harness human desires for sex and violence for their own ends. Individuals, if they wish to mature into productive and recognizable members of any society, must rise above their primitive instincts, redirect their desires toward acceptable goals and objects, and successfully manage the fluctuating psychological impact of repression.

Some philosophers argue against this view and claim that sexuality cannot exist outside of social meanings—what feels like a natural instinct, welling up from within an animalistic body, is itself a cultural construction. Often associated with the work of philosopher Michel Foucault, but actually having a robust history in sociological and feminist thought, this line of thinking suggests that there isn't an authentic sexuality to "liberate." For Foucault, the belief that we have repressed our natural sexual instincts is part of what makes sexuality so important to modern individuals as a source of liberation and identity. Doing something that *feels* rebellious—streaking through a crowded football stadium, dressing in drag for a BDSM-themed sex party, or having group sex—doesn't mean one is really escaping social control. Experiences of rebellion or freedom are just as much a part of the system as experiences of oppression. Similarly, even our most personal desires, which may feel natural, buried, or repressed, are created within cultural systems of meaning. Taken as myth, for example, Freud's ideas clearly inform the meanings of orgies discussed so far. Foucault points to the eighteenth century as a specific moment in Western history when sexuality came into focus as a dangerous and natural force that needed to be controlled for the good of the community. As sexuality became the object of multiple social discourses (psychology, medicine, self-help, feminism, etc.), new forms of legal, moral, scientific, and personal regulation were produced. These powerful forms of social control automatically generate resistance, however: medical categories such as "homosexual," for example, operate both as a means of pathologizing sexual behavior and as the basis on which people argue for rights and social acceptance. Further, sexual desire could now serve as an indicator of one's innermost self, or identity, and as an expression of truth.

The debate about the true relationship between sexuality and society continues, as philosophers split hairs on the meanings of "resistance," "identity," "self," "agency," and "desire." If you're interested in traveling further down that particular rabbit hole, pick up a book by Judith Butler, take two aspirin, and call in the morning.

What we talk about when we talk about orgies, then, is culturally and emotionally loaded. Orgies represent danger, an edge. Group sex is never the norm. While it is possible to unearth historical examples of societies where group sex was condoned at certain times, either in religious rituals or as a spontaneous reaction to certain crises or events, we have already discussed the problems with such excavations. Modern examples of such acceptance at a societal level are rare to nonexistent. We can find contemporary enclaves where group sex is regularly practiced, some of which are discussed in this book. We can find individuals for whom group sex is particularly arousing, fulfilling, or a preferred way to have sex; we can also find individuals for whom group sex is just one more way to "get off." But even in these cases, group sex involves transgressive elements, both personal and cultural; in fact, this is part of its appeal.

At the same time, however, the reality of group sex often seems worlds away from the imaginings put forth in this chapter.

Let's take a look.

Chapter Three

Becoming an Orgiast

The Social Organization of Group Sex

Tugging nervously on my cheap spandex dress, which got shorter with every step, I glanced back at my husband. He was clad more formally in a suit, following closely. He nodded.

Everything is okay. We're on the same page.

We trotted behind a gorgeous Brazilian couple through the winding halls of a Connecticut mansion. Futuristic erotic paintings lined the walls—a naked woman outlined in electric blue; a man's buttocks foregrounding two women on a bed; a prostitute reclining on a sofa, legs in the air, a red light above her head.

The music pumping so insistently outside grew fainter.

Though the property was used almost exclusively for sex-themed parties—swingers, BDSM groups, an all-women's pagan retreat—it was quite a few steps above the seedy sex clubs we'd tentatively explored earlier that year. But no matter how clean the venue or opulent the décor, places where people have a lot of sex have a seediness about them.

For a moment, I longed to be back by the pool, sipping another cocktail under the night sky and watching the mermaids. The beautiful topless women in glittery fishtail skirts were strippers from New York City. Prevented by their costumes from diving into the water or moving their feet, the women lolled on the rocks while guests swam out with champagne or appetizers. Other strippers, male and female, gyrated on pedestals scattered across the property, while couples mingled near the bar, kissed on the chaises, or stripped naked and dove into the neon- green water. A foursome embraced underneath the waterfall. Scantily clad waiters and waitresses offered body shots and drinks.

The Brazilian man glanced back at me, looking slightly amused. Perhaps he thought we were going to back out.

We're not exactly newbies. We know the ropes.

But we didn't know much about the couple we were trailing: they lived in the city, had been to numerous parties here at the estate, and spoke very little English. Long-haired and almond-skinned, they might have been fugitives from a romance novel. She was wearing a silvery gown cut so low in the back I could see the top half of her butt cheeks. He was wearing the required black suit but had skipped the shirt underneath, exposing his rippled abdomen. He carried a bottle of Cabernet, and four plastic wineglasses were threaded through his fingers.

They knew even less about us. Not that they seemed to care—in fact, they were clearly interested in isolating us as quickly as possible.

The couple had approached us poolside—it had been obvious to the regulars that we didn't know anyone. They asked a few questions about how we heard about the party, nothing more.

"Come on," urged the girl, reaching for my hand. "Join us for some wine. We've already reserved the room we want. They know us here."

Of course, we had all known what she was suggesting.

Although we'd been given a tour of the property when we arrived, along with four other sober and edgy new couples, I was now lost. The house was a dark labyrinth, featuring two group rooms with mattresses lining the walls and six smaller, themed playrooms stocked with sheets, soap, and condoms. Some of the doors to the rooms were open, allowing voyeurs to watch the action; other doors were shut. Though occasionally we heard a moan or slap as we passed, we were mostly enveloped by silence.

An attendant slunk toward us in the hallway, nodding and then diverting his eyes. Every staff member, we'd been assured, acted with the highest level of discretion. Guests were screened carefully and were expected to remain discreet as well. Our names were checked against a guest list, first at the wrought-iron gates framing the driveway and then at the front door. Our license plate number had been recorded. No cell phones, cameras, or video cameras were allowed outside the coat-check area—at least, not for guests. Several inconspicuous security cameras panned the pool deck and entryway.

Every time we lagged behind to peer inside an open room, the couple in front of us disappeared into the shadows. Low light, even in the nicest sex venues, is a gift, I reminded myself. We passed the "Cabaret" room, an exhibitionist's paradise featuring a stripper pole and stage, a glass-enclosed shower, and theater seating alongside the bed. The next room, labeled "French Kiss," was themed after the Marquis de Sade, with a dungeon wall—chains included—a whipping post, and a cage. It was notably empty— too kinky for the breed of swinger here tonight. A group of naked couples streamed into the hallway outside the "Taj Mahal" room, and the woman in front of me broke pace briefly to say hello to one of the couples. "Vanilla dinner next weekend in the city?" she asked softly.

We finally stopped at the end of the hall. "Rome."

"We love this room," the woman said.

The door clicked shut behind us. She locked it.

We stood in a Roman bathhouse, with a central hot tub and a rain shower. Towels were folded on the edge of the tub, and ceramic urns bordered the walls. The bed, nestled into the wall, was draped in layers of filmy fabric.

Here we are.

She stripped her husband of his tuxedo jacket. Wine was poured, but before I could take a sip, the woman led me toward the bed. She slipped off her dress and pushed me gently onto my back. We were partly hidden from the men by the gauzy drape, although I could hear them moving closer. I wondered whether this was a good time to go over our rules, to mention I was straight, not bisexual like so many of the women here, and to let them know we were still soft swappers, meaning we didn't have intercourse with other partners. And perhaps it would be smart to make sure that no one had been here before us and forgotten to strip the linens—

But it actually wasn't such a good time to get mired in details. I was already looking up at the writhing snakes painted on the ceiling. The alcohol was making me dizzy and peaceful, not interested in quibbling about my sexual preferences.

"Don't worry," she said. "No one else has been in here tonight."

Oh well. We were miles from home.

When in Rome . . .

Inexperienced orgygoers, as we saw in the previous chapter, tend to imagine scenes of chaotic decadence and sexual abandon that have a destructive domino effect on the social fabric. This chapter explores the ways that orgies actually unfold—at least some of them, anyway—or what could be called the social organization of group sex.

Now, it *is* generally true that people are more open to experimentation, sexually and otherwise, when freed of everyday expectations, roles, and responsibilities. When traveling, for example, people tend to do things that they wouldn't normally do—a reason many parents fear "spring break" even if they've never thought to call it carnivalesque. People may also be less inhibited during transitional periods or when the usual order of things breaks down—as during rituals, times of cultural change, certain types of play, or critical life stages such as puberty or the "midlife crisis." These are sometimes referred to as "liminal" or "liminoid" states. Liminality is typically used to describe the middle stages of formal ritual, when participants have left behind their prior identities or statuses but have not yet transitioned into their new ones. Liminoid states are experientially similar but found in complex and often secular social settings; the activities that produce liminoid states tend to be voluntarily undertaken, individualized, and associated with play or leisure. During such times, identities are in flux. Distinctions that ordinarily structure social interactions, such as social class or race, may be ignored or seem meaningless. Roles, norms, and beliefs usually accepted dutifully may be questioned. Liminal states are emotionally intense—disorienting, uncomfortable, and exhausting as well as exciting; liminoid states, while possibly less intense and not explicitly related to rites of passage, are still characterized by an experimental ethos. These states are temporary, however; afterward, people are expected to either return to their everyday lives or take on new roles or identities. Reality television shows, Outward Bound courses, and spiritual retreats frequently make use of these social psychological dynamics. Because the college years mark a transition into adulthood in many societies, one's identity is unstable during that time rather than fixed. The acronym "lug," or "lesbian until graduation," captures this temporary experimental ethos with regard to sexuality. At Burning Man, the harsh, unfamiliar environment coupled with an emphasis on radical self-expression and the stripping of everyday identities, roles, and expectations creates an experimental milieu. A woman who would never masturbate in front of her friends back home might be convinced to climb on the Orgasma-tron while wandering the desert in a pink wig and leopard boots, especially if the onlookers are sporting tutus and using "playa names."

Nevertheless, anthropologists have long pointed out that even during periods of sanctioned rule breaking or experimentation it isn't the case that "anything goes"; some limits, taboos, and norms are upheld. Sometimes new rules and expectations are formed. Take drunkenness. Alcohol is consumed in societies around the world. Drunkenness impairs people's sensorimotor capabilities and visibly changes their comportment; it also often constitutes a "time-out" from expected behavior. Yet beyond these generalizations, how people behave when intoxicated varies. Formosan aborigines, at least at one time, excused criminal behavior if drunkenness was involved. In Turkey, men act differently throughout the life cycle when drinking, even if the amounts consumed remain the same—young men "engage in brawls and other displays of bravado," as they build their reputations, but later in life they abandon such overly aggressive behavior.[1] Americans believe alcohol lowers inhibitions, using drunkenness to excuse some forms of sexual behavior. College students often preface "hookups" by overindulging in alcohol, for example. Studies have also found that people who *believe* they are drinking alcohol (but aren't) act differently from people who do not believe they are drinking alcohol (but are). Even during "time-outs," periods of carnivalesque inversion, liminal or liminoid states, or altered states of consciousness, then, people act in culturally patterned ways, observing certain rules and taboos while breaking others.

People *learn* how to act when drunk.[2]

People also learn how to act at orgies.

After years of working in strip clubs and visiting sex clubs in over a dozen states and a handful of countries, I've become familiar with red-light districts. Many adult establishments are located away from residential or mainstream commercial areas due to regulations. I've been to parties in abandoned warehouses and clubs on the outskirts of town, located in industrial parks where the large parking lots somehow always seem deserted. Many have inconspicuous, shadowy entrances or unmarked doors. To gain entry, I've sometimes had to jump through hoops: apply for membership online, submit photos, call a cell phone number to meet someone in a parking lot, give a password to a security guard. Walking inside an unfamiliar club, waiting for your eyes to adjust to the dim light, is a bit like walking into a haunted house—you never know exactly what, or who, is around the corner. On the other hand, some features of public sex venues and parties are relatively pervasive. Play spaces of all types must prevent hostile or accidental intrusions as well as quell the anxieties and fulfill the needs of patrons. Group sex participants break some rules but respect others, demonstrating concern with who sees what and with having orderly interactions. Participants may also reject certain types of partners or activities; in fact, the quickest way to get your orgy pass revoked is to assume that everyone equally desires to experience your sexual charms. Experienced swingers, for example, can recognize "newbies" at a sex party or share stories about the mistakes they made when starting out. Something understandable in a "normal" sexual encounter, such as professing love to the person one is having sex with or waxing eloquently about their physical charms, can completely disrupt a scene where couples are having recreational sex with their spouses present. Even gang rapes involve ordered mayhem: some victims are chosen while others are rejected (wrong sex, different ethnicity, too young, too old, "dirty," etc.); assailants take "turns" based on status within the group; and some types of violence are deployed while others are avoided. Organizing principles may be drawn from the broader cultural context or created within particular social enclaves—either way, the environment must *make sense* to participants.

"Outsiders" must be able to crack the code and become insiders.

Is group sex transgressive? *Yes.*

Random or senseless? *No.*

THREE WEDDINGS AND A FUNERAL (INTERVIEW, DAVID)

My partner and I started discussing swinging in 1993 and had our first experience in early 1994. We've now been playing for almost twenty years, since we were both twenty-two.

The past two decades have marked the swiftest evolution this scene has ever undergone, due to the Internet, and we've been there for it all. When we started swinging, people met at clubs (if you could find one), through ads in alternative weeklies like *The Stranger* in Seattle, or *City Paper* in DC, or through magazines like *Swingers Advertiser*. I still have the hard copy of the issue with our ad in it, along with an ad placed by former Nixon protégé Roger Stone, who was outed in the *Washington Post* and on Fox local in the late 1990s. People could join Usenet newsgroups, which were early online concepts working somewhat like Craigslist does today. In the mid-1990s, we also had BBS (bulletin board systems), small computer networks that you would call on your modem. A local BBS might have fifteen lines, and at times you couldn't get on. It was all text based, and while you had profiles that were not too different from now, stats and text, there were very few photos. It was primitive, but connections were made.

In the 1990s, the barriers to entry were significant. You had to work at finding your way into the community. There were fewer clubs, and lots of doors closed in your face. People were keen on discretion because they were vulnerable to persecution and prosecution—possibly losing jobs, friends, and family. By entering the community, you could explore your desires among people who protected you and your privacy, even if you didn't like each other. It was secret and special. We learned the ropes from older couples that had been around for years, basically apprenticing with them. We've done that for others since then, as we view passing on knowledge as key.

During those years, each city we explored had one main club. In Seattle it was New Horizons, a large on-premise[s] club with beautiful facilities that was open several days every week. In DC, it was Capitol Couples (later Starz, and then Crucible Lifestyle), which was only open one Saturday a month and hosted in a series of bar/restaurants. It eventually expanded to twice a month. Capitol Couples was supposed to be an off-premise[s] event, but a lot of sex transpired on the same tables where dinners were served the previous night. The owners of these clubs were older members of the community. Their businesses lacked competition, which meant little impetus for change. But the community had a central meeting point—if you went out, you knew where everyone would be. People came, met, and played. Some exchanged phone numbers or e-mails (still a fairly new thing). Since it was hard to find others, people were primed to play. Everyone was full swap. There was a lot of commonality—you didn't need to worry about what people were into because you knew they were looking for others to have sex with, that night or in the future.

The growth of the Internet in the new millennium triggered massive changes. Suddenly, previously hard-to-find information was at one's fingertips. Websites made searching for playmates easier; photos and eventually videos were added. You could literally see a couple having sex before you wrote to them. One could find the local swingers club in a few clicks and be there later that evening. As the barriers to entry dropped, the time from idea to action fell to almost zero. Newbies flooded the scene. Average ages fell, perhaps reflecting a more open mindset or simply the ease of finding information.

The swinging community grew more diverse. We started hearing about soft swap, a concept that made us laugh at first. Now, more people want to just look or talk, and much of what passes as swinging is about the atmosphere, the trappings rather than the sex. Different groups are pitted against each other, and the community feels more fragmented. A decade ago, you chose the people you played with—of course—but *everyone* who cleared the hurdles to get into the community was accepted, even welcomed. Age, size, and color didn't matter; a person could still be part of the collective. That attitude seriously eroded with the drive for "exclusivity." People became concerned about avoiding "less desirable" folks. I remember the first time I saw a roped-off VIP area at a swingers' event. I found it sad: Was it now us versus them? Or had they inadvertently put themselves in a pen?

In a way, these changes were inevitable: the scene became trendy, and party promoters look for an "edge" to sell events. Promoters toned down the sex—an erotic environment appealed to the raver/dance crowd, who weren't really swingers, but it couldn't go *too* far. The new promoters and entrants had no allegiance to the community and were quick to attack and ridicule "old-school" swingers as "fat and ugly." The new scene they wanted to sell was young, "hot," and "off the hook." Businesses began catering to niches instead of serving the broad community, slicing and dicing us for profit. Even websites adopted this "beautiful people only" mentality. Now we have a community without roots. Older businesses were swept away by the trendy new parties, but the trendy parties are just surface without depth. There is less respect for what came before or what will come after, only a focus on the individual. The embracing and tolerant community that we entered twenty years ago has changed radically.

The harsh reality, though, is that there is a finite swinger dollar. You can't be at three "off the hook" events at the same time, even if you constantly rush from one shiny new thing to the next. Combine that with the economic downturn and the aging of the Internet wave, and there isn't enough money to keep everything going.

Swinging mirrors patterns of broader society in other ways, too. Take porn. The lack of pubic hair in porn is now the norm in swinging also. In the mid 1990s, I had my first DP [double penetration], and it was a big deal. Now you see it everywhere. I'll admit that a few weeks ago I was almost pulled into one—a DP can be fun even if the logistics are challenging. But I don't like the arms race mentality on sex, the need to always look for the newest, hottest fad. Some people always played with kink, but now everyone seems to be heading that direction. It started with spanking, then hair pulling and choking (again emulating porn), and now people ask me about floggers and rope.

I'm still optimistic about the future, even if it requires regrouping. Yes, the swing scene has been invaded by a hoard of capitalists trying to sell us a certain vision of the lifestyle to make a buck. But in the end, the sex and the community—those like-minded people who enjoy pleasure with others—are still there.

This is at some level a hobby, sex for fun. As with any hobby, you will make friends, acquaintances and even enemies as you partake. Sex is easy—insert tab A into slot B—but friendship takes time to develop. I feel lucky that I can enjoy hedonistic fun with a couple we will never see again but can also develop deep friendships. We've been to three weddings and a funeral of friends in this scene. We have traveled with, loaned money to, and even cosigned loans with people we've met. I prefer to start with the sex and see if the friendship develops. If it doesn't, at least we have the experience to enjoy. And just because I enjoy group sex sometimes doesn't mean I can't have an emotional connection with someone or have great sex one on one, too. Some nights I eat steak; some nights chicken. Some nights, maybe I want both.

Group sex allows for variety, the spice of life. That part isn't going to change.

Accurate demographics are difficult to generate for alternative[3] sexual practices in most countries. Few nationally representative surveys address sexuality with much specificity, so researchers often settle for convenience samples, recruiting subjects who self-identify as participants in a particular scene or studying in a specific swingers' club, gay community, or BDSM organization. But convenience samples don't give us an accurate sense of how many people *overall* are having group sex, swinging, experimenting with BDSM, and so on and what their demographics are. Many people who swap partners, for example, do not call themselves "swingers"; some individuals who play with power wouldn't join an organization or consider themselves "into BDSM." Are people who take on an identity or consider themselves part of a community different from those who do not? And even if we could survey every single person in a given nation, how would we decide who *counts* as what? Is a woman who blindfolds and handcuffs her lover rightfully considered a BDSM practitioner? Is a man who has been to five sex parties counted as a "swinger"? What if those parties were all during the 1970s or all in the past month? What if he never got up the nerve to talk to anyone, much less have sex, but identifies as a "swinger" anyway? To produce demographics on group sex, would we include anyone who has *ever* had group sex, even once, or only those people for whom it is a regular or significant part of their current sexual experience?

Questions like these can be maddening. While they do not necessarily affect my overall inquiry as to the meanings of group sex for people who have it—a qualitative question—they impact the research available to me. Several communities[4] —such as swinging or the "lifestyle," organized BDSM, and gay male bathhouse or "circuit party" cultures— have been regularly studied by social scientists and thus appear in almost every chapter of this book. In each of these enclaves, multiperson eroticism is prevalent, involving complex relationships of witnessing and being witnessed.[5] In a global, Internet age, communities are not necessarily bounded geographically. Still, if enough people identify as something, researchers can locate and study them; because these particular groups also use public space for sexual activity (such as sex clubs and bathhouses), they are relatively accessible through physical field sites as well. These communities are briefly introduced below, although my investigation also extends to individuals who practice group sex in less organized ways—teen sex partiers, individuals seeking partners on Craigslist, "doggers," and people who go to gang bangs, bukkakes, or "mandingo" parties, for example—and to group erotic or sexual practices found in the anthropological literature.

SWINGING

In swinging, also called the "lifestyle," participants engage in recreational sex with outside partners while remaining heterosexually coupled or married and emotionally monogamous.[6] Couples have swapped partners throughout history, but the contemporary lifestyle is often traced to the sexual revolution in the United States during the 1960s and 1970s, becoming meaningful in the context of companionate marriage, a critique of monogamy, and a belief that recreational sex is possible for both men and women. Although swinging is generally thought of as Western, it has spread across the globe. On www.adultfriendfinder.com, one of the larger adult websites used by swingers, members from 178 countries have placed ads. In Ireland, more than Mass is attended on weekends; one of Ireland's swingers' clubs now boasts more than seventy thousand members.[7] Nonmonogamous couples do not always refer to themselves as "swingers"; I have heard terms ranging from "open" to "partiers" to "modern." Singles and dating couples may also be active in the "lifestyle"; single women, being relatively rare, are referred to as "unicorns."

Group sex is never essential for lifestylers, but most swingers have some experience with multiperson eroticism. Sexual encounters may be "full swap," involving couples in intercourse with another partner (or partners), or "soft swap," where touching, oral sex, "girl-girl play,"[8] or other activities short of intercourse occur. Lifestyle encounters usually involve no sexualized male-male contact, while women classify their sexual orientations fluidly— for example, as straight, bisexual, bisensual, bicurious, bicomfortable, biplayful, or even "bi-when-drinking-tequila." Most couples have rules and an understanding of the sexual and emotional boundaries that ideally govern their interactions with others (even if the rule is "no rules").

Sexual exclusivity remains the norm for committed couples in the United States, despite social changes making it difficult for some individuals: longer periods of singlehood and increased premarital sex, changing gender roles, more opportunities for meeting extramarital partners, and greater expectations for the role of sexuality in one's life and marriage. The lifestyle allows couples to negotiate conflicting discourses of sex and intimacy—for example, the belief that "casual" sex is possible before marriage but sex and love are inevitably linked afterward. Sex can thus be understood as an expression of love and commitment in the marriage but as "play" with other partners and in other contexts. Beliefs about sex, love, and marriage vary around the world and across social groups, however, which can impact the meaning of swinging. An Argentinean woman, for example, told me that "because all men cheat in South America," the lifestyle offered an opportunity to keep an eye on her husband.

Swinging is based on ethical ideals such as honesty, open-mindedness, discretion, respect, equality, and consent. Even if these ideals are not always actualized, the basic tenets of "ethical hedonism"[9] are fairly consistent—that is, lifestylers may argue about how much disclosure is appropriate and under what conditions, but the general impetus is toward transparency in motivation, identity, and anything else deemed important to one's sexual partners.

BDSM

BDSM (or SM) is an acronym for "bondage domination sadism masochism" and an umbrella term for activities revolving around "kink," fetish, or the exchange of power.[10] In addition to having developed specialized language, rituals, etiquette, and iconography, the global BDSM community includes networks of organizations throughout the world, festivals, conferences, and recognized leaders and experts. The majority of BDSM organizations are found in North America, with San Francisco and New York City forming important hubs, although organizations are found in other urban centers such as Amsterdam, Berlin, London, Rome, Sydney, and Moscow. Some organizations and events bridge sexual identities, while others cater primarily to either heterosexual or GLBTQ participants.

BDSM might not seem likely for inclusion in a book on group sex, as whether BDSM is "sex" is debated both within the community and outside of it. Some practitioners believe the sexualized image of BDSM in pornography and popular culture reduces the complexity of practices involved, which may or may not be organized around activities like oral sex or intercourse, and their overall aims. Sex may even be prohibited at some events. Still, BDSM involves many of the same boundaries as sex, such as between self and other or between the inside and the outside of the body. BDSM frequently focuses on the physicality and display of areas of the body deemed sexual—breasts, nipples, buttocks, genitals—and involves the cocreation of intense, arguably intimate, experience that many people interpret as sexual or erotic. BDSM practitioners have also written eloquently on the quest for transgression and transcendence through erotic activity, which is a central theme in this book. As one of my points is that all sex is about *more* than sex, especially when it involves witnesses and being witnessed, I hope the inclusion of BDSM here is seen as illuminating rather than offensive.

Although one might trace BDSM practices throughout history, my focus here is on present-day communities and on play occurring publicly enough that witnesses shape the meanings of interactions, such as at sex clubs, parties, and workshops. Not everyone who engages in BDSM plays in such a visible manner or identifies as part of a community. Professional "dominatrixes" who cater to paying clients engage in more private, dyadic scenes, for example. But for practitioners who do play publicly, watching each other in scenes is an important means of establishing hierarchy and reputation. An audience also lends authenticity to the scene for some participants.

Power exchanges can be enacted in numerous ways: for example, by controlling the body with bondage or restraints, by inflicting pain, or through domination, discipline, humiliation, or collaborative fantasy. Some BDSM "play" dramatizes inequalities embedded in roles or relationships: governess/child, doctor/patient, officer/prisoner, or horse/owner. Other scenarios draw on specific cultural and historical narratives of power and violence, such as Nazi/Jew or master/slave. BDSM can include fetishes or "kinks," such as rubber, leather, latex, fisting, "water sports," or manipulation of the breath or senses. While there is no standard length to scenes, there is preferably a buildup of intensity as players' limits are approached and explored. The relationship between the "top" and "bottom," whether long-term or transient, is ideally a source of arousal through the unfolding power exchange.

Consent is essential. The Marquis de Sade provides a wealth of ideas and fantasies for contemporary BDSM players, but given that the victims in his writing rarely consent, he was technically a "sadist" or a criminal rather than a "top." The emphasis on consent may extend to the prohibition of drugs or alcohol during scenes. Many practitioners uphold the standard of "safe, sane, and consensual" (SSC), a phrase associated with the organized BDSM scene. Players are expected to communicate and negotiate limits before each scene and to artfully respect the boundaries of others.

CIRCUIT PARTIES, SEX CLUBS, AND BATHHOUSES

Circuit parties are periodic dance events with a global presence, "revolving around music, drug use, and sexual pursuits." The parties are often themed— The Black and Blue Ball, The White Party, Montreal's Military Ball. While circuit parties appear similar to raves and other electronic dance cultures in music, style of improvised and individualized dancing, and substances used, there are important differences. Attendees of circuit parties are almost exclusively gay men; the DJs are often known personalities in the circuit party world. Circuit parties usually last more than one day, sometimes encompassing a long weekend with opening and closing parties. Many also have a historical importance in the gay community. The sheer size of the events, which could range from one thousand to ten thousand people, is important to many attendees. Attendees may also tend toward a preferred "look," for example, a masculine "gym" body.[11]

Even though most attendees at circuit parties do not engage in sex on the dance floor and many do not even do drugs, the events are *sexualized* in particular ways. Sociologist Russell Westhaver argues that circuit parties are "intimately linked to pleasurable bodily experience: prolonged dancing, the use of recreational drugs, the centrality of touch, the pursuit of sexual encounters, and the pleasures associated with sociality."[12] On occasion, sexual activity occurs on the dance floor or in designated areas of the venue; some attendees retire to "after-parties," hotel rooms, or private homes for sexual activity. Researchers have primarily paid attention to circuit parties as sites of both unsafe sex and drug use; a few have explored the positive side of events. Circuit parties can be considered "gay celebrations," for example, reactions against a "broader hostile or homophobic world" that allow gay men to take pride in their identity. [13]

More generally, bathhouses and sex clubs have also been of interest to both public health researchers and social scientists because of the possibility of unsafe sex and HIV transmission. Some sociologists and anthropologists have studied these venues as sites of socially deviant behavior or have explored the interactional patterns of patrons.

The following sections draw on the social science literature about the above enclaves, as well as my interviews and experience, to provide a general sense of both the way that people similarly organize group sex experiences and the specificity of different sites and practices. When people want to engage in transgressive behavior, they may purposely seek or create the kinds of temporary environments and interactions that make it more likely. The focus here is on contemporary, recreational settings, although some of the same strategies for distinguishing between everyday life and transgressive activity and transitioning between realms can also be observed in compulsory rituals.

THE RULES OF THE GAME (INTERVIEW, JAMES)

My favorite bathhouse is in Osaka, Japan, where I sometimes travel for work. I go to that bathhouse as much as humanly possible. Compared to bathhouses in the United States and Canada, the one in Osaka is immaculately clean. Nothing is dirty or dingy. It has marble countertops and is decorated with antiques, ornate statues, and crystal bowls. There are oil paintings on the walls. That was a shock, just how palatial some of the furnishings were, and that there even were furnishings. There's even nice carpet on the floor.

You don't see that everywhere.

But just like in other countries, you could easily miss this place if you didn't know where it was. It's in a gay neighborhood, but the door is barely marked.

When you enter, you're in an alcove with a giant Romanesque statue of a woman. She's holding a lamp, very baroque. Then another sliding door opens, and you see a sunken area for your umbrella. You take your shoes off and step up to a carpeted reception area. There is a row of lockers, and you put your shoes in a locker, insert ten yen, and take the key.

Then you pay for your visit using a vending machine. You pay different amounts depending on how long you're staying, whether it's just for part of the day or overnight, and based on your age. If you're over forty, you pay the most, though that's only about twenty-four dollars. The machine spits out a little paper ticket that you take to the reception desk. A young Japanese man takes your key and gives you another key on a wristband for a different locker, where you'll store your clothes. He also gives you a plastic bag with two towels in it, a facecloth-sized towel and a bigger one.

I figured out how all of this worked the first time, even though no one told me what to do. I guess I was motivated!

I remember heading down the hallway, past the antiques and oil paintings, and seeing a powder-room area with hair dryers, colognes, and a place to brush your teeth. I remember thinking, "This is unlike anything I've ever seen in North America."

There is a kitchen area with tables. You can buy grapefruit juice, sodas, beer, or liquor from vending machines, and they serve light meals. At the end of the hall, you come to two relatively large rooms with lockers where you undress and put on your towel. People hang out on couches and watch a large television. From that point, if you are less than forty years old you are allowed to go downstairs through a door with a special code. But even when I was less than forty years old, I didn't know enough Japanese to ask for the code! Occasionally a man I was with brought me down to that area, which I found a little boring. People seemed more inhibited. There were semiprivate areas to escape to, maybe because the younger guys were shy. It was very dark. There were showers and a big room with bunk beds. There were even three or four rooms where you could lock the door. I have no interest in that whatsoever. I prefer to see what's happening. There was also a little theater showing anime or monster movies—not porn—and a reading area with couches and Tiffany lamps and comic books. You'd see guys reading the comics.

I'd think, "I didn't come here to read comics!"

So I prefer other areas of the club. There are two staircases leading up to the next level, and one is narrow with a very low ceiling. I'm the big white guy who has to duck to get up the stairs. I'm often the only white guy in the club. Everyone else is Japanese. But standing out and appreciating their difference and my difference is part of my experience. Before I went to Japan, Asian guys weren't on my erotic radar. But then I found myself in a sea of Asian faces, and all of a sudden, I started to see variation. I started to think, wow, there are some Japanese guys who are fucking hot. I'm into beefy guys, and here are these Japanese "bears" with hot bodies, goatees, and shaved heads. Very beautiful.

Anyway, upstairs you put your larger towel in *another* set of lockers—there are lots of lockers!—and keep the smaller "modesty towel." You cover your genitals with this when you walk, out of "respect," but lots of guys don't, and so much the better, I say. There is a steam-room area with two types of wet saunas. One is the kind we're used to in North America. The other is this strange sauna I've never seen anywhere else in the world. It pelts water at you forcefully, like you're in a hailstorm. The tiny droplets of water are like pinpricks on your skin.

Maybe six people can fit inside—everything tends to be small in Japan.

You clean yourself before playing or going into the sauna. There's an area where you wash Japanese-style, sitting down on a stool. You soap yourself up and rinse off with a handheld shower, or you can put water in a plastic pail and pour it on yourself. I prefer this ritual to the Western-style showers. When I get overheated in the saunas, I'll come out here to the Japanese-style shower area and just pour cold water over myself, again and again and again. And I know I must be quite a sight, because I'm large in comparison to them, and my skin gets really pink when I'm hot. While I'm washing, I look in the mirror and see guys staring at me. Some men are erotically interested in me, the "potato queens," but I'm sure many think I'm disgusting. "Sticky rice boys" are the Asian guys that only like other Asians.

I sit there in my own zone, pouring cold water over myself, not feeling any pressure to hurry. It's about relaxation. Sometimes I realize I've been sitting there for a long time. Just being—but in a very corporeal way. There are so many sensations. On your skin, you have warm and cold, and pools of water, pelting drops of water, poured water. I'm usually there in the winter, and Japan is a humid cold. I never get warm except in the sauna. So I revel in the hot water on my body or the heat in the sauna—-it feels like the first time I've been warm in ages. And everything is beautiful. You're just surrounded by the beauty of the setting and the bodies. The lighting is low, and when you lack visual information, corporeal sensations are heightened even more. The goal is ultimately to hook up, I guess—that's my expectation. But sometimes it doesn't happen, and then there's still this whole other sensual aspect to it.

My favorite time to go to the bathhouse is on Sunday afternoon. Most people in Japan have that day off, so the bathhouse is busy and people aren't drunk. I'm not a late-night person, and I don't derive pleasure from staying up into the wee hours waiting for people to get uninhibited enough to have sex. Occasionally, I'll go on a Saturday night after going to my favorite bar. Sometimes, instead of taking someone home to hook up, I take him to the bathhouse. Mostly, though, I prefer meeting guys in the bathhouse, not in the bars. There just seems to be so much less game playing in the bathhouse.

My favorite room has mattresses on the floor, with duvets and buckwheat pillows. Can you imagine? Duvets? Soft lighting. There are Kleenex and trash cans, and it's very clean. For me, it's a peak erotic experience in the sense that I can have group sex, be watched having group sex, and watch people around me having group sex. In some places, like in a Western bathhouse, you get a room and it's one on one, or you can invite more guys and lock the door. They might have an orgy room, but it's not filled with futons like in

Osaka. You're standing up in a group, not lying down. In Osaka, I can be having sex with three or four guys, but I'm always watching who walks through that door. There's something about these random guys who wander through while I'm having sex—it turns me on. Sometimes they come over and look at me. Sometimes, I touch them and then they join us.

I also like bathhouses because knowing everyone is there for sex is a turn-on for me. The possibility of someone else walking in is not.

In Osaka, I recognize that even though everyone is there for sex, they don't all want sex with me. Only a minority likes white guys. Because Japanese culture is so ordered and polite and rule bound, I'd rather not offend anyone. So I go into my favorite room, stand against a wall, and wait. Maybe that's part of the appeal for me as well—I don't have to do any work. All I do is stand there, and I stand out. I usually don't have to wait very long. Often I am approached within minutes. People walk right up to me and touch me, usually, and then we start. If I tap their hand twice and turn away slightly to signal I'm not interested, that's the end of things. If I'm already having sex, a guy might squat next to me. If I stroke his lower leg, then he'll join in.

Part of what's exciting is someone new, so after a while, if you want to move on, you do. In North America, I always say, "I need to take a break." In Japan, I might just say, "Arrigato," "Thank you," and move on. There isn't much conversation in the group sex room. If you want to talk, there are other areas to go to. In other areas of the club, you can share information, what you do for a living, what they do. I give my first name but not my last name. It just doesn't seem necessary. I might give an e-mail.

People who are into group sex, I think, are very well behaved. I've been having group sex for many years. I can remember saying "no" when people, usually older guys, were groping me. They stopped—you usually don't have to say "no" forcefully. Only once in a bathhouse I had to say, "If you don't stop, I'm going to yell." But that was exceptional. I'd never experienced anything like that before because 99.99 percent of people are very polite. My attitude is that if you're in a space like that, you're signaling that you're open to being touched. I wouldn't be offended if someone touched me, but I reserve the right to say no, thank you, and I respect it when someone says it to me.

No Talking in the Orgy Zone: The Organization of Space

Social scientists Martin Weinberg and Colin Williams compared five gay baths in cities across the United States and conducted informal interviews with patrons. They determined that there were ideal conditions for what they termed "impersonal sex": (1) "a safe setting with low public visibility and with arrangements that inhibit intrusion and facilitate anonymity"; (2) access to numerous attractive potential partners; (3) clear and simple "road maps" for interaction to minimize conflict or stress; (4) bounded experiences so that relationships are primarily limited to sex; (5) a congenial atmosphere that masks rejection; and (6) convenient, relaxing settings.[14] Not everyone is seeking "impersonal sex" when they visit a public sex venue; some visitors come with friends or spouses or hope to make enduring connections. Still, Weinberg and Williams's ideal conditions are useful for thinking about other places where group sex occurs than bathhouses and for other participants than gay men.

Dutch researcher Maurice van Lieshout studied "the Mollebos," a rest area that became one of the most popular cruising spots in the Netherlands in the 1990s. On Monday nights, gay men interested in "leathersex" and S/M gathered at the Mollebos for "leather nights in the woods." Many of these men preferred a style of masculine comportment and dress, such as tight leathers accentuating the penis and buttocks, borrowed from American imagery of cowboys or bikers. Leather nights provided an opportunity for men to meet others with similar interests in an outdoor location. One informant said: "It gives me a special thrill to see other guys with a similar image, to know I'm part of this group of horny leathermen." Some men, Lieshout found, sought an audience for their scenes, such as the man who liked to walk his "slave" like a dog, leading him by a leash and collar, or the army officer and his younger "soldier." Others wanted to cruise new partners for sexual activity and BDSM play.[15]

The Mollebos was naturally segmented into two zones, "an exploration or social zone and a sexual and orgy zone." Leather night participants parked their cars close to the parking lot exit, which differentiated them from visitors actually using the rest stop. Before cruising and during breaks, men socialized in the parking lot. At a gap in the fence, men entered the woods using a path. After their eyes adjusted to the darkness, men could catch glimpses of potential partners as they walked up and down the path. Many men made this trek several times each night. Several groves could be reached from the path; these became sexual zones. Two sexual areas were also used for cruising; men who had already found partners could have sex in a third clearing. Another path led into a more heavily wooded area. This served as the "orgy room." Lieshout writes: "At night it is very difficult to see anything there, and it was necessary to use other senses in order to track other people. In trying to manoeuvre in the darkness, often the best thing to do was to walk until you bumped into another guy. Hands grasping at you, sensual sounds, the smell of poppers, and a vague visual sense of moving figures made it clear you were not alone." Patrons interested in anonymous sex with multiple partners used this space. Afterward, they exited out the other side, either returning to their cars or circling around to cruise again along the path.[16]

The Mollebos area, Lieshout argues, showed striking similarities in spatial organization and behavioral expectations to other leather bars in Amsterdam with backroom facilities, such as the Argos, the Eagle, the Web, and the Cuckoo's Nest. "Generally speaking," he writes, "the further one penetrates these leather bars, the less talking takes place, the less lighting is installed, and the more sexual activities can be expected."[17] Similar patterns exist at other kinds of sex clubs, outdoor public sex locales, bathhouses, and parties.

Anthropologist William Leap suggests that "rather than assuming that interpretations of public or private space are locations, fixed within local terrain," we might treat the terms as "attributes of landscape which are assigned to particular sites by particular social actors and for particular reasons."[18] The same might be said of distinctions between social and sexual space. Zones, for example, serve several purposes. An exploration zone that precedes sexual zones protects against intruders, whether accidental or hostile. Entrances to sex clubs tend to be inconspicuous, and reception areas have a gatekeeping function. At the Club Baths in New York City during the 1970s, visitors entered through a number of locked doors, which "delayed possible intrusion by an unwanted guest"; they were then asked to sign a registration form before they were buzzed inside. This movement "from a more public space to a more private space, from outsider to participant," writes sociologist Ira Tattleman, "established one of the clearest boundaries in the baths."[19] At contemporary lifestyle clubs, patrons may similarly be asked to cross such physical thresholds, provide identification, and sign a waiver acknowledging that they are entering an environment where they might see sexual activity. Patrons may also be asked to become "members" or to commit to certain rules, making it more difficult for undercover police to argue that they were unwittingly exposed to lewd behavior. (Requiring membership may also be used as a legal shield, identifying the establishment as a private venue subject to different regulations.) People posing security risks can ideally be identified before penetrating too far into the space. Employees may deny entry to people who seem unfamiliar with the environment or who refuse to cooperate with regulations such as removing clothes before entering certain areas. Spatial segmentation is also a way participants can protect themselves by monitoring their visibility. One will rarely gain entry to a sex club and be immediately exposed to the most extreme behaviors or specialized environments offered ("dark rooms" for anonymous sex; dungeons for BDSM play; orgy rooms; etc.). If a venue is raided or an intruder does gain access, participants engaged in the most transgressive activities have more protection if they are situated farther from the entrance.

An exploration or social zone also provides a transition for patrons. Group sex participants eschew some norms of sexual privacy but may have an increased interest in anonymity, especially in relation to the broader community. As patrons change out of street clothes and don towels, costumes, or specialized attire such as fetish wear, they become less recognizable. Costumes and masks have long been used during rituals and celebrations to help participants break with the everyday. As people shed outside markers of identity and conform to the norms of the space, they become less inhibited and are implicated as participants. (If you run into a coworker, at least you *both* have some explaining to do if you're each sporting togas.) Even private parties may require guests to change clothes once inside. Some venues offer showers, saunas, or hot tubs for relaxing and preparing the body. Patrons may socialize before progressing to sexual activity; some venues provide opportunities to eat, drink alcohol, listen to music, dance, compete in contests or games, and converse. Some venues display pornography or allow patrons to flaunt themselves on stages or stripper poles.

Conversation usually diminishes as one moves toward the sexual zones, as many participants find it distracting. As an interviewee stated, "It can be rough to maintain an erection while listening to folks across the room chatting about their kids." Lighting often grows dimmer as well. Some venues require full nudity before entering designated play spaces, which serves as a further transition and boundary. Exploration zones thus also allow participants to evaluate potential partners before moving into areas offering more relative privacy and anonymity.

Patrons who use space inappropriately—having sex in socializing areas or socializing in sex areas—face censure. One couple, new to the lifestyle, told me of being chastised at a party for having sex under a blanket on a lawn chair. When they then moved to the pool, they were asked to leave the event. The hosts found their behavior rude and dirty, asking, "Are you going to cum in the pool?" This same couple had locked a bedroom door earlier in the evening during a threesome, also raising the ire of the other guests. Although sexual activity was supposed to be limited to the bedrooms, the doors were also expected to remain open so that everyone had access to play space. The couple had incorrectly assumed that being at a "sex party" meant that the other guests would not be offended by them having sex wherever they chose.

Darkness offers anonymity, and for some participants, the greatest loss of inhibitions. Weinberg and Williams write of a club with a dark corridor known as "Pig Alley," where "the old and unattractive" could more easily find partners; sexual excitement was generated by the anonymity of exchanges rather than the physical attributes of participants.[20] It is not just participants who have difficulty finding partners who find such exchanges exciting, however. Many sex clubs and parties offer "dark rooms" and entry into such areas is rarely accidental. Held in San Francisco, "Darkness Falls" is a safe-sex party for couples and single women that takes place in complete blackness. Transsexuals are welcome, although pre-op trans women pay the rate for single women and trans men are charged as biological men. Both are required "to bring a biological female partner"; even in pansexual, sex-positive San Francisco, there seems to be a gender imbalance in the desire for group sex. (Working the door on those nights, I imagine, poses unique challenges.) Participants remain completely anonymous except to the organizers; the only time they risk seeing one another is upon arrival. Couples check in, undress as desired, and then are instructed to carefully crawl into the play area, as standing could be dangerous given the lack of visibility. When the party begins, organizers suggest that participants gently touch others and ask, "Would you like to play?" If one hears, "No, thank you," or one's hand is removed, this signals a lack of interest that should be respected. "Room monitors" reprimand "bad behavior" and are available to help participants with anything they need.[21] Even in a setting where encounters might be anonymous, then, group sex remains organized, monitored, and patterned.

Not every location where group sex occurs can be mapped neatly onto exploratory and sexual zones. Layouts vary. Facilities may offer different amenities, from baths and saunas to a dance floor. Borders between zones may blur, depending on the needs of participants and their familiarity with each other. Doggers, for example, arrive in cars and primarily remain in or around their vehicles; in this case, the inside of the car becomes an inner sexual zone, as some individuals are invited to watch more closely or participate and others are not. In some countries, even mixed-sex socializing is transgressive and may need to be shielded from hostile intruders; multiple inner zones may be necessary. Gay men had public sex before commercial venues were legal, in parks, public washrooms, and alleys, and they continue to do so today.[22] Climate, amount of police or security surveillance, and the lack of other sexual outlets in a given neighborhood can make some spaces attractive for group sex even if the layout is not ideal. In the 1960s, gay men frequented the ravine in David Balfour Park, Toronto, because it was quickly accessible after making an initial contact, but the steep slopes and dense underbrush provided enough coverage for sex acts. "Orgies easily start and continue with changing personnel," one man recalled. "It is really quite civilized." The ravine was comparable to an inner sexual zone: "nearly complete silence is observed—except for 'thank you' at the end. . . . The exchange medium is touching and sex. You don't become raucous, wild, and wooly. The rule is to be well-behaved, the code is silence."[23]

Experienced participants may be able to pinpoint locations used for sexual activity by paying attention to these characteristics. An interviewee explained: "I've had enough sex in public places that I can look at a place and think, 'Guys have sex there.' Once I was visiting a new city and there was a park across from my hotel. Just looking at how it was laid out, I knew guys would be having sex. The park had meandering roads and little parking lots that were completely surrounded by trees, so there was privacy. It was dark, far enough from the busy city streets so that the lights didn't bother you. I watched a car drive into that park from my hotel room, and thought, 'Those people are going to have sex.' I don't need to seek out information on the Internet about where to go now because I literally see space differently."

When participants cannot manipulate the layout or control entry to a space, gatekeeping functions can be performed in other ways, such as through signals (foot tapping; gesturing; positioning), roles ("lookout"), or modifying behavior in the presence of suspicious individuals. If sexual intentions are concealed or activities cease, a sexual zone is temporally rather than spatially distinguished. An interviewee described his experiences in a "tearoom," or public restroom that men used for sex: "You never knew who was going to come through the door, but nine times out of ten, it wasn't a guy going in to pee. We would wait in the stalls. When someone new came in, we'd let a period of time go by and then give a signal, a foot tap, or people would start cracking the stall doors and looking out. Soon, you could have ten or twelve guys having oral sex or jerking off." Some venues or parties use time limits as part of the structure—after midnight, for example, all participants may be required to remove their clothes or leave.

Despite variations, then, one usually finds a segmentation of space for social and sexual purposes, a progression through space or time toward increasingly explicit sexual activity, and norms that reflect a trade-off between privacy and anonymity.

PLAYING TOGETHER (INTERVIEW, VICTOR)

My partner and I are very much in love, but neither of us is monogamous. At the beginning of our relationship we decided to try being open. When we are in the same country, we always play together, but he lives in South America and I live in the United States, so sometimes we go to sex clubs alone.

At some point, after we started bringing one person or a couple home together, we talked more deeply about what we each liked. He was surprised to hear that I enjoyed fisting someone. I explained to him that I had physiological reactions from fisting someone that were ten times more intense than fucking someone. There's something about driving someone else crazy with pleasure that really turns me on. He hadn't thought about that, and he was worried that it would cause damage and that a guy wouldn't ever be tight again. I explained guys could be very flexible that way.

For our first experience with it together, we went to a bathhouse in South America where we'd played before. There was a room with a sling and a toilet that the bartenders would let you have for fifty minutes. They also provide gloves and lube. We found a hot guy and brought him and his partner into the room. We fisted him, played with him, sixty-nined him, and other things. My boyfriend never thought he would enjoy fisting, but now he does. One thing we've noticed is that men who are really hung, the guys who tend to be "tops" in the clubs or on sites like Man Hunt, flip nine out of ten times when they realize we will fist them. They get used to playing that same script—other guys see how big they are and just expect to be fucked. But we give them something different. I find it erotic to take them out of their comfort zone.

My partner is more of an exhibitionist than I am. In the bathhouses, he puts on a show. He finds a lot of power in that, and says it's the best of both worlds: he's in a committed relationship and also experiencing this freedom he's never had. I'm over that part of it, but I have more experience in sex clubs. I understand he's had boyfriends cheat on him in the past and is really thrilled about having this other milieu to experience things without guilt and secrecy.

Whenever I'm playing with him and another guy, I'm cautious. I don't want someone just connecting with me so that he gets frustrated, or vice versa. We've had it happen where someone connects more with one of us. Sometimes those people function like ghosts—they remind us of the rules and force us to work things out. We have a range of what is acceptable. If the person is attracted to us 50-50 that's ideal; if it's 65-35, we've learned to manage it. If it's not working, we decided I'd signal by biting his left ear. Or if we're in a bathhouse, we just tap each on the shoulder twice and move on. It's a simple code. You take your towel and keep walking. You learn how to communicate nonverbally to make sure you're not hurting each other.

If a guy doesn't understand what we need in terms of balance, we won't play again. Once, we brought a young guy in, for example, but he was connecting more with me as a daddy figure. Afterward, I explained it had to be more balanced. He and my boyfriend started communicating online, and to me, that meant that he understood and was willing to explore. It's not someone else's fault if they just like one of our bodies more, but I need it to be balanced or I won't even get hard. I also want my boyfriend to enjoy it—I love this guy. I don't want him depressed or resentful. When men leave, we give them a score and decide whether we'd repeat the experience or not. There are plenty of other men out there to choose from. Of course, there are some moments during group sex when we aren't all engaged together. Sometimes there's a small pocket of time where I notice that he has a great connection with someone. If I get over my threshold of jealousy, I can pause and then watch them kiss and tell them, "That's hot." Or sometimes we've had guys who sit on my cock and he sits behind them to watch, saying, "Wow, that's incredible." Sometimes when you're fisting, it is just two people who are intimate even if others are watching—that's understandable.

Then, there are also times emotions get the best of me.

I've explained to my partner that when we bring people home, there are three sides to the bed. The headboard is against the wall. If I need to stand up and walk around the bed to join them, I am not included enough in the dynamic. He's had experiences where another guy sort of pushed him out of the way to get to me. Those are things we have to negotiate. We have different styles because when that happens, I just stop the sex. Once, I even got out of the bed and said, "Dude, if you're only playing with him, wait until I'm out of town. It's not going to work tonight." They were shocked at my directness. My partner would have tried to make it work without saying anything. But I was direct. I said, "I'm not having a good time." And so the other guy said, "Let's play together." It actually ended up being a very open and pleasurable encounter. But we need to always communicate, and if we need to restructure, we should do it right away.

"So, Do You Come Here Often?" The Organization of Interaction

All members who attend our events, especially for the first time MUST follow all the guidelines listed below, to protect the comfort, well-being, and integrity of all our erotic guests.

The goal here is to feel safe, sexy and liberated!

We all know that we are RESPONSIBLE for our BEHAVIOUR . . . "NO" means "NO"! Club Bliss was created to allow like-minded people to meet in a safe, friendly and sexy environment.

If you arrive TOGETHER, play TOGETHER, exit the venue TOGETHER and NOT alone. We encourage a space for Ladies to tease, flirt and play! *** LADIES RULE MEN FOLLOW ***All members must be RESPECTFUL toward all parties. ASK before initiating. Remember: Some members are exploring certain areas for the first time and are at a voyeuristic stage. [24]

When it comes to behavior, a "road map," or set of shared norms and expectations, exists in bathhouses and other sex venues. [25] Some groups are highly organized, with explicit, formal rules, as in lifestyle or BDSM communities; others are more informal. Some individuals or couples play at home, where they might design their own rules or import ideals from a broader social milieu. The purpose is similar, however: a road map helps participants avoid conflict or awkwardness when approaching potential partners, negotiating sexual activity (which acts will be engaged in, with whom, for how long, when it is acceptable to join in or watch, etc.), and disengaging when necessary or desirable. Some sex clubs post rules and give tours of the space during off-hours; some offer introductory lectures or classes for newcomers where expectations are discussed. Tales of sex club woe can often be traced back to confusion about the rules of engagement in a particular locale. Making the process additionally difficult is the lack of verbal communication in sexual zones. Many sex clubs or event organizers monitor substance use, as misunderstandings are more likely when participants are intoxicated. Sexologist Charles Moser wrote retrospectively about his visits to BDSM parties over twenty-five years, some of which were held in private homes and others in commercial spaces. The number of guests ranged from just a handful to over five hundred. Although he found the specifics of the etiquette to be variable, such as when and where other participants could talk to submissives, all of the events had rules and expectations that were usually made explicit. Sometimes participants were asked to sign an acknowledgment of the guidelines upon entry. Many newcomers did not play immediately but became accustomed to the group first. [26]

Norms arise around the types of conversations and sexual activities expected. In general, it is best to avoid asking intrusive questions at sex clubs, although definitions of intrusiveness vary—offense might be taken at questions about someone's occupation but not at inquiries about their favorite sexual position. Full names are not routinely shared among new partners; swingers joke about showing up for a date and not knowing the last name of the other couple on the dinner reservation. "Um, have Sam and Gina arrived?" "Outing" someone by revealing an identity, occupation, or other information without consent would always be inappropriate. In lifestyle settings, it is rare to find people evaluating others' ongoing sexual performances, although such commentary might occur in more discreet conversations or at a later time. At BDSM play parties, on the other hand, Moser and others have noted that practitioners tend to discuss others' scenes, comparing skill and technique and evaluating their erotic appeal. Moser also found that even though most of the private BDSM parties he attended did not prohibit explicitly sexual activity, guests often limited themselves to fondling the genitals or oral sex, if anything. Guests considered themselves "sexually adventurous and open" and may have even had experience in other group sex settings, but the play parties were focused on nonorgasmic sensation (even if some continued the experience in private after leaving). At many lifestyle venues, one finds genital sex but very little (or light) BDSM play. While there may be no official prohibition against certain activities, whether anal sex or spanking, groups tacitly encourage some behaviors and discourage others.

Negotiating sexual activity is relatively straightforward in some settings—people just *ask*—but more complex in others. In lifestyle situations, for example, women often, but not always, verbally negotiate for the couple; negotiations may involve back-and-forth exchanges as consent is secured from multiple individuals. Lifestyle couples can set limits ahead of time by identifying as "full swap," "soft swap," or "girl-girl." Negotiation also takes place through body language and behavior—sustained eye contact, repeat looks, smiles, and brief touches. Dancing, when possible, allows people to approach others in a noncommittal manner, although positioning or progressive movement into sexual zones may indicate preliminary consent. If a couple plops down on the main mattress in an "orgy room," for example, they reserve the right to reject any particular individual but shouldn't get too worked up if others continue to approach. People who want to join a scene may position themselves near the individuals they are interested in and wait for a signal rather than diving headfirst into the pile. Voyeurs may instead hug the walls, watching but avoiding eye contact. The way one dresses or undresses can also signal interest and even which acts are acceptable. Some lesbians and gay men have used "hanky codes"—colored handkerchiefs indicating interest in particular fetishes or activities depending on where they are worn. A black hanky denotes interest in S/M, for example, and wearing it on the left side of the body signals that one is a "top" rather than a "bottom." Hankies aren't a foolproof method, however. Colors vary across regions, and even if your hankies match, it doesn't mean you're destined for the back room unless other forces align. At swingers' clubs and parties, leaving on one's bra or underwear can mean that one does not wish to be touched in those areas. The guidelines for Darkness Falls suggest using clothing as a tactile guide to where one does or doesn't want to be touched.

If an individual has decided to forgo selecting his or her own sex partners or activities, this deviates from the norm to such an extent that it often requires either a partner to support this intention—as when a "master" orders a "slave" to service patrons—or necessitates special positioning, such as when an individual requests to be tied to a table in a "gang bang" room.

Couples seeking sex together must also communicate with each other, occasionally nonverbally. One couple told me they decided to squeeze each other's leg if they were uncomfortable with whatever was happening. Unfortunately, it took a few misunderstandings to realize that they inadvertently squeezed each other when feeling pleasure as well. A feeling of "having each other's back" is important to many couples who play together, however they communicate their needs to each other and regardless of sexual identity.

Differences in communication styles can be found between gay or "straight" (heterosexual or couple-based) settings. Men in gay bathhouses, for example, might communicate sexual interest and availability by "simultaneously gazing at another while manipulating [their] genitals."[27] In a heterosexual sex club, however, staring and masturbating often appears aggressive to both other men and women. (In fact, being hounded by strangers grasping their penises, even if rare, is one of the main reasons I've heard women give for disliking sex clubs). A lifestyle couple might instead use a more subtle approach, perhaps beginning oral sex with each other and then glancing at others they wish to join them. According to Weinberg and Williams, gay men can also signal interest through a form of touch where "one partner explores the other with his fingers, which the latter removes from those areas he does not want stimulated or penetrated"[28]—a move usually referred to as "groping" by nonacademics. This tactic is less welcome with heterosexual women, who tend to interpret it as aggressive and invasive rather than experimental. Similarly, one would not test whether someone was interested in BDSM by swatting him with a cat-o'-nine-tails as he walked by; in BDSM play, the roles (top/bottom), implements (crop, bondage, etc.), and limits of the scene would ideally be discussed ahead of time. Positioning also works differently in BDSM scenes, where observers may be welcome but expected to remain distant and silent.

Differences can also be found between gay men's and lesbian's expectations. In contrast to the silence of men's sexual encounters, for example, women's public group sex has been described as "celebratory" and even loud. Women at bathhouse events in Canada were encouraged by the organizers to negotiate verbally, laugh, and express pleasure audibly if they desired. And while touching in a male bathhouse usually signals sexual interest, touching at these women's events indicated "flirtation, indulgence, and a way to take advantage of the carefree environment" rather than sexual availability. Rather than occurring between strangers, touch was often used by women who already knew each other or who had set up dates ahead of time to play at events.[29] This resonates with patterns I've observed at lifestyle events where women set the tone of interactions. At circuit parties where some sexual activity takes place on the dance floor, brief encounters may be acceptable, but more sustained interactions are expected to occur in areas designated for sex.[30] Men may also be expected to remain upright and mostly clothed. As one man suggested, there is a difference "between just sort of innocent sexual play—like checking out each other's dicks and stuff like that on the dance floor—and having your pants around your ankles. You wouldn't want to be naked on the dance floor having sex with somebody."[31] Participants learn to scan a new environment for clues to how acceptable sexual interactions will unfold.

Cultural differences and ambiguities can cause interpretation problems: Does a smile indicate sexual interest, or is it simply a gesture of friendliness? When does watching become "creepy"? People who do not know or respect the codes of conduct of a setting draw attention to themselves—researchers included. Lieshout mentions noticing "suspect visitors" one evening at the Mollebos: "three boys about twenty years old who arrived together—a fact which is in itself reason for suspicion—talked too loud, and were not familiar with the layout of the area."[32] Some breaches of behavioral codes are relatively benign, such as talking loudly while others are having sex. Participants in a group encounter may be expected to finish as a group, especially if couples are involved or if the space is small; it would be a breach of etiquette to continue having sex if others were saying goodbye or waiting on a spouse. Other breaches are considered more serious and can result in violators being asked to leave the venue, such as removing a condom without permission during intercourse or ignoring a safe word in an S/M scene. Occasionally, whether something constitutes a minor or serious breach varies by the setting. In some lifestyle settings, couples are expected to play only together and at the same level; that is, the woman can't hide in the lounge while her husband lurks around the orgy room, and if she has indicated that she is only soft swap, he should not pursue intercourse unless everyone agrees on it ahead of time. This varies by gender and according to the law of scarcity, of course: if *he* were the one hiding in the lounge, her participation as a "single" woman would likely be encouraged rather than problematic.

Even outside of sex venues, individuals interested in alternative sexual practices are attuned to subtle cues that signal like-minded others. What is sometimes jokingly called "gaydar" or "playdar" is not ESP but a way of knowing based on subtle, occasionally unconscious, observations of verbal and nonverbal cues such as appearance, use of language (calling sex "play," for example), or means of positioning or signaling.

Anthropologist William Jankowiac argues that spouse exchange around the globe is "seldom based on spontaneous choice but rather is organized around a *ritualized* code of conduct that highlights each spouse's authority to approve or reject the transaction." Among American lifestylers, the couple becomes more valued as a unit rather than as individuals to protect against jealousy and promote emotional fidelity. Spouses ideally "remain acutely conscious of one another's needs, interests, and desires" as they move through three distinct action phases: preparation, participation, and rejuvenation of the pair-bond.[33] In each phase, couples verbally and nonverbally reassure each other of their commitment. The specifics of ritualized codes of conduct vary among group sex participants, but the existence of such ordered phases of involvement can be widely observed. While a roadmap helps individuals negotiate group sex activity, ritualization helps participants integrate transgressive activity with, or differentiate it from, their everyday lives.

This brief discussion in no way does justice to the complexities and variations in the spatial and social organization of group sex across venues and sexual identities. Generalizations such as the ones found here can be challenged by counterexamples, although my bet is that the counterexamples will point toward a *different* social order rather than a lack of order. Far from being a "free-for-all," group sex is highly negotiated. When humans breach norms of sexual privacy—even as they aim for transgression—they do not do so in random or senseless ways. Thus, even if some of these particular organizing principles do not hold at, say, a nightclub in Nairobi, where being gay is illegal and LGBT individuals are banned from public places, other norms could be expected to arise in those back rooms. Because group sex is social and ordered, outsiders can eventually become participants.

One should be suspicious of accounts of group sex where participants are described as having completely thrown off the shackles of custom, "extinguished all power of moral judgment," or lost all sense of discrimination between sexual acts or partners. In many cases, it is just as likely that the observer was so shocked by the things he thought were happening that he paid no attention to the multitude of things that were *not* happening. One should also be suspicious of theories produced by "armchair orgiasts" who posit a singular or ultimate effect of orgies on societies or individuals—whether the result is destruction or liberation. Most American swingers congregating on Saturday night for group sex in suburban hot tubs are back to work on Monday morning, perhaps saving for a trip to Hedonism in Jamaica but not plotting to overthrow the government or bring down capitalism. Some French teens drink themselves silly before group gropes, but it seems unlikely that *Le Skins* parties are destined to end in insanity, animalistic consumption of the family dog, or suicide. The very banality of group sex, in fact, may be somewhat disappointing. Even libertines who *try* to harness the power of the orgy, believing that participation is a route to social transformation or that it leads to experiences of the sublime, can find that a sudden stray foot to the face or accidentally falling off the bed are the most immediate sources of jeopardy to be faced.

Orgies do not bring about the end of civilization as we know it. Yet neither have they become mundane. Although *some* people in *some* places have experimented with the extremes of sexual behavior to an extent that a deep ennui saturates their adventures, I would wager that their ranks are small. In fact, it is because taboos still exist that participants attempt to regulate sexual encounters and conceal activities from accidental or hostile intruders. In part because of the sediment of meanings discussed in chapter 2, group sex is different from masturbation or dyadic sex. When people have sex in groups, they do not do so arbitrarily but instead to achieve personal and social ends, from enhancing arousal to creating community bonds. Before delving into what group sex *does*, however, examining the human emotions of disgust, shame, and guilt will take us deeper into our exploration of its symbolic and emotional potency.

Chapter Four

Disgust, Shame, and Guilt

The Primordial Soup of Desire

Human eroticism differs from animal sexuality precisely in this, that it calls inner life into play. In human consciousness, eroticism is that within man which calls his being into question.
—*Georges Bataille*

Man is the creature who blushes.
—*Friedrich Nietzsche*

"UNE MÉMOIRE DIABOLIQUE"

In 2001, a petite, middle-aged, married art critic and magazine editor named Catherine Millet shocked French society with the publication of *La vie sexuelle de Catherine M.*[1] In the explicit memoir, Millet reveals—among other things—a taste for being the center of attention at sex parties and gang bangs. A lifelong exhibitionist, she becomes more daring in the company of a regular lover who offers her to anonymous men in restaurants, parks, art galleries, parking garages, a swingers' club called Chez Aimé, and anywhere else he decides to lift her skirt and invite a stranger's hands to wander. "In the biggest orgies in which I participated," Millet recalls, "there could be up to about 150 people (they did not all fuck, some had come to watch), and I would take on the cocks of around a quarter or a fifth of them in all the available ways: in my hands, my mouth, my cunt and my ass."[2] She occasionally admits to feelings of uneasiness or hesitation before such an event or of succumbing to exhaustion afterward but nonetheless jumps in without complaint. She even catalogues her battle wounds with pride—scrapes,

85

bruises, rashes, soreness, or stiffness in her legs "after being pinioned sometimes for four hours."

Millet refuses, both explicitly and through her adventures, many of the
sexual narratives available to contemporary women as well as taken-for-
granted explanations of cause and effect in erotic life. Rather than character-
ize herself as damaged by a grandfather's inappropriate touches in her youth,
for example, Millet casts it as a coming-of-age experience, disconcerting but
valuable. As an adult, she claims more embarrassment at being caught with
crumbs on her mouth than being seen naked or having sex in public. Groups
of men preparing to take her sexually, one after another, inspire in her not
fear of potential violence but an appreciation for the kindness they show her.
Millet also resists defining sex as either inherently repressive or revolutionary: living one's live in a sexually open manner, as she most certainly did,
does not guarantee either positive or negative experiences. [3]

Hailed as the "most explicit book about sex ever written by a woman,"
The Sexual Life of Catherine M inspired both admiration and animosity.
Many critics were disturbed by Millet's matter-of-fact, emotionally detached
style, decrying the book as "boring," "not sexy," or "explicit without being
erotic." One reviewer, pronouncing the writing "dreary" and "dull," suggests
that for Millet, sex "is as simple as eating a bowl of soup."[4] It is no surprise
that many readers expecting titillation are dissatisfied. The pages are filled
with orgies, but also with the unappealing realities of human bodies—cellu-
lite, "drooping guts," "balding heads, and jowly faces." There are bad teeth
and bad smells. Every body fluid makes a cameo appearance, although something about Millet's reactions to these close encounters with humanity calls
to mind St. Catherine of Siena, drinking pus from the sores of her plague-
ridden patients, instead of Lisa Sparxxx, the "world gang bang" record holder
and star of *Gag Factor 13*.

Millet is neither insane nor lusty, but otherworldly.

She might, in fact, actually like the soup-eating metaphor. After all, she
claims that she "never really thought about my sexuality very much" before
writing the book. Fucking is "like breathing" for her. Uncomplicated. She
avoids flirtation, which makes her awkward and uncomfortable, and prefers
to hasten on to the main event wherever it might occur, no matter how public
or proscribed: "If it were possible for the thronging crowds at a train station
or the organized hordes in the Metro to accept the crudest accesses of pleasure in their midst as they accept displays of the most abject misery, I could
easily undertake that sort of coupling, like an animal."[5] She also claims
"indifference to the uses we assign our bodies," offering every bodily orifice
to the group "without hesitation or regret" and "with a totally clear conscience."[6] This indifference extends to her sexual partners—who might be
male or female, washed or unwashed, of any height and weight, or even
indistinguishable from one another, a parade of anonymous appendages.

Even in her fantasies, Millet is available to all—a "vulgar fat man," business-men with "saggy" faces, the kitchen boys, or very old, dirty men who haven't washed "for so long that they'll have scabs on their skin."[7]

I wouldn't say that sex is *simple* for Millet.

"I sweat very little," she writes,

> but sometimes I was drenched in my partners' sweat. There would also be threads of sperm that dried along the tops of my thighs, sometimes on my breasts or my face, even in my hair, and men who are into orgies really like shooting their load into a cunt that's already dripping with cum. From time to time, on the pretext of going to the toilet, I would manage to extricate myself from the group and go to wash.[8]

Millet takes satisfaction in having "no feelings of restraint" in the moment, in pursuing "the contrasting intermingling of experiences of pleasure, which projects us outside ourselves, and filth, which belittles us."[9] "You don't have to be a great psychologist," she admits, "to deduce from this behavior an inclination for self-abasement." Her inclination to find "appeasement in filth" was coupled with feelings of "extraordinary" freedom:

> To fuck above and beyond any sense of disgust was not just a way of lowering yourself, it was, in a diametrically opposite move, to raise yourself above all prejudice. There are those who break taboos as powerful as incest. I settled for not having to choose my partners, however many of them there may have been (given the conditions under which I gave myself, if my father had happened to be one of the number, I would not have recognized him).[10]

Unsurprisingly, she admits to reading Bataille.

Her indifference, in fact, is calculated transgression. After all, if one is truly indifferent to the uses to which the body is put, why repeatedly use one's body for orgies? Why get into a taxi sent in the middle of the night to be whisked away to a gang bang? Why expend the energy to appear "tire-less" or "uninhibited" in front of the throngs of people gathered around waiting for their turn? And if one "hates to feel wet anywhere other than under a shower,"[11] why bathe in the effluvia of others—their sweat, semen, urine, or feces? Millet's indiscriminate sexual partnering is not the spontane-ous result of a loss of self or morality, as in the orgy stories of chapter 2; rather, it is deliberate and premeditated. Edging against the boundaries of personal and social acceptability is part of the erotic appeal of her adven-tures.

Her "open mind"[12] in such matters, Millet believes, was partly because she "had not imagined" that her own pleasure could be the aim of a sexual encounter until around the age of thirty-five, although there is clearly more to the story. The pleasure she does experience is incidental and vicarious:

"First, I had to . . . literally abandon my whole body—to sexual activity, to lose myself in it so thoroughly that I confused myself with my partner."[13] She becomes exhibitionist and voyeur as her erotics focus either on herself as the center of the activity or on the body "left behind" when she fantasizes her sense of self as displaced. During sex, Millet often imagines herself as less than human, taking on an "animal identity": a "spider in a web" when surrounded by men, a "waddling duck" when being asked to walk while being penetrated from behind, and something "between a frog and those upside-down insects that beat the air with their short legs" when lying on her back on top of a man. This fantasy of animalistic indifference alternates with self-conscious transgression. Millet writes of seeing her reflection in the mirror while masturbating, of avoiding her eyes yet watching her body as others might:

> I cannot recognize myself in such a state of release; with a feeling of shame, I reject it. That is how pleasure stays on a knife edge: just as the multiplication of two negative numbers gives a positive number, this pleasure is the product not, as is sometimes said, of an absence from oneself but of the bringing together of this perceived absence and the feeling of horror that it provokes in a flash of conscience.[14]

Millet delights in such exposure, although it is unclear whether she has more erotic investment in her actual sexual adventures, in her "*mémoire diabolique*" of those adventures,[15] or in the narratives she creates for others. She details her escapades for friends, "savoring" their disgust at specific acts or partners, evoking "dirtiness" and a "contagious ugliness."[16] She also enjoys her reputation. "I was seen as someone with no taboos, someone exceptionally uninhibited," she writes, "and I had no reason not to fill this role."[17] Writing a memoir, of course, prolongs the pleasure of both "wallowing" in the muck and throwing handfuls of it at the crowd gathered to watch, fascinated and repulsed. As Millet indulges readers with intimate details many would rather not think of, much less expose, she once again leaves herself behind:

> Because . . . the same woman whom I described as uncomfortable under someone's insistent gaze, and who hesitates to wear suggestive clothes, the same woman in fact who partook blindly in sexual adventures with faceless partners, this same woman, then, takes indisputable pleasure in exposing herself on the condition that the exposure is distanced at once, by a narrative.[18]

"DO IT LIKE THEY DO ON THE DISCOVERY CHANNEL"?

In a 2006 news story shared widely on the Internet, pandas became pornography's most significant new species of consumer. The Chiang Mai Zoo in

Thailand borrowed two giant pandas from China, hoping they might mate successfully in a warmer climate. They hadn't done so well in China. Pandas are reclusive creatures in the wild, with little experience interacting with each other. They are also notoriously poor breeders. Captivity exacerbates the situation: the already finicky pandas have fewer sexual partners to choose from, and the sedentary lifestyle makes them lazy.

These two pandas—Chuang Chuang and Lin Hui—were no exception.

Tired of watching the platonic pandas putter around their leafy habitat, showing no interest in copulating, zoo officials decided to be proactive. First, they separated the pandas, hoping that distance might kindle desire. Next, the male, Chuang Chuang, was put on a diet, as zoo officials worried that he was too portly to mate without injuring Lin Hui. Then Chuang Chuang was given a big-screen television, some low-calorie bamboo, and a stash of panda porn.[19] The pandas' cub, Lin Ping, was born in 2009 as a result of artificial insemination.

No one ever promised that porn helps you mate with . . . your mate.

Still, panda porn has since been used successfully back in China, at the Chengdu Research Base of Giant Panda Breeding, where scientists find "that the combination of porn, exercises, and the occasional ménage à trois" at least stirs up curiosity about sex for young male pandas, an important first step. Zhang Zhihe, the director of the research institute, reports that "more than 60 percent of his pandas are now capable of having sex on their own— up from just 25 percent twenty years ago."[20] Journalists compared the pandas' sexual dysfunctions to those of humans—"sometimes married couples just need to add a little spice to their love lives."[21] The difficulties of "mating in captivity," actually the title of an internationally popular book on monogamy,[22] may be shared among mammals.

Zookeepers in India scrambled to find a film of chimpanzees having sex when faced with a similar situation. It wasn't just that the primates were unimpressed with the human performances in *I Dream of Jenna*, but that young chimps learn the facts of life by watching adult chimps. Unfortunately, there were few other chimps to watch and very little live action in their habitat. Instead of spending all their time "eating and playing," zookeepers hoped males that watched a chimp sex flick would show more interest in females who approached them.[23]

Now, we cannot make too much of these stories. Who knows what wild pandas or chimps really need to get them in the mood? Perhaps zookeepers created desires for sexual imagery rather than stimulating existing desires to watch other animals having sex. Even if pandas had opposable thumbs and mirror neurons, for example, they might never develop the Qinling Mountains as the *Ailuropoda melanoleuca* version of "San Pornando Valley."

How people learn about sex in modern societies is a controversial topic. Humans are social animals, not reclusive loners like pandas. But unlike

chimps or their bonobo cousins, widespread norms of privacy during sex—
and often, actual laws against public copulation—mean that most of us don't
learn how to have sex by watching our elders and relatives. Aside from porn,
the average person knows little about what sex looks like for other people
once they stumble home from the neighborhood pub. In rural areas around
the world, children observe animals mating; urban parents with National
Geographic on their cable lineup know that city kids show interest, too.
Youthful curiosity doesn't stop with animals. Anthropologists occasionally
witness young children engaged in sexual play with each other with no adult
reprimands, although this is rare in Western societies. Other times, due to
close living quarters, as in cases of whole families sharing a bed, kids learn
about sex inadvertently. In some societies or groups, "apprenticeships" or
coming-of-age ceremonies still impart sexual knowledge to young adults;
young men may still be taken to a brothel by relatives for their first sexual
experience, for example.

Many American parents wish sex education could occur through osmosis;
others want control over how—and what—their kids learn. Contemporary
youth may learn about sex from peers, educators, pop culture, and personal
experience. In some countries, such as Switzerland or the Netherlands, com-
prehensive sex education is offered in public schools beginning at an early
age. In the United States, public sex education programs are often pressured
to maintain an abstinence-based approach.

Mainstream sex education doesn't even usually include photographs,
much less action-focused instruction. Watching others have sex, however, is
still a way of obtaining information—whether live or recorded, "educational"
or "pornographic." A 2009 study of fourteen- to seventeen-year-olds in England found that many admitted to learning about sex from pornography, even
though they realized it might "give boys or girls false ideas about sex."[24]
New York teenagers credit Google and YouTube as sources of both useful
and "inappropriate" information about sex.[25] ProFamilia, a German social
work organization that teaches about sexuality in middle schools, found that
new questions were spurred when teens educated themselves using porn. One
young girl, for example, worried she was "turning into a man" because she'd
found a hair growing in her armpit—she'd never seen women with underarm
hair in the porn she viewed on the Internet.[26]

In 2011, after one of his human sexuality lectures at Northwestern University in Chicago, Professor Michael Bailey allowed two guest speakers to
perform a live demonstration of a female G-spot orgasm. The six hundred or
so undergraduate students were informed that the demonstration was optional
and would be sexually explicit; around one hundred remained. The woman
took off her clothes and lay on a towel on the auditorium stage. Explaining
that she had a "fetish for being watched by large crowds while having an
orgasm," she then proceeded to indulge this desire with the help of her fiancé

and a sex toy.[27] Although one student expressed surprise at how explicit the demonstration became, most supported it as educational, and none filed complaints with the university. Still, the incident became a national scandal, which Bailey realized when he received a call from Fox News. Reactions both on and off campus ranged from "troubled and disappointed" to utter panic. Bailey was rebuked for poor judgment. Clinical psychologist and sexuality expert Judy Kuriansky told Fox News that the demonstration was inappropriate, aiming at "shock value more than educational value." While educating about sexual behavior, even "kinkiness," is important, Kuriansky insisted, "talking about it can show you just as much."[28] Some critics couldn't even explain *why* they believed the incident was so harmful but responded with revulsion anyway. That the guest speakers used a motorized sex toy called a "fucksaw" didn't help Bailey's case. Bloggers and journalists sprang on the term, reporting on "fucksaw-gate," Northwestern's new "minor in fucksaw sciences," and "Professor Fucksaw." "Fucksaw fallout" spread beyond campus: after the scandal, students on spring break from Northwestern who were supposed to build a nature trail in Hixson, Tennessee, were prevented from camping on the nearby property of the Community Baptist Church while they did so. The pastor, Clifton Roth, had stumbled onto the story, decided that God meant him to see it, and resolved not to have his church "associated with a university that would condone a live sex-toy demonstration."[29]

With a "fucksaw," no less.

In response to the controversy, Bailey explained to the media that one of his primary research areas was sexual diversity. Previous guests in his sexuality course had been swingers, transsexuals, and convicted sex offenders.[30] His students were consenting adults, he emphasized, not "fragile children." Eventually, Bailey issued an apology for his decision though maintaining his stance that the demonstration had not caused harm. As he told his class: "Sticks and stones may break your bones, but watching naked people on stage doing pleasurable things will never hurt you."

Witnessing and being witnessed in erotic activity, however, can trigger intense and ambivalent emotional responses. Group sex can have educational aspects for humans, as participants are exposed to the many ways people express or experience pleasure as well as how bodies look and move during sex. But sex education of any form is rarely just about techniques or facts—those of us who teach about sexuality grow accustomed to the predictable silences or nervous giggles of the audience. After all, long before we become interested in the mechanics of intercourse, reproduction, or motorized dildos, we've absorbed a great deal of critical information about sex.

THE RAZOR'S EDGE: DISGUST, SHAME, GUILT, AND
SEXUALITY

Disgust, shame, and guilt are the basic social emotions that Freud called "mental dams," focusing intently on the orifices used for sex, elimination of waste, and eating. At the same time as they "dam" unconscious and potentially troublesome sexual desires, however, disgust, shame, and guilt can also be implicated in arousal.[31]

Studying emotion across cultures, like studying privacy or other concepts, presents philosophical and methodological difficulties.[32] While it would be impossible to do justice to the intricacies of the debates raging through the vast literature on emotion, the question of universalism versus particularity must be addressed. Although all languages have a word for "feel" and ways to describe feelings as "good" or "bad,"[33] terms about emotion that exist in one language do not always have direct equivalents in others. Some extreme cultural constructionists or relativists argue that this proves no emotions are universal; other thinkers believe this to be an example of how cultures distinctly elaborate on human emotional experience, not that people actually *feel* differently. An equivalent of the German word *Schadenfreude*, for example, does not exist in English. Still, the regularity with which celebrities such as Britney Spears or Kim Kardashian end up on the cover of *People Magazine* for failed relationships or weight gain shows that Americans can "derive joy in others' misfortunes," regardless of whether the experience is recognized or labeled. For my purposes here, disgust, shame, and guilt are explored in terms of their mandatory, minimal meanings—that is, as abstract concepts pertaining to potential human capacities and experiences across cultures, regardless of which terms exist in a given culture's language.[34] Those minimal meanings, of course, are always fused with more specific cultural and personal meanings. (Many thinkers believe that shame and guilt require uniquely human capacities for symbolic self-awareness and self-reflection, although there is evidence that some animals, especially those who live closely with humans and must respond to human emotional states, may be developing these capacities.)

Disgust is a prime example of a universal human response—strong aversion involving withdrawal from a person or object—that is triggered and expressed in culturally and individually variable ways. Although humans have an innate capacity for disgust, the triggers are not necessarily instinctive, as any mother who has found her infant drawing on its body with feces can attest. Disgust can also be overcome, as the same mother then demonstrates by washing her baby. *That's Disgusting* is a popular book that teaches some rules of disgust to children. Illustrations of various actions, such as sticking your hands in the jelly jar, eating hair, and pooping in the bathtub, are followed by the refrain, "That's disgusting!" My daughter loved the book, especially when we yelled the refrain together. Unfortunately for me, she also began replicating each scenario, one by one.

What did I expect from a researcher's child?

Had she not gotten in trouble for doing so, however, I believe she might have found some of the results more amusing than disgusting. My responses, I was highly aware, likely shaped her future experiences of those disgust rules as either fun to break or horrifying to encounter.

Sexual contact requires "boundary crossings"—both the boundaries of the body and the boundaries of the self—that are invested with intense psychic meaning: *Me. Not me.* Because sex requires intimate contact between bodies, disgust rules come into play—consciously or unconsciously; culturally and individually. Genitals mark a boundary between the inside and outside of the body. Body fluids, one's own or those of other people, are often seen as contaminating, dangerous, or powerful; contact with body fluids may be subject to a variety of taboos. A video used to teach abstinence in American schools asks teenagers to chew cheese snacks and then spit the chewed-up crackers into glasses of water. The dirty water represents body fluids that the teens then "share," simulating sex by pouring the concoctions into one another's glasses.[35] Although viewers are indeed disgusted by this exercise, as are participants, the video misses an important point. Certainly, it might turn your stomach to think of someone's spit in your mouth, much less other body fluids. This is why the cheese-snacks exercise worked in generating disgust—at least at that particular moment. This is also one of the reasons that sex can be so traumatic when used as violence. But what about your *lover's* spit? Does anyone really think these young viewers were plagued by visions of soggy Cheez-Its during their next backseat Twister session?

William I. Miller, a law professor who writes on emotions and human culture, points out that a person's tongue in your mouth "could be experienced as a pleasure or as a most repulsive and nauseating intrusion" depending on your relationship with the tongue's owner.[36] The thought of a stranger's invasion of one's bodily boundaries can cause disgust; so, too, can the touch of someone too familiar. (One therapist I know asks troubled couples to kiss—with tongue—for five minutes a day. The most common response she hears? "Yuck!") Although disgust rules may be relaxed or overcome in certain situations, then, the fact that they exist can add to the arousal of those breaking them. When we are in love or want to have sex, Miller argues, we will do things or let things be done to us that "would trigger disgust if unprivileged, if coerced, or even if witnessed." If one never overcomes disgust in certain situations or with particular partners, one's sexuality may be experienced as too inhibited. If one never feels disgust over boundary transgressions, others may wonder about his or her sanity.

Miller argues that semen is perhaps the most polluting body fluid, with "the capacity to feminize and humiliate that which it touches."[37] A niche

genre of gonzo pornography[38] involves group sex where a "money shot"—
the standard male ejaculation scene—is not the erotic conclusion. Instead,
semen and other body fluids such as urine, saliva, enema fluids, or vomit
from multiple actors are collected. All these fluids have the power to disgust
and pollute, especially when externalized from the body (even our own saliva, for example, which we swallow hundreds of times a day, becomes disgusting once put in a glass, and most people balk at reingesting it). The scene
culminates when an actor (gay male porn) or actress (heterosexual porn)
either enthusiastically or reluctantly ingests the fluids. This is usually done
creatively: a film in the *Perverted Stories* series shows a woman using the
concoction on her breakfast cereal instead of milk; other films feature fun-
nels, straws, or bowls. Fluid ingestion is viewed as a means of challenging
limits, both social and psychological. The incorporation of foreign body
fluids (or body fluids made "foreign" by their externalization from the body,
such as spit in a glass) into one's own body violates the integrity and the
boundaries of the body onscreen but also jeopardizes the viewer vicariously.
At least some of the erotic power of pornography emerges through the graphic transgression of taboos, although there are cultural and historical patterns
in what is considered "hot" and individuals respond differently. In gay porn,
fluid ingestion carries additional erotic meaning as visual proof of unsafe
sex. In the film *Fucking Crazy*, bottom Max Holden retains the semen from
gang bang participants in his body overnight and ingests it the next day.
Some viewers find these scenes arousing; others find them disturbing.[39]

There is a fine line between disgust and desire.

A fine line, like Millet's knife edge.

Miller's analysis is culturally specific, however, as the meaning of body
fluids, and the taboos surrounding them, vary across time and place. An array
of practices sometimes collectively referred to as "ritualized homosexuality"
was reported in about 10 to 20 percent of Papua New Guinea cultures, although no longer practiced consistently today. In these societies, vaginal
fluids were believed polluting—adult men would often spit after saying the
word "vagina" and would try to avoid inhaling "vaginal smell"—but semen
was viewed as powerful. Young boys were required to leave their mothers
and transition into "men's houses" at around ten to thirteen years of age,
when they also began having sexual contact with an older male or series of
older males. Semen was believed essential in order for boys to mature into
men; same-sex contact was believed to build up semen in the body, while
heterosexual contact was thought to deplete it. For this reason, many taboos
existed on heterosexual intercourse but far fewer on same-sex activity.
Among some groups, such as the Marind-anim, same-sex activities continued
until marriage or the birth of a child; among other groups, same-sex practices
were primarily limited to rituals and initiation ceremonies. Initiation ceremonies might involve oral sex, anal sex, masturbation, or, as found among the

Kimam, collective intercourse with women, after which the semen was gathered and rubbed on the men's bodies.[40] Although these practices were rooted in the specific cosmology of each group, men's sexual activities were generally kept secret from women; being witnessed by a woman potentially undermined the entire social structure by exposing the source of male strength and dominance.

Anthropologist Gil Herdt points out that these New Guinea men were not "homosexual," even though they engaged in powerful, secret homoerotic relations; eventually, they took up exclusively heterosexual relationships.[41] Anthropologist Deborah Elliston disagrees with Herdt that the relations can consistently be termed "homoerotic" or even erotic, arguing that "erotics and sexuality are not central—and probably not even relevant to the meanings of these practices."[42] Instead of "ritualized homosexuality," Elliston uses the phrase "semen practices."[43] She points out that boys initially responded with "revulsion and significant fear" upon learning that initiation entailed fellatio. Initiations also unfolded within hierarchical structures of age and gender— boys are feminized and positioned as inferior to older bachelors, who are inferior to the male elders, in a transition to manhood. Although fear and revulsion arguably play roles in many societies when youth are introduced to sexuality—in the United States, for example, girls may be taught that losing their virginity will be painful, and both sexes are warned about the dangers of disease (pollution)—Elliston's aim of sidestepping the question of homoerotic or heteroerotic motivation is important.

In societies without a concept of "essential sexual orientation"—for example, where all boys progress through age ranks first associated with same-sex and then opposite-sex activity to become "men"—the possibilities and dangers involved in contact with body fluids differ from Western scenarios. Practices such as cane swallowing, which causes vomiting, and induced nosebleeds expurgate female substances from the men's bodies, illustrating how the categories of masculinity and femininity are seen "as permeable and subject to change through contact with other substances."[44] Semen and breast milk are linked in many societies with semen practices, and women were also sometimes believed to benefit from the ingestion of or contact with semen. In initiations, Sambia boys were told that breast milk is created from the transformation of semen in the mother's body (the women, however, challenge this belief).[45] Elliston points out that the Kaliai even have a term to designate "those liquid substances which have the capacity to create social ties"— which are semen or male substance, breast milk, and "the fluid of the green coconut."

The plots of *Perverted Stories* and *Fucking Crazy* would surely fail in such contexts—the jeopardy experienced by viewers of consumption porn is unintelligible if the actress's breakfast of semen-cereal is interpreted as enhancing her reproductive potential or siphoning male strength or if Max

Holden's ritualized semen ingestion is not a mark of his willingness to push the edges of sanity but a necessary part of becoming a man.

Nonetheless, fluids remain powerful, subject to taboos and implicated in the boundaries between self and other, and disgust becomes a sliding indicator of how these boundaries are conceptualized within and between groups. According to anthropologist Raymond Kelly, the Etoro of the Highlands area believed that heterosexual relations depleted male virility, but did not necessarily find women themselves to be polluting. The Kaluli, on the other hand, more rigorously enforced segregation between men and women and believed that menstrual fluid was so polluting that if a menstruating women cooked or stepped over food, those who ate it—and in particular, her husband—could fall ill and die. And while the Etoro practiced oral insemination, believing it produced strong men, they reviled Kaluli anal insemination initiation practices, which were "regarded as totally disgusting." Not surprisingly, the Kaluli and Etoro considered themselves enemies.[46]

Shame is a close relative of disgust and a means by which disgust rules and other social norms are taught and enforced. As social and reflexive beings, humans objectify and compare themselves with others. Anthropologist Richard Shweder suggests a minimal conceptualization of shame as "the deeply felt and highly motivating experience of the fear of being judged defective." This might involve either a "real or anticipated loss of status, affection, or self-regard that results from knowing that one is vulnerable to the disapproving gaze or negative judgment of others." Shame often focuses on four key evolutionary areas: sexual behavior, prosocial behavior (failures to meet obligations), conformity to rules, fashions, or traditions, and "resource competition (failure to compete competently for resources and/or being seen to lack the abilities to competently do so)."[47] Cultures may focus more attention on any given domain, depending on other beliefs, meanings, and circumstances; the emphasis can change over time. Children learn cultural norms, such as how to respond to their bodily functions, through the attention, facial expressions, and encouragement or discipline of parents, other adults, and peers. A capacity for shame, Shweder believes, is necessary for social life, and "shame-like feelings of one sort or another are probably found everywhere in the world, at least among 'normal' or non-psychopathic members of human social groups." Still, the abstract fear of being judged defective takes specific cultural and historical shapes; it would be incorrect to say: "The word for shame in the such-and-such language is X."[48] Shame—at least in the way that Shweder is interested in it—is not a "word" in any language; it is a universal abstract concept.

Psychiatrist Michael Lewis similarly argues that universal and relativist approaches are not antithetical when it comes to shame, although he defines shame differently, as "self blame following an important failure of the self." Both shame and guilt are "negative feeling states meant to interrupt actions violating either internally or externally derived standards or rules," although these standards and rules vary over time and place.[49] As an evaluation of the self, shame is more intense than guilt, Lewis believes, so aversive, in fact, that "humans everywhere attempt to rid themselves of it" using a variety of techniques to dissipate their feelings, such as forgetting or denial, laughter, or confession. If shame is too painful for an individual to acknowledge, it may be "bypassed" or transformed into sadness or anger. If someone is shamed frequently or intensely and unable to recover, that person may exhibit the more extreme parallels of these emotions, depression or rage.[50] Individuals may be more or less vulnerable to shame or guilt due to personality differences, the nature of their relationships, their experiences of child rearing and punishment, and their social positions (sex, social class, race, religion, ethnicity, etc.).

Psychoanalyst Joseph Lichtenberg defines shame even more broadly, as an emotion that blunts initiative and curbs excitement. He views shame as the primary dividing factor between sensual and sexual experience. Sensuality is soothing, pleasurable, unconflicted, and related to our attachments to others. Sexuality, on the other hand, arises when a child's pleasure seeking is inhibited by caregivers; these activities then become tense and conflict laden, representing a struggle between bodily pleasure seeking and shame. Constraints and prohibitions introduced by caregivers are reinforced in various forms by authorities and institutions over the life course. Sexuality thus has an edge that sensuality does not, he writes, "and that edge is itself a stimulus" to excitement, involving elements of power and transgression.[51] Shame, for Lichtenberg, is instrumental in creating the prohibitions and boundaries that we later find arousing; it is also a key element shaping the experience of boundary crossings as disturbing, subversive, or rebellious. Because shame is a threat to the self, the precise ways that shame interacts with sexuality depend on how the self is conceptualized in relation to others in any given belief system. Still, shame animates *all* expressions of human sexuality to varying degrees.

Each of these thinkers conceptualizes shame slightly differently. Shweder, for example, avoids the term "self," a concept which some anthropologists deem ethnocentric. Lewis retains the concept of the self but argues that his definition holds even if we recognize multiple selves—shame arises in relation to the failure and blame of any of them. Lewis also provides a way to distinguish between shame and guilt, at least phenomenologically, and recognizes that when shame is unacknowledged or too intense for an individual to bear, it may be transformed into other emotions. Lichtenberg's shame is more primal, as consciousness of a "self" is not necessary in his approach; one can observe aversive responses to the dampening of pleasure-seeking behavior in infants and toddlers. Although there are implications to choosing among these definitions, each way of theorizing shame highlights these crucial aspects: shame is experienced in relation to real or imagined others, inhibits us from violating norms, is an aversive experience, and is implicated in erotic life.

Some thinkers classify societies as either "shame" or "guilt" cultures, depending on which emotion dominates their moral systems, although such a distinction is problematic. Guilt is minimally conceptualized here as a self-reflexive acknowledgment that one's behavior does not conform to known standards, rules, or goals. Guilt can have immediate effects, causing us to cease a given behavior, or more long-term impacts, preventing us from doing something again. Guilt can also become intertwined with arousal when we break rules. Some individuals come to feel more "turned on" when violating prohibitions. Guilt might be thought of as that voice in your head saying, "You shouldn't be doing this," as you either shift your actions in line with social expectations or grow more excited about doing exactly what you aren't supposed to be doing.

A preference for relative sexual privacy can thus be widespread among humans, bolstered by our emotional capabilities for disgust, shame, and guilt, and at the same time rooted in specific beliefs. Being "caught in the act," then, does not happen the same way, have the same meanings or repercussions, or generate the same emotional experience across contexts or individuals. In cultural contexts where nakedness is viewed as shameful, for example, preferences for sexual privacy may be related to, though not completely explained by, desires to manage bodily exposure. Nudity is not necessary for sex (just think—"lights out, under the covers"), but the human body is highly symbolic; the way one's body is displayed and the "uses to which it is assigned" are often intense emotional matters. Just ask the stripper whose next-door neighbor has unexpectedly appeared at her stage, or consider Millet's discomfort at being seen with crumbs on her lips but not with her lips on others' genitals. One might feel "naked," in the sense of being shamefully exposed, regardless of one's state of dress. The meaning of bodily exposure also varies, depending on who is interpreting it. While a young Canadian girl may be embarrassed if a stranger catches her dressing, the experience does not necessarily shame her entire family, as it might in Afghanistan. And even though Captain Cook wrote that "these people are Naked and not ashame'd," the Tahitians might have thought otherwise—about the nakedness, at least. What a British trader interpreted as sexual exhibitionism—a Tahitian woman who several times "unveiled all her charms" before him, even turning around several times to give him "a most convenient opportunity" to admire her—was quite possibly a display of her tattoos rather than her genitals. Tattoos were a reassurance that she was a mature adult, safe to barter with, and a sign of status.[52]

In contemporary Western cultures, nudity has conflicting meanings. In Hellenistic traditions, nudity is revered as truthful and natural; in Hebraic traditions, being clothed is a mark of humanity.[53] Because prohibitions on nudity can thus be figured as either necessary for civilization *or* as the repression of a "natural" humanity, the naked body stirs up ambivalent emotional reactions. Nudity can produce desirable feelings of exposure, as between lovers, or shameful ones, as when stripping is used as a punitive measure. Those who willingly or purposely shed their clothes in public—"streakers" or nudists, for example—are often viewed as disrupting the social order and are criminalized, pathologized, or stigmatized.

But preferences for sexual privacy are not always related to feelings about one's exposed body. The Yanomami of Brazil, who live in *shabanos*, or group houses, use the word *soka sokamou* for crude or impolite sex. Acceptable sex occurs in relative privacy, in the rainforest or their gardens, and preferably in the morning. If a couple have sex in the *shabano*, they should remain quiet.[54] While the same fear of being judged defective and suffering a social loss because of one's inappropriate sexual behavior could be said to underlie both the Yanomami concept of *soka sokamou* and the American idea of "sluttiness," the words do *not* mean the same thing. Rather, they are culture-specific manifestations of shameful behavior in particular contexts. "Being walked in on" or "being heard" during sex—experiences for which middle-class Americans do not have a specific word, perhaps because they are relatively infrequent[55] —is closer to *soka sokamou* in terms of actual meaning. Sluttiness, on the other hand, is a negative evaluation of behavior tied to beliefs about gender and sexuality.

Disgust, shame, and guilt are never the entire story in sexuality; other emotions, experienced and interpreted within interpersonal, social, cultural, historical, political, and economic contexts, play supporting roles. Gender, class, race, age or generation, educational background, religious identification, and other social positions also influence the realm of sexuality and erotics. Part of what makes group sex so powerful even across these differences, however, is that it violates even more disgust rules, psychic boundaries, and cultural prohibitions than dyadic sex—and it does so in front of witnesses.

"TAMING WITH THE BANANA": GANG RAPE AND SOCIAL HIERARCHIES

Gang rape is a particular kind of group sex.

Experiences of extreme disgust, shame, and guilt can be produced through forced sex. When disgust is *not* overcome by desire, transgressions of one's bodily boundaries are not arousing but shattering. If shame spreads too far, putting the self in more jeopardy than can be sustained, the subsequent annihilation is not exciting but terrifying. Guilt can continue to punish after the fact, leading to cyclical self-blame. An exploration of violent group sex, then, provides a dramatic entrée into some of the social reasons for breaching norms of sexual privacy and the emotional impact of doing so.[56]

Randy Thornhill, an evolutionary biologist, argues that rape evolved as a form of male reproductive behavior. Sex that looks less than consensual, or "forced copulation," has been observed in the nonhuman world. Male scorpion flies offer females "gifts" of dead insects or saliva before mating, for example. But if the male scorpion fly arrives without a gift, he may use another strategy: he chases the unwilling female, clamps her with a "notal organ" so that she cannot resist, and mates with her. Forced copulation also occurs among some mammals and birds. Sea otters and dolphins, marine mammals with devoted human followings, have reportedly taken part in "gang rapes," occasionally leading to the death of the female. And although mallard ducks are put forth as paragons of social monogamy, unattached males sometimes aggressively coerce females into sex. Groups of male ducks have been observed pecking at a female until she submits, occasionally killing her in the process. Female ducks have resisted forced mating over the centuries by evolving spiraling vaginas to counteract the corkscrew-shaped penises of male ducks. When an uninvited male "explosively extends" his penis—which by the way, is large enough to make him the John Holmes of the bird world—he may ejaculate into a cul-de-sac. Most forced matings, then, don't end in fertilization, leading one writer to quip: "Clearly, it's not size that matters, but what she lets you do with it."[57] In each species, different pressures have led to the evolution of forced copulation as a reproductive strategy. Thornhill believes that forced copulation in humans similarly evolved as a response to the mating strategies used by men and women. Human females are not willing to mate with any or all men; they consciously and unconsciously discriminate among potential reproductive partners. But human males have been selected to mate with as many females as possible. Because of these differential sexual adaptations, Thornhill argues, mating becomes a game. Men gain access to women by possessing physical traits that women prefer or by competing against other men for power, resources, social status, and so on. Rape, according to Thornhill, is a strategy that an "inferior" male can use when a female is not willing to mate with him or when the costs of forcing a female to copulate are low.

Simplistic evolutionary theories of rape have been soundly challenged. First, interpreting observations across species presents hurdles. Even granting that forced copulation in the animal kingdom doesn't look enjoyable, how might one measure "consent" in waterfowl? Second, among humans, rape serves purposes far beyond reproduction. Critics point out that women who are of nonreproductive age are still raped, as are men. Some men rape their wives, with whom they may have consensual sex. Patterns and definitions of rape also vary across cultures and time periods, suggesting social and historical influences. Most importantly, when looking at rape in human populations, we must examine the *meaning* of the behavior, not just what is observed. Rape can be traumatizing for humans, even more so when involving multiple participants and witnesses.

Some historians argue that the assumption that rape causes psychological trauma is relatively recent. In nineteenth-century Great Britain and the United States, the legal and medical focus was on the physical pain and bodily injury of victims, for example; even when the notion of psychological trauma finally entered the picture, it took years to become mainstream.[58] Distress can also be conceptualized differently across contexts. For example, a Western psychologist sent to Bosnia to treat rape and torture victims for PTSD was told: "*We* have fear in our *bones*." The victims' emphasis on "collective solidarity" and on somatic fear rather than mental distress meant that few wished to pursue individualized therapy. After electing one woman to speak for all of them, the entire group met together.[59] Trauma is also influenced by cultural and personal definitions of rape: Is forced sex with one's husband rape or "part of being a woman"? Is unwanted sex more or less traumatizing in a context where it is thought to be "just the way things are"? Still, the efficacy with which forced sex is used as a weapon or form of social control reveals this variability as primarily one of degree rather than substance.

My aim here is not to answer ultimate questions about forced sex in human populations. Instead, the focus is on patterns of social, psychological, and symbolic meaning and motivation that emerge across situations.

Gang rape can punish gender transgressions and establish, display, or maintain social hierarchies. The anthropological record provides several examples where gang rape was *institutionalized* for these purposes. Thomas Gregor's research on the Mehinaku of Brazil is one such case. The Mehinaku historically used gang rape to punish women who dared to peek at the "sacred flutes," instruments infused with spirits and stored in "men's houses." Rather than being an impulsive group assault on a woman caught eyeing the flutes, a gang rape was publicly announced and justified by the village leader. Men's participation was expected and symbolized "the men's loyalty to one another, and their willingness to betray the ties of affection, kinship, and economic dependence" linking them to the punished woman. A woman's gang rape, then, is significant for the men she is related to, who may feel shamed both by her behavior and by their inability to protect her from punishment. Not every Mehinaku man took part enthusiastically; in fact, Gregor writes that some men resorted to "magical methods of inducing an erection."[60] (Viagra had not yet been introduced at the time of his research.) Gang rapes serve as warnings to other women who witness them or when they become public knowledge through stories told by the victim, witnesses, or perpetrators.

Among the Mundurucu, another Brazilian Indian tribe, a similar myth explains that women once controlled the "sacred trumpets" housing ancestral spirits. At that time, women were the sexual aggressors; men were sexually submissive. But because the spirits of the ancestors demanded ritual offerings of meat and because men were skilled hunters, women's dominance was eventually overthrown. Men stole the trumpets and hid them; threats of gang rape, supposedly, kept women from attempting to regain control of the instruments and restoring themselves to power. Threats of gang rape, however, were also used in more everyday situations to control female behavior. Gang rape could be used to punish women who intruded on men's spaces—the sexes were even separated for sleeping—or who threatened male status. A young Mundurucu woman who did not conform to gendered expectations of subservience—for example, by failing to cover her mouth when laughing, looking directly at a man, seeking the company of men, or in other ways failing to act demurely—might also risk gang rape.[61]

"We tame our women with the banana," one Mundurucu man said.[62]

Even where gang rape is institutionalized as a form of social control, however, power structures are complex. Yolanda and Robert Murphy, anthropologists who studied the Mundurucu, note that despite threats of gang rape, women rarely expressed curiosity about the sacred trumpets and "were obviously less impressed with male prowess and its props than were the men." When talking with a female anthropologist rather than a male one, Mundurucu women did not necessarily cast themselves as inferior and were sometimes openly contemptuous of men's rituals of separation and dominance.

"There they go again," a Mundurucu woman commented.[63]

Gang rape as revenge for female adultery is found in both Mehinaku and Mundurucu history, although in less institutionalized forms, and is reported elsewhere around the world. The Cheyenne of the Great Plains allowed the husband of an adulteress to "put her on the prairie," for unmarried men to rape her. For the Omaha, also a Native American tribe, a woman's adultery or sexual aggression could similarly be punished by gang rape and abandonment.[64] Bukkake, a type of pornography where a woman is covered in the ejaculate of multiple men, is supposedly based on a feudal Japanese punishment for adultery. After bukkake victims were ritually covered in semen, they became literal untouchables. (This history may or may not be important to those who eroticize modern bukkake as a genre of porn or sexual practice.)

Forced sex is still meted out as punishment for infidelity today. In 2005, Kate Wood, a researcher studying in the Transkei region of South Africa, collected stories about group rape, locally referred to as "streamlining," from young men and women involved. While some assaults were considered criminal, especially when involving weapons or resulting in injuries, other scenarios were viewed more ambiguously, as when a group of friends took advantage of a girl who was drunk or sleeping or punished a girl who had been unfaithful. One man told Wood:

> This girl . . . say she's a bitch and sleeps around, and you think you should discipline her. You call maybe two of your friends and you tell them you want to deal with that girl—this is what we'll do. I'll go in the room, have sex with her, fuck her and fuck her—and then leave the room as if I'm going to pee, switch the light off, then the next one follows, fucks her, and then the next one will go in and do the same. Even if the girl has had enough, she won't be able to do anything because she's naked at that time. [65]

The young men argued that a woman "deserved" to be raped if she had consented to at least some sexual activity, had a bad reputation, was "asking for it" through her attire or behavior, or "should have known better" than to put herself in such a situation. While many young women disagreed, they were reluctant to report streamlining because they feared that others might think they *had* actually done something to deserve it or that their reputations would be further damaged. [66]

Men are also the victims of gang rape by other men (and, very rarely, women), which similarly works to punish gender transgressions and establish, display, and enforce social hierarchies. Men who do not conform to a society's expectations of masculinity are particularly at risk. Gay men, transgendered individuals, or men not deemed masculine enough in how they dress, walk, talk, or behave risk rape and murder by homophobic gangs around the world. In 2008, European papers reported the gang rape of a Sicilian man by eight men because he wrote poetry in prison. An anti-Mafia prosecutor linked the attack to the Mafia's emphasis on a traditional masculinity that set it apart from a liberalizing society. [67] In US prisons, the situation for trans people is often grim, as they may be housed according to biological sex rather than gender identity, even if they have secondary sex characteristics such as breasts or facial hair that do not match their official identification. [68] The 1999 film *Boys Don't Cry* was based on the story of Brandon Teena, a transgendered man from Nebraska. When he was arrested for forging checks, a local paper reported the arrest using his birth name, Teena Renae Brandon, outing him as biologically female. Two acquaintances publicly forced him to display his genitals and raped him; they murdered him after he reported the rape.

Although sexual violence toward female military personnel is a familiar issue in the United States—women are more likely to be assaulted by fellow soldiers than killed in combat—men are also victimized. Assailants target men they believe are gay, who are young, or who are of a lesser rank in an attempt to drive them out or to intimidate them. One recruit reported being attacked by a group of soldiers who "shoved a soda bottle into his rectum, and threw him backward off an elevated platform onto the hood of a car." He was warned that "they were going to have sex with me all the time" and that they would shoot him once they were deployed to Iraq.[69]

Punishment for gender transgressions could be inflicted, hierarchies could be enforced, and physical submission could be compelled through other, possibly simpler means. But gang rape violates both personal and cultural boundaries, producing intense emotional responses that directly impact a victim's sense of self. Experiences of disgust, shame, and guilt are key to this process, though not identical across cultural boundaries. Marian Tankink, an anthropologist working with refugees from South Sudan, argues that Western concepts such as trauma and posttraumatic stress are not applicable to understanding the women's responses to sexual violence. The women she interviewed were most distraught about their "shattered social lives." They did not necessarily feel guilty about being victimized and "their internal sense of dignity and integrity seemed not to have been irretrievably damaged." Their reluctance to talk about their experiences was based on the need to prevent "social death" in a context where silence was valued, especially in relation to sexuality, and where daily life revolved around one's family and community relationships.[70] Dinka people, Tankink explains, have a "we-self" rather than a sense of self that emphasizes "I," and they exhibit a strong identification with the values of their families and ethnic group—talking about one's experiences thus also affects one's broader social network.[71] Like the Bosnian victims who wished to meet as a collective with the psychologist rather than individually, South Sudanese women, Tankink suggests, have a need for a social or community healing that is more important than an exploration of personal well-being.

Regardless of the sex of the victim, gang rape also dramatizes the victim's lower status in relation to both each perpetrator and the group as a whole. While other punishments also physically or symbolically mark victims, the conscious and unconscious mobilization of disgust and shame for perpetrators and witnesses in addition to victims makes gang rape extremely powerful.

Me. Not me.

BLAMING THE VICTIM—CONTAGIOUS DISGUST, INFECTIOUS SHAME

On March 6, 1983, two brothers, Daniel and Michael O'Neill, along with a friend named Bobby Silva, were driving home through the North End area of New Bedford, Massachusetts. Suddenly, they saw a girl run out of Big Dan's Tavern and into the street, directly in front of their car. At first they thought she was naked but then realized she was wearing only a brown coat and a sock, even though it was a cold night. When they stopped to help the terrified young woman, she grabbed onto Dan's neck "so hard that police would have to pry each of her fingers off him hours later." The men covered her with their jackets while she told them she had been raped on a pool table in the bar, a claim they believed when they saw a few men from Big Dan's "hastily make their way to their cars."[72]

The young woman was a twenty-one-year-old mother named Cheryl Araujo. The drama unfolding that night became the basis for the 1988 Hollywood film *The Accused*, for which Jodie Foster won an Academy Award for best actress.

The ensuing legal case was controversial. All the defendants were Portuguese immigrants, and despite the fact that Araujo was also Portuguese, local ethnic tensions in New Bedford led some people to believe the accused men were scapegoats. The O'Neill brothers received death threats from citizens who sided with the accused men but nevertheless testified on Araujo's behalf. The "Big Dan's case" also incited debate about the relevance of women's sexual history, appearance, and behavior in rape accusations. Araujo was not the first—nor the last—woman to be blamed for having been raped. However, as the accuser in the first nationally televised criminal trial to receive so much attention, Araujo was subjected to scrutiny by the media and the American public. Defense attorney Frank O'Boy said the trial drew "a firestorm of publicity" from the very first day. "Tens of thousands" of protestors for both the defendants and Araujo, he remembers, marched through New Bedford and Fall River while the trial was being held. Most news stations ran short pieces on the trial; others gave it "gavel to gavel" coverage.[73]

Though witness testimony varied, Araujo did not fit the model of an "innocent victim"—something the defense team attempted to use against her. She had gone to the tavern alone, leaving her children at home. Strike one. She bought a drink at the bar. Though she claimed to have had only one drink, one of the defendant's lawyers alleged that her blood alcohol level was at least 0.17 when the attack occurred, almost twice the legal driving limit.[74] Strike two. She also interacted with some of the male bar patrons. Strike three.

Accounts differed as to what occurred next. According to Araujo, she watched a group of men play pool and then was approached by two strangers. When she refused to leave with them, another man seized her from behind and carried her to the pool table. Her clothes were stripped off. Men took turns raping her as others held her down. Araujo later testified: "I could hear people laughing, cheering, yelling. . . . I was begging for help. I was pleading. I was screaming."[75] Defense attorneys, on the other hand, suggested she "willingly engaged in sex on the pool table with one of the suspects before the others joined in." Despite Araujo's testimony and the testimony of her rescuers, one of whom said he had "never seen anyone as scared as she was,"[76] she was portrayed as "a whore" and as if she were "looking for trouble" by being out alone, at night, drinking in a tavern.

Four of the six defendants were eventually found guilty of aggravated rape. Even so, Araujo was ostracized in New Bedford and moved to Miami with her children.

Rape victims have more legal protections in the US courts since the 1980s but still find their appearance and behavior dissected in the media and by the public. More than twenty-five years after Araujo's assault, in October 2010, newspapers reported that an eleven-year-old girl in Cleveland, Texas, was gang-raped in a dilapidated trailer. Once again, the case sparked racial tensions in a town that is half white and half African American and Hispanic. And once again, victim blaming emerged as part of the public response. The eighteen alleged assailants, who ranged from fourteen to twenty-seven years old, initially found more sympathy and support than might be expected: "These boys have to live with this the rest of their lives," one hospital worker mused. The young girl, however, became the focus of "anger" and "vicious remarks" from community members. She was criticized for not resisting her attackers or reporting the incident to the police herself—the investigation began after a cell-phone video of the assault was given to authorities—despite her statement that the men threatened to beat her and told her she could not return home if she didn't cooperate and even though an eleven-year-old child cannot legally consent to sexual activity. One news report insinuated that the girl courted danger through her behavior and appearance: "Residents in the neighborhood where the abandoned trailer stands—known as the Quarters—said the victim had been visiting various friends there for months. They said she dressed older than her age, wearing makeup and fashions more appropriate to a woman in her 20s. She would hang out with teenage boys at a playground." The girl was taken into custody after her parents were implied to be neglectful: "Where was her mother? What was her mother thinking?" a neighbor asked.[77] Shortly afterward, Republican Florida state representative Kathleen Passidomo defended a Florida bill legislating "proper" student attire, suggesting that the young girl was raped because "she was dressed like a 21-year-old prostitute," and that such a bill was warranted "so what happened in Texas doesn't happen to our students"[78]

As the investigation proceeded, authorities learned that the girl was raped on at least six occasions over a three-month time period. Used condoms were recovered from the trailer containing the victim's DNA, along with that of some of the accused men; two additional suspects were eventually charged. Although one defense attorney likened the sixth-grader to a "spider" who lured unsuspecting men into her web, the first two men who went to trial received a ninety-nine-year jail sentence and life in prison without the possibility of parole, respectively. As of January 2013, thirteen of the other defendants had settled their cases with plea bargains, with seven juveniles receiving probated sentences and six adults receiving fifteen-year jail terms. [79]

Why are victims of gang rape so often disparaged? Miller argues that disgust and its "cousin," contempt, are emotions with intense political significance because of their role in maintaining social hierarchies. "Disgust," he writes, "evaluates (negatively) what it touches, proclaims the meanness and inferiority of its object." For victims, shame can be triggered by seeing themselves as an object of disgust for others. At the same time, however, the "polluting powers" of that which has been deemed low make claims to superiority vulnerable. [80] Shame and humiliation are "the emotions that constitute our experience of being lower or lowered," and they "exist in a rough economy with those passions which are the experience of reacting to the lowly, failed, and contaminating—disgust and contempt." [81] The need to disidentify with victims can trigger violence, be used to justify it, and even underlie the responses of unrelated individuals. Victims of gang rape elicit multifaceted, often unconscious fears of pollution in assailants and witnesses, fears that are defended against by seeking social and psychological distance from the one who has been lowered—the exclusion of the victim.

Photographing or videotaping sexual assaults is surprisingly common where mobile technology permits. Why would participants in a crime take and distribute visual evidence helping to identify them? Some participants do not believe a crime was committed, justifying the attack as something the victim consented to or deserved. Such documentation may also be part of the process of distancing from and excluding the victim, a process that begins with the attack but continues afterward in a variety of ways. What, exactly, runs through a teenage boy's mind when he posts photos online of his friends gang-raping a drugged sixteen-year-old girl? In fact, in 2010 such an incident occurred at a rave party held in Pitt Meadows, a city near Vancouver. Not surprisingly, conflicting stories are told about the incident. A young woman "became separated from her friends" and was taken to a nearby field. Initial reports suggested that seven young men then raped her. Later witness statements indicate that while up to a dozen people may have watched, not all participated in the assault. Regardless of the actual number of assailants, the victim's physical injuries were substantial and required medical attention. At least one witness documented the rape on his cell phone and uploaded photographs to Facebook. Some reports state that the victim had no memory of the events of the evening until she saw the pictures on Facebook. Other accounts suggest that someone who knew the victim saw the images on Facebook and reported them to the police. [82]

What captured the media's attention is that a witness took and distributed photos so casually. Why didn't the young photographer intervene if it was an assault? Was he afraid of retaliation or becoming a victim himself? Did he realize he had done anything wrong, either by witnessing the incident or sharing the photos? Did he know the girl would be recognized or that the photos would "go viral" on the Internet? And what about the other teens who downloaded, forwarded, and commented on the Facebook photos? Were they troubled either by the rape or by their part in consuming it? Some students reported being upset after seeing the images, but others vilified the victim online and in the press, suggesting she must have been a willing participant despite her age, injuries, and intoxication.

As the drama unfolded, the victim dropped out of school due to harassment. The youth who posted the photos online, also sixteen, was initially charged with making and distributing child pornography and with distributing obscene material; when he pled guilty to the latter, he was sentenced to twelve months of probation and ordered to apologize to the victim.[83] Several other men pictured in the photos were investigated, and an eighteen-year-old man was charged with sexual assault. When the sexual assault charges against him were dropped because of a lack of evidence, the girl and her father pleaded with witnesses to come forward. Thus far, however, any remaining witnesses have maintained a "code of silence."

Police warned that possessing and redistributing photos of the incident is a crime. A young man who attended high school with the victim seemed less distressed about the rape than about the possibility of child porn charges being brought against students: "No one realized that at the beginning and now everyone's freaking out," he told a reporter.[84]

Well, maybe not everyone. A blogger who posted his thoughts about the Pitt Meadows incident made an interesting discovery. His September 17, 2010, post received more than two thousand hits, one-fifth of his total hits ever. Yet although tempted to "pat himself on the back" for his "tremendous writing skill," he writes, "the stats show something different." In fact, when looking at the search terms that led people to his blog, he found that most people were looking for the actual photos and video of the incident, not for information about it. Further, many of these browsers then continued on to www.pornhub.com.[85] Interest in this story, he believes, was less about concern over sexual violence—gang rapes happen frequently, though we hear only about a small percentage of them—and more about voyeurism.[86]

After all, this incident made Facebook.

The Pitt Meadows case raises issues about the legal culpability of bystanders. Although the patrons of Big Dan's Tavern who cheered on Araujo's rapists were not prosecuted, the idea that they potentially *could be* became the plot of *The Accused*. The Pitt Meadows photographer received a light sentence, but the case still sets a precedent for similar incidents where witnesses photograph or videotape sexual assaults without joining in or intervening. Participating as a witness—even as a secondhand witness who downloads or forwards photographs—can become a way of distancing from someone who has been marked inferior, aligning oneself with the more powerful side. This is part of the reason why gang rape victims often evoke scorn and hostility rather than sympathy. The escalation of violence that sometimes occurs during gang rapes can similarly be related back to these dynamics—the victim is lowered with each assault while the group becomes more cohesive, resulting in progressive dehumanization.

In some cultural settings, the ostracization of the victim extends to her entire family. On June 22, 2002, in Meerwala, a rural village in Pakistan, Mukhtaran Bibi (now known as Mukhtaran Mai) was gang-raped by four men after her twelve-year-old brother was accused of fornication with a Mastoi woman, who was from a more powerful caste.[87] Because of the woman's higher social status and local beliefs that justice required "an eye for an eye," village elders punished him by ordering Mai's rape. Tricked into thinking she was expected to publicly apologize to the offended family, Mai attended a local gathering with her father and her uncle. After she apologized and one of the elders declared the dispute settled, Mai was abducted at gunpoint and gang-raped in a nearby stable. Mai was then marched naked in front of the villagers until her father was allowed to take her home.

Instead of killing herself—as is foreseeable in such cases due to the unbearable shame associated with rape—Mai filed charges. Pursuing rape cases in the legal system is difficult in Pakistan; Mai's illiteracy made it even more so. Police may refuse to investigate if the accused are of a higher caste than the accusers. Assailants may threaten their victims (or their families) with further violence if an attack is reported. Further, the Hudood Ordinances, Pakistani laws enacted in 1979 to punish *zina*, or extramarital sex, in accordance with Islam, make such cases complicated. Married Muslims can be sentenced to death by stoning, while unmarried couples can be sentenced to one hundred lashes. The maximum sentences require four eyewitnesses to the crime. Unfortunately for a woman who is raped, and even those who are gang-raped, finding four witnesses to testify on her side is difficult. If she does not succeed in proving rape, she can be punished for *zina*. Campaigns by international and Pakistani human rights organizations to repeal the laws have failed. Amnesty International reports that 88 percent of the women currently jailed in Pakistan are held under the Hudood Ordinances.[88] It is not surprising, then, that the Pakistan Human Rights Commission estimates that a woman is raped every two hours in Pakistan and that a gang rape occurs every eight hours[89] —the costs of forced copulation are low for perpetrators.

In a noteworthy turn of events, newspapers in Pakistan picked up Mai's story, spreading it around the world. The international media attention helped her case, and the perpetrators were eventually tried in court and sentenced to death. In March 2005, however, another court overturned the convictions of five of the men and reduced the death sentence of another to life in prison on the basis of "insufficient evidence." On April 21, 2011, the Supreme Court of Pakistan upheld the acquittals. Mai has remained in Meerwala, where she runs a school. Her notoriety grants some degree of protection—the eyes of the world are on her, at least occasionally—but also a great deal of persecution. Over nine years of court battles and publicity, she has faced continual harassment from both the government and villagers, along with recurring death threats. She now fears the acquitted men will return and harm her or her family.

Journalist Bronwyn Curran has questioned the dominant narrative surrounding the case. Although Curran admits that a crime was committed and that Mai set a precedent for women in rape prosecutions, she points out that Mai did not originally register the case herself and that the publicity surrounding the case may have both detracted from the technical aspects of data collection and warped the story in the media. She further suggests that Mai was delivered to a Mastoi man by the men in her own family, a traditional practice known as *vani*, or offering a woman in marriage to compensate for a crime. Curran also questions reports that Mai was raped by multiple men and paraded in front of bystanders.[90] Other voices have raised dissenting opinions about specific "facts" in the case—discrepancies occur in dates, descriptions, number of assailants, witness testimony, and so on. Some have even accused women's rights groups of inventing the story of a "poor tribal woman" facing violence and humiliation for their own purposes. International pressure led Pakistani president Musharraf to offer Mai a payment of 500,000 rupees within three days of the breaking story, which was an unprecedented move (about $8,300 at the time and 160 times the average monthly wage).[91] Although Mai used the money to start her school in Meerwala, her acceptance of the payment has been used to discredit her version of events. In an interview with the *Washington Post*, Musharraf commented that rape accusations were a "money-making concern" in Pakistan: "A lot of people say if you want to go abroad and get a visa for Canada or citizenship and be a millionaire, get yourself raped."[92] He later retracted the statements, but the interview had been taped. His statements are illustrative of not just misogyny but a system of global inequality where even if Mai had been paid one million rupees and saved every penny, she could not expect to enter Canada at even the poverty level if she were to immigrate.

The lesson here is a familiar one: out of all the stories that might be told, we must always bear in mind that the stories that *are* told and circulated strike a chord with the audience consuming them. Who "tricked" Mai into thinking she was simply expected to apologize to the tribal council? If Mai's own male relatives were indeed involved in transacting a secret "exchange"—a "marriage" to atone for her brother's wrongdoing—their actions would have been illegal in contemporary Pakistan, but not unheard of. Of one thing there seems to be no doubt—Mai did not want the sex that occurred on July 22, 2002. Her case, no matter how convoluted, highlights issues around sexual violence in places where the shame of the victims extends to families, relatives, and even acquaintances.

Gang rape can be used as vigilante punishment when perpetrators are unlikely to face repercussions, and when gang rape shames not just the victim but also a wider social network. The exclusion of the victim is thus taken to a further extreme: in addition to figuring her as an outsider to the perpetrators, the violence can destroy her social ties. This is different from the victim blaming that occurs in Western countries. Mai has been photographed only in modest dress and headscarves and was never personally accused of sexual impropriety. While women everywhere experience distress after gang rape, possibly facing rejection from husbands or families, the aftermath is even more difficult for women living in societies that associate women's chastity with family honor and future marital options. With little economic security and severe limitations on their mobility, women do not have the option of starting a new life somewhere else. Occasionally, relatives even enact vengeance by murdering a woman who has shamed the family. Some victims thus decide to live with rape as a secret rather than face the future as irrevocably marked and isolated, bringing shame and financial ruin on their families.

Gang rape, then, marks and excludes victims in multiple ways, impacting their past, present, and future social relationships. Victims, perpetrators, witnesses, and even those hearing the story have complicated conscious and unconscious emotional responses to the violence, especially as it symbolizes contagious inferiority.

"IT'S LIKE COMING HOME": AFFIRMATION AND BELONGING

Even if watching panda porn had excited Chuang Chuang enough to shuffle over to Lin Hui with amorous intentions or clarified what he was supposed to do when he got there, he probably wouldn't have first hurled his bamboo shoot into the air and yelled excitedly, "Yes! This is what it means to be a *panda*!" But for humans, the process of self-reflexive comparison that keeps us in line through shame can also generate feelings of recognition and affirmation. Some thinkers argue that the links between sexuality and the sense of an inner self, or identity, stem from relatively modern Western discourses. My point in this section is not to essentialize the relationship between sexuality and identity, but instead simply to illustrate how witnessing and being witnessed in transgressive sexuality becomes meaningful to some group sex participants, some of the time.

Betty Dodson is a sex educator and artist who has taught courses on masturbation for decades. That story you heard about naked women sitting in a circle and examining their genitals with a makeup mirror? It was probably inspired by one of Betty's "bodysex" classes, which began in her living room during the 1970s and required doing just that. Annie Sprinkle is a former porn performer turned sex guru who has taught a variety of classes on sexuality that include the audience in hands-on exploration of her body. In "Public Cervix Announcement," Sprinkle reclines, inserts a speculum, and allows audience members to view her cervix using a flashlight. She has masturbated onstage and taught vulva massage. Carol Queen, a former sex worker and writer, has offered workshops through the sex toy store Good Vibrations and the Center for Sex and Culture in San Francisco. Barbara Carrellas, author of *Urban Tantra* and a well-known tantra instructor, "thinks" herself to orgasm in front of her classes using her breath and "energy." While you might not learn how to "think-off" from watching her demonstration, there are still some things you should *see*.

For each of these American activists and educators, live group demonstrations do more than disseminate information—they also help combat sex-negative beliefs, banish feelings of shame and inadequacy, and nurture an acceptance of sexual variation. Similarly, in early academic work on swinging in the United States, participants reported that observing others in the nude and having intercourse was "a significant growth experience."[93] Some contemporary lifestylers similarly talk about group experiences as a lesson in overcoming shame about sex and the body: "The advantage of [swinging] is that it allows for sexual freedom, instead of shame and repression. Our society is ashamed of our sexuality. Swinging has allowed me to let go of that shame and really embrace my sexuality."[94] Both women and men, gay and straight, told me that seeing others have sex—live and up close—made them feel "normal."

At a sex party I attended, a porn star demonstrated his nearly fail-safe method for inducing female ejaculation, or "squirting." His girlfriend served as a responsive and patient model for the "students" until other women volunteered. Female ejaculation is a misunderstood phenomenon, and the fluid is often erroneously thought to be urine expelled from the bladder during sex. Some women find ejaculation unpleasant; for others, it offers pleasure superior to orgasms or accompanied by them. During his demonstration, couples in various states of undress ringed a queen-size bed, shifting positions to better view the action. Serious anatomical explorations, during which the instructor would actually guide someone's fingers into a woman's vagina to help locate and stimulate the Skene's gland, were punctuated with moments of humor.

"Wear goggles if you want a closer look."

"Best to do this in hotels so you don't have to do the laundry."

For the seasoned orgygoers in attendance that evening, the lesson offered an opportunity to increase their repertoire of party tricks. For women who previously felt ashamed about ejaculation, the lesson was also comforting.

In 2009, Josefine Larsen conducted interviews with young women in Rwanda about *guca imyeyo*, or labia elongation. The practice of stretching the labia minora, which is also reported across Africa in Uganda, Burundi, the Democratic Republic of Congo, South Africa, and Sudan, among other countries, was once categorized as a form of "genital mutilation" by the World Health Organization, but was dropped from this category in 2008. In Rwanda, labia elongation is relatively common, often beginning at puberty and continuing until a girl's first menstruation. Bonds formed during this time, however, last far longer. As it is considered inappropriate for mothers and other family members to be involved, young girls turn to their peers for information and instruction on "pulling." "Teams" of five to ten girls meet in the bushes in rural areas or at each other's houses in urban areas to practice stretching techniques, which they learn verbally, by watching other girls, or through demonstrations on their bodies. Some girls pull daily, others only once or twice a month, attempting to obtain an ideal length of around 8 cm, or the length of a middle finger.

Labia elongation has normative aspects. Traditionally, *guca imyeyo* was considered "decent" because it provided coverage of the vagina during child-birth or when women were unclothed. A woman who had not elongated her labia might be disgraced or sent home when she married. Labia elongation is still believed to enhance attractiveness, but in contemporary times it is also believed to increase sexual pleasure for both men and women. The labia swell during intercourse, providing additional friction, and elongation is also believed to encourage female ejaculation, which is highly desirable during intercourse. The exchange of fluids has symbolic importance in Rwanda, especially in sexuality. Women who cannot ejaculate are considered "empty," and compared to "hard, dry, infertile land"; there are special terms for the children of women who were unable to ejaculate, evidence of the social aspect to sexual performance.[95] Women thus believed that labia elongation was necessary to keep a man faithful. Girls who did not pull could find themselves ostracized among their peers and rejected as marital partners. Still, Larsen argues that the practice of *guca imyeyo*, which was seen as part of becoming a woman, has positive effects. *Guca imyeyo* offers a chance to acquire social capital and respect from older relatives, but also to talk to each other about femininity, marriage, sexual health, childbirth, and pregnancy. During pulling sessions, girls become more comfortable with their genitals and more aware of their sexuality. At the beginning when they are still adjusting to the pain, for example, girls pull each other's labia and scrutinize each other's progress. Girls developed bonds with each other through their "intimate secret"—"We have all seen each other naked so we share some-thing strong," one interviewee said. Another participant claimed: "Women come together, shape each other and make a special relationship through the practice. This is special because Rwandese people normally keep secrets: we are not open. There is a certain confidence between us, sometimes it comes naturally, but whenever someone helps another with *guca imyeyo* this kind of relationship is made." "Labial elongation," Larsen argues, "is fundamental to the communal construction of female identity, eroticism and the experience of pleasure, reinforcing feelings of pride."[96]

Feeling affirmed in one's sexuality can occasionally be a step toward identifying with or feeling part of a larger group. Sociologist Corie Hammers studied two Canadian lesbian/queer bathhouses, the Pussy Palace in Toronto and SheDogs in Halifax. One of the organizers of the Pussy Palace events stated: "I continue to be appalled at the amount of shame women have when it comes to their sexuality and desire. The bathhouse is a place where people can come to counter that negative social conditioning."[97] The Pussy Palace featured a "G-spot room," where women learned to find and stimulate their G-spots, along with demonstrations of fisting, strap-on play, and female ejaculation.[98] The organizers believed in creating a "safe" place—all female, with explicit and implicit rules of etiquette—where women could explore and educate themselves: "There are still so many myths and misunderstandings when it comes to the G-spot, or fisting, or S/M. We are attempting to provide accurate information, [to] allow queer women to know their bodies in a way that is genuine, real and sensual."[99]

For the patrons that Hammers interviewed, bathhouse events also provided a "fat-positive" and queer-friendly space: "Two butches having sex, a butch in femme lingerie giving a lap dance, and two fat and proud femmes having loud sex are there to be seen and heard."[100] One woman explained that the bathhouse was one of the only places where she didn't feel judged for her appearance; attending the events, she said, "has made me feel more comfortable about my body and my sexuality, with myself and how I relate to others."[101] Another said: "I am seeing people like myself. Fat people, weird people. There are large women here who like themselves and are carrying themselves in a way that says, 'Look at me, I am beautiful.' . . . I come here feeling quite good in my skin. I also feel revitalized sexually."[102] Other women found the bathhouse to be a safe place to be witnessed as desiring and experiencing sexual pleasure. One interviewee, for example, found that after being watched while she had an orgasm in the sauna, she felt "alive and desirous," finally accepted by others—and herself—after years of self-loathing.

Gay male circuit partiers express similar sentiments. One of Westhaver's interviewees commented: "There's a freedom in knowing that you're a subgroup that does this; you're unique . . . we can celebrate our uniqueness, but in a room with 5000 other people that are, you know, doing the same thing . . . there's an excitement to that."[103] Although not all of the attendees participated in sexual encounters on the dance floor, many did. Encounters ranged from "playing with someone's dick" to "a standing-up-not-quite-naked-orgy" where mutual masturbation, oral sex, and, more rarely, sexual intercourse occurred.[104] Witnessing and being witnessed in erotic activity, regardless of how explicit, generated feelings of self-acceptance: "When you see people who are having no issues with being gay, no problem at all . . . well, you just get right into it, you just feel so good about yourself";[105] "I finally saw something that I could see myself being. . . . I saw what I understood to be gay, that was what I wanted, what I knew I wanted to be"; "It's like a feeling of coming home in a way."[106] Another man felt "blessed" for the first time at a circuit party: "I can remember feeling proud of being gay, proud of being myself, and feeling really lucky to be who I was—like not wanting it any other way, never wanting to be straight. I'd never thought like that about myself before."[107] The events allowed the men to "differentiate themselves from a larger heterosexual order" as well as confirm and celebrate community: "When straight boys go out they beat the shit out of each other and trash the place. When we go out, we take our shirts off and hug each other."[108] One man said of having sex on the dance floor: "Well, this is what it means to be gay, I was just being gay, and I just did it."

Not everyone feels affirmed during or after group erotic experiences (and, as we saw with gang rape scenarios, the possibility for emotional vulnerability and devastation after such exposure is one reason why group sex as violence is so effective). Some participants already feel positive about their sexuality; self-acceptance, then, is not necessarily a need fulfilled by group settings. Other individuals feel insecure after comparing themselves with others in group sex situations, possibly shamed for not responding the way they think they should. Several women told me that they disliked the emphasis on female ejaculation at some sex parties because it made them feel inadequate or pressured to participate. "Yes, I *know* that 'every woman can do it,'" one woman said. "I've done it, I don't want to do it again, and I don't find it pleasurable." Dominant standards of attractiveness are also difficult to escape. Lifestylers complain about pressure to look like "Ken and Barbie." Circuit partiers spend hours in the gym trying to achieve "the look"—muscled with low body fat, tan, dressed (or undressed) appropriately. One man described "the look" as a celebration of masculinity: "That's where the facial hair comes in; chest hair is coming back, the big muscle, the cock rings make your genitals protrude: everything that can epitomize male sexuality and being a man."[109] Other men describe "the look" as a form of competition and feel pressure to be "beefy, tough, and macho."

Although some environments are more competitive than others, some male interviewees, both in heterosexual and gay group sex scenes, occasionally struggled with performance anxiety. Performing well sexually during group encounters was a way to display skill, dominance, and stamina. Penis size was valued and compared. Some gay men sought to impress others by the number of partners they took on or the extreme acts they engaged in when bottoming. Participants enjoyed "watching someone taking it" and challenging themselves, "How much can I take?"[110] Male sexuality, the men believed, was "active and agentic," "natural and primitive, wild and outrageous."[111] This ideal, however, could generate insecurity as well as pride or excitement.

UGLY, TACKY, AND HUNGRY: REPRESENTATIONS OF SWINGERS IN THE MEDIA

The 1970s are over, but some things seem to be making a comeback: lava lamps, wallpaper, Donna Summer's concert tour and . . . swingers. The fascination with "the lifestyle" (as swingers fondly call it) is seeping into suburban, upper-middle-class social scenes.[112]

The living room . . . is where the swingers reenergize between strenuous "sessions" on the spread. This consists mostly of cheese, peel-and-eat-shrimp and bowls full of potato chips. Hard to stomach a plateful of pickled mushroom as an old guy with a flabby ass parades around wearing a G-string with a chicken on the front. I don't want to touch anything (peel-and-eat shrimp, potato chips, Oreo cookies, old man cock).[113]

What *is* it about swingers?

While researching nonmonogamy in the United States, I noticed that swingers were rarely portrayed favorably in the media. In itself, that isn't surprising, as monogamy is a deeply held ideal (even if many people deviate in practice), and swinging challenges traditional models of marriage. But what particularly fascinated me was the repetitiveness and homogeneity of the physical descriptions. Swingers are overwhelmingly portrayed as ugly—unattractive, overweight, aging—and as tasteless—gluttonous, working class, or hopelessly out of date. At the same time, however, they are repeatedly likened to people who might just be your neighbors or coworkers.

Two documentary films, *The Lifestyle* (1999) and *Sex with Strangers* (2002), garnered reviews exhibiting this pattern. Film reviewer Stephen Holden writes: "What sort of people engage in recreational group sex on a regular basis? David Schisgall's documentary *The Lifestyle* provides one answer: mostly cheerful, but paunchy, suburban couples who have either slipped into middle age or are starting to advance past it."[114] The film, according to Holden, is "disquieting": "Although some may be stimulated by the movie's fleeting glimpses of gray-haired, potbellied, cellulite-jiggling, over-60 orgiasts lustily going at it in their suburban living rooms after an evening of barbecue and California dip, many more will probably be repulsed."[115] Another reviewer calls *The Lifestyle* "the most persuasive argument for pornography in all of its unrealistic depictions of sexuality" because "watching forty and fifty-somethings participating in group sex (in between trips to the buffet table for jellied salad) is a truly bizarre and extremely non-erotic experience . . . it seems as if the filmmaker searched under every rock in the country to find the most narrow-minded individuals possible."[116]

In a review of *Sex with Strangers*, Phil Villarreal writes: "Swinging, the film makes it seem, is not a hobby that attracts the young and fit. Or intelligent."[117] Another reviewer laments of the characters, one of whom he describes as a "leathery lizard," that "None of them is particularly attractive or interesting; indeed, their sexual predilection would seem to be the only thing which makes them special, and they wave their incessant horniness like a banner. One featured couple actually trolls for sex in their motor home, parked outside discos. The epithet 'white trash' unfortunately fully applies."[118] The descriptions slide into an almost visceral disgust: "James and Theresa are the most secure in their deviancy. Despite Theresa's sagging chest and the apparently unnoticed tastelessness of James' body piercings (think Anthony Hopkins with a southern accent and pierced ears), they've kept at it, bagging three, sometimes five partners in a weekend, and enjoying every minute of it."[119]

Journalists and bloggers get their hands dirtier by actually visiting swingers' clubs, though all the while assuring readers that they have no real interest in participating in any sexual activity and relaying their trepidation at each step along the way. Blogger India Nicholas writes of a visit to a swingers' club, for example:

> I will admit, I was a little nervous when I walked into the club. . . . Not because of the handful of grandma's walking around in stripper heels and garter belts, but because of how badly I stuck out in my seven layers of sweaters and Keds. I tried to look casual; I leaned against the bar, sipped $3 champagne, and tried *so damn hard* not to look directly as an old woman's naked breasts get fondled in the corner. *Oh god*, I thought embarrassed, *what if I see someone I know?*[120]

Smoking Jacket blogger and writer Harmon Leon posed as a couple with a female friend to gain access to a swingers' house party. On the drive, he wonders: "Will I end up having sex with someone's wife? Will someone's grandmother hit on me? Will images from this evening cause me to wake up screaming like a traumatized Vietnam vet?" On entry, he notices "a dank smell" and "seedy lighting." Blogger Erin Mantz visited a swingers' club in Maryland with the aim of confronting couples to ask, "Why do you do it?" and "How can you do it?" Because she didn't actually talk to participants—her husband was anxious to leave before anything started happening—she instead chronicles her own apprehensive emotional state.[121] "A bit shaky as I climbed the steps of the building," she writes, "I braced myself for what I might find." Although the owners looked like people she "might run into at a health club or local take-out joint," she feels nervous as she follows them down "a well-lit but long and narrow stairway full of fear." She imagines what she might see at the end: "Some kind of orgy? Group sex rooms in full force? Whips and chains?"

Their lack of desire, as these writers tell the tale, is justified. Attendees at swingers' clubs and parties are repeatedly described as past their prime and, given their propensity to snack in between bouts of stomach-slapping sex, they care little about the fact that they fail to meet cultural standards of attractiveness. Such people have no right having sex, the writers imply, much less sex in public or with anyone other than their equally old and unattractive partners. Leon, for example, encounters lone men in towels, "trolling the party for fresh newbie meat" and "a skeleton-skinny old woman in her sixties, drunk out of her head," who "tries to tantalize" him by showing him her "turquoise old-lady panties."[122] The orgy room, he writes, is "full of naked unattractive couples, some to the point of plain obese, with rolls of flesh one could get lost in, twisted into a variety of random sexual positions."[123] (Leon is a humorist, so one might expect outlandish embellishments, but his tactics are eerily similar to those found in ostensibly serious accounts.) A writer from *Details* magazine makes no effort to disguise his contempt for swingers at a "mandingo" party, where white women congregate to have sex with single black men:

> These women resemble Kathy Bates more than they do Kathy Ireland. As they hover around the snacks on the kitchen island, the Mandingos mill among them in silk pajamas. And almost instantly, while the women's mild-mannered husbands chat about real estate and the PGA, the games begin. Hands rove from chicken wings to breasts, from chips to hips, from guac to cock. One couple grinds by the sink and feed each other meatballs. Husbands and wives start slinking off with their chosen Mandingos. The party has begun its carnal ebb and flow, between nookie in the bedrooms and foreplay in the kitchen.[124]

Swingers, their attire, and their surroundings are described as "cheap" and "sleazy." A woman from Mississippi has "an uncanny resemblance to Roseanne Barr."[125] Participants drink "$3 champagne" or use "beer cozies," eat naked from buffets, and live in motor homes. A Florida sex club is described as "a pleasant snapshot from 1978," with "turquoise walls, a red pleather couch and chair," and "paintings that would not look out of place at your grandmother's house." The men have "slicked-back" hair and wear tacky jewelry like "a large dragon medallion" or "thick gold chains."[126] The pictures of swinger couples on websites are described as "standard hardcore amateur smut; women naked, men naked; women on men naked, all taken from a terrible angle from a Kodak that was spanking new when the Brady Bunch was still on in prime time."[127]

Granted, the furniture probably *is* "pleather"—as it should be in a public venue daring to provide couches—and not everyone who participates in the lifestyle is conventionally attractive. Swingers come in all ages, shapes, sizes, and fashion sensibilities. Let's also grant that if someone has never before seen other real, live, nude people having sex—we're not talking about porn performers here—it can be a shock to the senses. Bodies move in unappealing ways, and there is no director to filter what the audience sees. Real sex scenes hit a bit close to home, one writer suggests: "People who pay for the Spice channel pay to see breast implants, hard bodies and flawless sexual choreography, not stretch marks, wrinkles and other human imperfections; they're not paying to watch themselves."[128]

But are swingers really more unattractive than the average person? The next time you're standing in a grocery line, bored, try imagining everyone in view, including yourself, naked. How many shoppers are "Ken and Barbie" material? Now, mentally dress them again. What's the group level of fashion sense? Do you prefer them clothed or unclothed? (Your response will probably have something to do with how you feel about your own naked body.) Aside from college campuses, where participants in rampant hookups are at least still young, or in those few social enclaves where the "beautiful people" congregate into later decades, most people out there having sex are probably somewhat paunchy and middle-aged, a fairly common demographic in modern America. So why even mention it—*over and over and over*?

Seeping. Trolling. Jiggling. Sagging.

Where is Catherine Millet when you need her to step out of the shadows and start gleefully flinging muck?

It doesn't matter that these representations focus on only a small subset of people engaged in swinging. Many people refuse to burden themselves with the label of "swingers" and thus are passed by when writers seek their next sensational topic. Others escape the notice of voyeuristic journalists because they patronize private parties, invitation-only circuits, or expensive retreats instead of public sex clubs. A reporter would need more gusto to access these spaces, as well as meet the standards of attractiveness required. But these representations aren't about facts in the first place—they are about disavowal and distancing. *Not me.* Even granting that sex clubs might inspire nervousness in first-time visitors, it's not as if these writers are truly afraid of sexual assault or other types of violence. They are, instead, expressing, or catering to, a fear of contamination.

As Miller notes, some perceived vices and "moral failures" trigger disgust: "Disgust is more than just the motivator of good taste; it makes out moral matters for which we can have no compromise. Disgust signals our being appalled, signals the fact that we are paying more than lip-service; its presence lets us know we are truly in the grip of the norm whose violation we are witnessing or imagining."[129] Unable to denigrate swingers directly on their morality, which would seem prudish rather than liberated, these writers tell tales of a descent into the depths of a dark world full of unsavory individuals and strange practices. They bravely resist both the sexual advances and the buffets—if six pomegranate seeds enslaved Persephone, one can only imagine the penalty for chicken wings—eventually reemerging into polite society physically unscathed but psychologically unsettled. The desire, and even need, these writers have to distance themselves from swingers is palpable in their descriptions; as witnesses, they have been implicated in social transgression and are seeking escape.

If middle-aged James were only "bagging" Theresa, would they arouse such revulsion as a couple? If they were monogamous, might he instead be exhorted to "accept her changing body" and work at keeping sex hot despite culturally dominant depictions of the only desirable bodies as young, tight, and beautiful? Would her "sagging chest" have even been mentioned?

The real problem with swingers is that they transgress norms of monogamy, public nudity, and dyadic sex. Often, they do it all at once, "cheerfully." They initiate "newbies" into deviant practices. They laughingly tell stories that make "normal" folks cringe, like about digging through a trash bag filled with used condoms looking for a lost ring.[130] They feed each other meatballs in the kitchen before "slinking off" for a threesome. Certainly, other lovers eat together—who could forget the blindfold, cherries, and honey in the film *9 1/2 Weeks*? Swingers, though, move too comfortably "from guac to cock." They barbeque in the buff, forgetting they're naked (with a journalist in their midst).

Naked swingers peeling shrimp become the new millennial version of the maenads, the female Dionysian celebrants whose loss of sexual self-control morphed into the desire to tear apart animals with their bare hands, devouring the raw flesh.

Well, maybe not quite *that* bad. But the principle is the same. Once a mental dam bursts, contamination will seep into *your* secret gardens. Eventually, we have a flood on our hands and no ark in sight.

Are they already your neighbors?

How would you know?

Once they've tucked their tawdry medallions inside their shirts or swapped stripper heels for granny flats, these people might be sitting next to you at the monthly PTA meeting. Holden writes: "For the most part, [swingers] look like normal workaday folks, and could even be your neighbors." And for all her anxiety, what does Mantz find inside the club? "Nicely dressed women." A woman who looked "like she could have been a parent volunteer at my son's preschool." A women's bathroom that "could have been the washroom at Nordstrom's where moms say hello and commiserate with toddlers in tow," except that "some women looked at me a little longer than, well, normal." This scares her: "I left pretty quickly."

Mantz and the others survive their symbolic journeys into nonmonogamous debauchery; some writers even end their pieces with measured comments about how swingers obey the rules—"no means no"—or seem "harmless" as long as they are allowed to channel their "obsession with sex" into the lifestyle. Contemporary swingers aren't portrayed as murderous criminals, like the Bacchic worshippers of Rome; most educated readers wouldn't buy that as fair or balanced. Still, moral lines are subtly drawn as a sense of corruption is deflected into the physical world—the swingers' bodies, attire, and preferences.

It's not just swingers. When English footballer Stan Collymore was caught "dogging" in 2004, he was denigrated in the press as a pervert. The headlines were relentless: "Former star in sex shame"; "Collymore: My shame over 'dogging' sex"; "Collymore's arrest shame"; "Dogging shame of soccer star"; and "Collymore plea over sex shame." Doggers were labeled "sexaholics and sociopaths," at risk for STDs.[131] Collymore even referred to himself as "disgusting." But he also questioned the hypocrisy and maliciousness of his treatment by the media: "Why are some infidelities accepted and brushed swiftly under the carpet while others are judged to belong to some dangerous twilight world . . . ?"[132] As one journalist noted, even years later Collymore hadn't completed the usual tabloid cycle of public exposure, remorse, and redemption. Some of this is perhaps related to his personality, as Collymore seems to court controversy. But a special kind of vitriol, it seems, is reserved for people involved in consensual group sex. Had Dante known of swinging, dogging, and mandingo parties, he might have added a special ring of hell.

Yet there is an intriguing flipside to this phenomenon. Consider the response to a 1995 article, "D.C. Swings! Couples Meet for Cocktails, Hors d'Oeuvres, and Blowjobs at a Washington Restaurant," in Washington, DC's *City Paper*. The story focused on a local lifestyle group called Capitol Couples. Attendees were described as "mostly lumpy, middle-aged, white: drab men with har-har laughs wearing country-club sweaters, painted women with Jell-O breasts in plus-size garb à la Frederick's of Hollywood." The sex is similarly portrayed in language chosen to repel rather than titillate; the author observed "groping hands," "dangling tongues," and a blow job given by a woman with "frightening, pendulous breasts."[133] The following month, however, the *City Paper* reported that they hadn't received a single complaint related to the article. Instead,

> Much to our surprise, both *City Paper* and the article's author have been inundated with calls and e-mails from men and women seeking to join the sex club. A man from upper Northwest was the first to call. "Uh, I read your article and thought it was real interesting," he said nervously. "How can a person find out where these activities are going on?" Though we initially feared the caller might be a law enforcement official, we soon realized he simply wanted the club's phone number, as did dozens of others, including one elderly Potomac woman who said, "It's my husband's birthday this weekend. I want to surprise

him." For all you wannabe swingers out there, Capitol Couples' number is
. . .[134]

Terry Gould, a journalist who wrote *The Lifestyle: A Look at the Erotic Rites of Swingers*, tells a similar tale. Admittedly, when he was given the assignment of writing about a Vancouver swing club in 1989, he approached it as an "investigation into the dark world of organized sex" and then "rang the warning bell of disease and degeneracy" by writing a "scathingly condemnatory" piece. Then, he writes, "something odd happened": "I got more telephone calls from curious readers—both male and female—than I'd had for all my articles on the Chinese mafia, Sikh terrorists, and gun-running Nazis combined." He provides a partial transcript of a typical call:

Caller: Is this the same Terry Gould who wrote "A Dangerous State of Affairs"?

Gould: The very same.

Caller: I couldn't believe my eyes. I had no idea that the health department or police would even allow that kind of thing.

Gould: Well, it's apparently not against the law.

Caller: It should be. . . . My husband and I were sickened. Either the women must be lesbians or I don't know what their husbands have done to them. Are most of the women lesbians?

Gould: I guess you'd say some are bisexual.

Caller: So this is their outlet then. . . . Okay, I'm sorry to take your time. But just—I thought something should be written more on the subject. Are you permitted to give me a telephone number for this so-called swing club?

Most of the callers, he realized, eventually asked for the phone number, and the Vancouver Circles club saw an increase in membership. Gould became suspicious that publications condemning lifestylers "were actually capitalizing on the vicarious needs of their readers."[135]

This wouldn't surprise Michael Bailey, who pointed out that the live sex demonstration at Northwestern was one of the top news stories for several days, even "during a time of financial crisis, war, and global warming." Moral outrage, agitated curiosity, or *both*? In addition to producing anxieties, swingers and others who transgress social norms around sexual privacy and monogamy will continue provoking interlopers, at least until those norms substantially relax. *The Sexual Life of Catherine M* sold millions of copies and has been translated into forty languages. Critics can say what they'd like about the artistic or masturbatory limits of Millet's prose, but she clearly sensed the potential for disgust, shame, and guilt to fascinate and attract as well as repel.

Case Study: The "Dark Orgies" of the Marind-anim

The Marind-anim live on the southern coast of New Guinea, or what was Indonesian Irian Jaya, now Papua. Today, most are Catholic or Protestant. Of their current culture, little seems to be written. Marind-anim are said to "keep to themselves." They obtain around 97 percent of their needs from the forests, swamps, rivers, and sea—even if by design, other options would be limited. The area they inhabit is marked by lack of transportation, poor road conditions, and scarce access to medical care and educational resources. Continuing isolation from the larger market economy indicates marginalization, and disputes regularly arise over fishing and land rights.

At one point in history, the Marind-anim were known as ruthless headhunters with an occasional proclivity for cannibalism, roaming hundreds of miles to raid other Papua New Guinea groups. Since calling people "cannibals" can be as incendiary as accusing them of having orgies, the Marind-anim developed a harrowing reputation. That feasts, weddings, and dances were accompanied by group sex made matters worse, eventually exposing the group to heavy-handed colonial intervention.

Jan van Baal, a Dutch cultural anthropologist and the governor of Netherlands New Guinea from 1953 to 1958, is one of the primary ethnographers on the Marind-anim. His 1966 publication, *Dema: Description and Analysis of Marind Culture*, synthesizes his observations with an analysis of existing Dutch and German sources, primarily focusing on the coastal region. The book, which is 988 pages in length, describes a world that was fairly incomprehensible to those who came into contact with it and raises complex questions about the impact of European colonialism on native life.

The Dutch settlement of Merauke was established as an administrative post in 1902 to control Marind-anim headhunting raids, which had been

125

ranging into British New Guinea and drawing complaints. Clashes in world-view were immediate. Marind-anim disliked colonial impositions of territory, and Dutch officials found even their basic assumptions about social organization challenged. Administrators had concluded that each "long drawn out series of often miserable huts, built on the low ridge high on the beach, where the vegetation of coconut palms begins" was a village. "It seemed all very simple," Van Baal writes, "the villages stretched in one long row all along the coast, waiting as it were to have their names noted down in a register and their chiefs recognized as village chiefs." The trouble was that there were no "village chiefs." (Though traditional authority figures existed in Marind communities, they were not recognizable as such to the colonials.) In 1914, the administration, "disgusted with natives who had no chiefs," finally began appointing village chiefs. Although the "villagers" were consulted during the process, "the institution never became a success," and the chiefs continuously lacked prestige.[1]

If the Dutch were surprised at the lack of an administrative framework and an attitude toward authority so very different from their own, one can imagine their surprise at other aspects of Marind life.

By 1905, the Missionaries of the Sacred Heart had descended on Merauke. Due to a lack of training, linguistic difficulties, and "puritan ethics," Van Baal explained, early missionaries focused on isolated aspects of Marind culture in their writings and interventions—not surprisingly, headhunting, cannibalism, and orgies—without really understanding or contextualizing these practices. As such, they may have been deceived about the true prevalence of ritual cannibalism; some stories and myths were specifically told to throw "the uninitiated" or cultural outsiders off the scent of the real secrets underlying their rituals. Van Baal believed that early rumors about ceremonies where young women were raped by groups of male initiates and then eaten were false, for example, although he acknowledged that Indonesian hunters and traders could tell "impressive stories." He had been "taken" himself with a trader's tale of encountering "a woman who was pent in a cage in the forest, ostensibly for the purpose of being fattened to make a better meal." Van Baal first surmised that the woman was menstruating but began to doubt the story entirely after conversations with Father Jan Verschueren, a missionary who had done extensive research on Marind customs and rituals.[2] More measured reports, however—such as that the arms and legs of headhunting victims were occasionally eaten—Van Baal believed to be true. Instead of being ritualized or linked to spiritual beliefs, though, these episodes of cannibalism usually occurred among "medicine men" who believed that human flesh had magical properties or supplemented the community's diet during difficult times.

Yet even if cannibalism was more a myth than a reality—or practiced only in hard, hungry times—other customs, such as burying elderly relatives alive when they became a burden, using cadaverous fluid in initiation rituals, or naming people after "captured skulls" (using the last word the victim uttered before being beheaded), prove the memory of the Marind-anim as one to be reckoned with from the days of colonial rule to the present. Head-hunting served as a marker of manhood. Obtaining "head names" was one of the primary reasons for headhunting expeditions, although the raids also provided an opportunity for Marind-anim to kidnap children—between 10 and 20 percent of the Marind population was estimated to be of foreign origin, although kidnapped children were raised as their own.[3] Colonial officers instituted penalties for headhunting and began confiscating the evidence—one raid yielded ninety "fresh heads."[4]

Then there was *otiv-bombari*.

During his time living among the Marind, van Baal developed an appreciation for some of their cultural beliefs, gestures, and rituals but admitted to being disturbed by the "dark side" of their sexuality—men having anal intercourse with very young boys (referred to as "homosexual" intercourse by van Baal, "ritualized homosexuality" by later researchers, and "semen practices" by others), heterosexual defloration rituals and fertility ceremonies "perpetrated upon 'very young girls' by groups of men," and regular extramarital "promiscuity." An unmarried man risked being seen as a "poor wretch," and most Marind-anim were "heterosexual," but as with certain other Papua New Guinea groups, same-sex relations were prevalent and linked to intricate cosmological beliefs. Marind-anim believed that semen, or *sperma*, was the essence of life, health, and prosperity. Young boys began initiations into adulthood between seven and fourteen years of age, moving into men's houses for up to six years, learning the *Sosom* myth and the symbolism of bullroarers, and engaging in anal intercourse with older men. Although most groups engaging in semen practices required the activities of the men's houses kept secret from women, Marind-anim required women's participation in some of the rites (even as other myths and sacred objects, such as the bullroarers, were kept hidden). *Sperma* was necessary for women's fertility and was also believed to feed the fetus in the womb. Food mixed with *sperma* was served on special occasions. For all these purposes, *sperma* obtained from the vulva of a woman after copulation was preferred over that obtained from masturbation; for van Baal, this male dependence on females became a source of underlying conflict and aggression.

Van Baal defines *otiv-bombari* as "promiscuous sexual intercourse"— *bombari* meaning "ceremony," *otiv* meaning "numerous" and referring to the men's house. *Otiv-bombari* did not involve a general exchange of women but instead comprised a group of many men and "usually not more than one woman—sometimes two but never more than three." Some writers classify *otiv-bombari* as a fertility rite, as it was practiced at age-grade ceremonies, weddings, in the years before a woman had children, and when a woman began menstruating again after childbirth. Van Baal questions this as the sole explanation, though, pointing out that the ceremony was performed at other times as well, such as after the completion of a new garden. This feast, or *wambad-bombari*, was classified "as a compensation for services rendered."[5] Ceremonies were also held to collect *sperma* (semen) to mix into food or rub on the body for medicinal or magical uses; *sperma* was even applied to plants. In these cases, a limited number of women "would have intercourse with as many men as possible, while the excreta are collected in a coconut-bowl."[6] Given that "wife-lending" was practiced as a form of hospitality and payment and the host of a feast was responsible for ensuring that women were sexually available, van Baal argues *otiv-bombari* might have been "an attraction as well as a ritual act," sometimes serving as a form of "prostitution" and sometimes to enhance the festive character of the occasion."[7] The festive mood—at least for men—was also heightened by drinking a "liberal dose" of *wati*, made from the kava plant. Kava has narcotic properties similar to muscle relaxants and benzodiazepine; it can reduce anxiety and produce mild euphoria or "exhilaration." Women did not usually drink *wati*, believing that it caused infertility.

The most common use of *otiv-bombari* was in the wedding ceremony. Once a couple decided to marry, the ceremony began with the bride donning a new "apron," which attached to a string around her waist. She received gifts of food from relatives and then presented offerings to the groom's parents, including a sago loaf to his mother "signifying that, from now on, she no longer needed to cook his meals." At nightfall, "a few old women led the bride to a spot in the bush behind the village, where some sheets of eucalyptus bark are spread out." She then had "intercourse with all the members of her husband's clan or phratry, perhaps even with all the local members of his moiety." After the ceremony, the bride was included in *otiv-bombari* more generally and took up residence in her husband's mother's house.[8]

Previous European observers had been captivated by *otiv-bombari*, but van Baal identified "astounding gaps" in their knowledge of the rules participants followed—clearly, he knew enough not to believe it was a free-for-all. Van Baal claimed that the order of participants was established ahead of time; in the wedding ceremony, for example, the inmates of the husband's men's house went first.[9] How women were chosen for center stage in other *otiv-bombari* was less clear. But just because previous observers "failed completely" in recording the rules, he warns, one should not assume that patterns of mutual obligation did not come into play. "The Marind," he points out, quickly learned that *otiv-bombari* was "behaviour which the whites condemned as immoral" and "wisely managed to avoid making these [rules] a subject of discussion."[10] Van Baal also doubted the "physical feasibility" of stories that the bride had sex with as many as thirty to one hundred men (although some of today's "gang bang" stars might beg to differ). He trusted the more measured accounts, which declared that "not more than five or six claimants were allowed to have access to the bride during the first night; if there were more, intercourse was resumed the following night." Men's same-sex anal intercourse, though embellished as "unrestricted sodomy" in some reports, was subject to many of the same rules as *otiv-bombari*.

We cannot infer much about individual experiences of *otiv-bombari*, whether pleasurable or distasteful. Reliable subjective accounts were challenging to obtain in such a setting, given colonial power relations, language barriers, and patterns of sexual segregation. But, for Marind-anim, sex was not primarily about desire or pleasure, anyway—part of the reason that van Baal disliked using the word "orgy" to describe *otiv-bombari*. Neither men nor women, van Baal observed, were necessarily sexually satisfied by *otiv-bombari*. Even if spread out over several nights, *otiv-bombari* could be a "traumatic" physical experience for women: "They were said to be in fairly bad shape after such a night. The next day they could hardly walk, sometimes they could only move crawling on all fours, so the women told the interviewers. On the whole, it was a burden to them. Nevertheless, several female informants confessed that they participated, not primarily because it was their husbands' wish, but because they felt it was a necessity."[11] Women worried about becoming ill or infertile if they refused. While men might have received more gratification on the whole, some expressed conflicting feelings or were opposed to *otiv-bombari*. During the ceremonies, most men "committed the sexual act in the natural way but some had to give up and achieve emission by masturbating." Ambivalence even arose in the term itself. Van Baal also notes that an early interpreter used the term *otiv-bombari* only for the wedding ceremony, designating all other promiscuous intercourse as *dom-bombari*; *dom* meant "ugly" or "bad in a moral sense." As this use of the word *dom* was recorded before missionary influence had "sufficiently asserted itself to make the Marind condemn one of their most cherished customs as morally reprehensible," van Baal interprets it as an indication that *otiv-bombari* was not "a pleasure rite, but an obligation" for both sexes, perhaps even reflecting men's distaste for having sex with women.[12] Other evidence came from their myths and religious beliefs. It is impossible to even summarize here the many detailed myths that van Baal and others collected, though it is worth noting that one of the most important and prevalent images was of a couple stuck together in copulation; there are many variations on the theme, but often the penis must be severed to free the couple and later extracted from the woman's vagina by a stork.

The existence of extramarital sexual rites did not mean that Marind-anim took a liberal approach to sexuality in general. Premarital pregnancy was discouraged, and children born before marriage could be killed. To "avoid shame and humiliation," a young girl who became pregnant might "try to bring about abortion by such means as leaping from a tree or being dragged over a forked tree."[13] Men might "lend" their wives to other men as a form of payment or hospitality, but women's infidelity could be punished with homicide.[14] Children were indulged in sexual play when they were very young, but such contact became subject to numerous taboos as they aged.[15] Cultural contradictions also arose in relations between men and women. The symbolic inferiority of women did not necessarily mean overall devaluation. Van Baal argued that despite women's heavy workloads, ritual subordination, and tendency to be beaten by their husbands, women were not simply slaves to men and readily defended themselves. Further, he noted that if a wife fulfilled her many duties, she would not be discarded for a younger women even "when her good looks fade"—"of this more decent sin, popular in many civilizations, we do not hear in Marind-anim society."[16]

The story of *otiv-bombari* takes an ironic twist with regard to fertility. Contact with Europeans had sparked several influenza epidemics and introduced venereal disease, both of which impacted the size of the population and the birthrate. When a medical study conducted in 1920 found high rates of sterility among the Marind, a "depopulation team" was sent to determine the possible causes. Around 25 percent of the Marind were found to be affected with donovanosis, or venereal granuloma, a bacterial infection that causes genital ulcers. The disease, which had been first identified in 1896 in Madras, Queensland, and New Orleans, was possibly introduced to the Marind-anim at a festival in Merauke occurring in 1905 or by the Australian laborers used to construct the outpost. Venereal granuloma was believed to be sexually transmitted and highly contagious (although van Baal observed that it spread more slowly among Marind-anim than should have been expected given their sexual practices). Venereal granuloma provided an urgent reason, officials believed, to clamp down on native promiscuity. Efforts to control infection throughout the 1920s and 1930s led to a medical campaign requiring "an almost complete change of the native patterns of life."[17] Authorities banned feasts and dances, along with *otiv-bombari*. "Model villages" were set up, requiring families to live together, as boys' and men's houses were also associated with sexual license. Sexual practices continued in secret, often at the urging of the elderly women, although there were fewer opportunities for Marind-anim to participate in the ceremonies that had been so central to their social life.[18]

These measures brought venereal granuloma under control, although the birthrate remained low. Women who were not infected with venereal granuloma were also found to have high rates of infertility, and both van Baal and the depopulation team noted that precolonial Marind-anim women faced similar problems. Historically, the low birthrate was perhaps why Marind-anim obtained children by abducting them during headhunting missions or purchasing them from other tribes. Although recognizing that the evidence was correlational, the depopulation team believed that *otiv-bombari* played a significant role in infertility, writing that "the absence of pregnancies is probably due to chronic inflammation of the *cervix uteri* and chronic irritation of the female genital organs in consequence of excessive copulation." Because of the supposed curative powers of *sperma*, *otiv-bombari* had intensified after contact with Europeans when fertility further dropped, becoming concentrated on young women having difficulty conceiving and exacerbating the problem. Van Baal tentatively agrees, pointing out that the generation born after 1913—those whom had been indoctrinated by the missionaries, educated in schools, and no longer practiced *otiv-bombari*—showed a decrease in sterility.[19]

In 1937, the Roman Catholic Mission sent van Baal to Bad, a community that had recently held a *sosom* celebration, to crack down on participants. Van Baal had mixed feelings—the rituals were prohibited, but the legal justification for doing so was tenuous, and although homosexual promiscuity was "obnoxious" in public health terms and venereal granuloma was still present, he had long desired a more "humane policy" on native feasts. He decided this aim would be better accomplished if he did not start feuding with the mission over "sodomy," however, and headed up the river to seek witnesses to the event and reprimand the community. In his ethnography, he recounts the trip "as an illustration of the dangers of interfering with other people's religious life." Although everyone in Bad must have known about the ceremony, he writes, people feigned ignorance until he threatened to reveal their secrets, including the bullroarers, to the women. "Exploding a bomb could not have had a more dramatic effect," he writes:

> All the kind black faces suddenly turned ashen and haggard, and Pandri put a trembling hand imploringly on my arm: "No Sir! please Sir! you can't do that. We shall all die!" he whispered. "All right," I said, "just tell me what happened," and they told me all I already knew, taking care to add very little to my knowledge. They swore that they had not committed sodomy, because, they said, "We are afraid of the awful wounds the disease may inflict on a boy's anus and buttocks."

Van Baal sentenced the men to fourteen days' detention, which was not harsh enough in the eyes of his superiors but only the beginning of the calamity from the Marind-anim perspective. Afterward, everywhere he went van Baal saw "old men sitting by the side of the path, with dejected faces consulting each other on the disaster which had befallen them." Several weeks later, they showed the women their bullroarers, because the "Big Man at Merauke knew everything."[20]

To fully understand *otiv-bombari*, we would need to dig deeper into Marind-anim history, myth, religious beliefs, political relationships with neighboring groups and colonial powers, kinship structures, and so on. It is difficult to do so, however. "Marind-anim culture," van Baal writes, "belongs to the past."[21] The participants, along with most of the individuals who wrote about them, are dead (Van Baal died in 1992). By the 1940s, nearly the whole of Marind-anim life had changed. Warfare and headhunting were still forbidden and penalized harshly. Feasts remained banned, and marriages had to be registered with the administration. Living arrangements had been altered. The idea of a husband, wife, and children living under one roof may have been the most desirable model for the Dutch, but to the elder generation of Marind-anim, it was "completely immoral."[22] People stopped gardening and growing vegetables, as they were forbidden to engage in *wambad-bombari*, and the government discouraged leaving their villages. According to a report from YAPSEL, a nongovernmental development organization started in 1987 with the aim of helping contemporary Marind-anim become economically self-sufficient, a "moral depression" had developed in their communities. Later missionaries to the area reported "inertia" and "general indifference" toward almost everything in their environment, and this difficulty in "acculturating" has continued to the present day.[23] In a 1993 report, YAPSEL argued that rebuilding a "healthy socio-cultural base" among the Marind was essential for economic change. They suggested that development workers encourage "activities in the cultural field," such as "writing up folk tales," reconstructing "traditional dances," and "saving and continuing skills regarding traditional material culture (musical instruments, weaponry, plait work)."[24]

Although *otiv-bombari* was suppressed over a hundred years ago, the custom remains intriguing to westerners because it presents such a contrasting view of sexuality. The Dutch regulation of Marind-anim rituals wasn't the first campaign waged against certain forms of sexuality in the name of public health but with an underlying moral aim, nor was it the first time that contradictions in how a group conceptualized and practiced sexuality produced ironic or unintended effects.

In the years since the depopulation team's tentative conclusion that "excessive copulation" was causing chronic irritation, a medical link was found between pelvic inflammatory disease and infertility. Even before venereal granuloma was observed in the population, anthropologist Bruce Knauft points out, Marind-anim women's sexual practices could have caused tissue damage. In a tropical climate, even slight skin wounds can quickly become infected; vaginal tears or trauma could thus trigger a worsening chain of infection. Chronic vaginal infections could eventually lead to pelvic inflammatory disease and permanent sterility.[25] Later research also found donovanosis to be less contagious than originally assumed—perhaps accounting for van Baal's observation that it was *not* spreading "like wildfire" even though it was indeed endemic to the population. Racism, according to medical anthropologist Lawrence Hammar, led to constructions of donovanosis as a disease of persons who were poor, dark-skinned, lived in tropical areas, exhibited a lack of hygiene, and were sexually promiscuous.[26] Thus, even though an etiologic agent was found in 1905, both Dutch and German interventions among the Marind-anim focused on "moral education of the people," inciting them to monogamy "by building houses according to a given model and by combatting superstition and sexual excesses."[27] As in other colonial settings, medicine and morality intermingled such that practices already disturbing to Europeans could be controlled, even eradicated, in the "best interests" of the native population.

This official history, still frequently told, has the flair of a redemption narrative: although the campaign initiated against Marind cultural practices by the colonial administration was intrusive, even devastating, to their traditional way of life, it was ultimately justified and successful in eradicating the disease and restoring fertility—indeed, a *future*—to the Marind-anim. An alternate narrative, perhaps, would not deny that donovanosis was found in the population. But as infertility was a more long-standing issue, the threat was not one of rampant contagion. Interventions might still have been warranted but could have proceeded more humanely, as van Baal suggested.

Both narratives raise questions. Were the Marind-anim saved by colonial intervention, given that their population was declining? Were they on a fast track to self-destruction before the Dutch even set foot on the beaches, or to use van Baal's words, were they already "up against a wall" because of the many contradictions in their beliefs and practices? And if the Dutch indeed "saved" them, what exactly was saved? Are folktales, "traditional dances" (minus *otiv-bombari*) and "plait work" *enough*? If bullroarers are no longer powerful symbols linked to living myth and ritual but simply "musical instruments" purchased by tourists and New Age hippies, might we not expect a level of moral depression?

What if a bacterial infection were just a bacterial infection, without a lesson in morality embedded within it? What if, instead of imposing monogamy, the colonial administration had worked imaginatively with the Marind-anim to manage the spread of bacterial infection without a sea change in social life? On the other hand, what if restrictions on *otiv-bombari* were welcomed by some Marind-anim? Could the practice have continued on an optional basis, or would it have lost its power and mystery in the process?

What if . . .

Chapter Five

From the Coolidge Effect to Cosmic Ecstasy

Group Sex as Arousal and Transcendence

THE "GANG BANG GIRL" (INTERVIEW, BRIANNA)

For a few years, I was the "gang bang" girl in town.

It wasn't like it suddenly happened one day—*voila*! But it also wasn't something I pursued, a lifelong fantasy or anything like that. A number of forces just came together at a particular time and place. I was getting divorced. I was working too hard, supporting myself and my soon-to-be-ex-husband. I was restless. I wanted adventure. And I really needed sex. There hadn't been much sex during my marriage.

One night, a married man I was having an affair with shared a fantasy he had of me getting gang-banged by five guys. A gang bang hadn't ever occurred to me as exciting before that, but he planted the seeds of curiosity. Okay, that sounds interesting. I started looking at websites that were used for hooking up and fantasizing about anonymous partners. One night, I hooked up with a random guy and then went home and wrote my boyfriend about it, thinking it would turn him on. But it didn't. He got very upset. After he calmed down, though, he asked me to do it again—this time with a girl. So I did. He got upset again.

That relationship didn't last.

By the time I met Sam, I was ready to have my sexual boundaries pushed, and he was the perfect person to do it—he hosted sex parties and fetish events, was in an open relationship, and had an intellectual side that appealed to me. Beyond that, our physical chemistry was intense. We had anal sex the first night we were together, in a dirty public bathroom. Our sex life heated up over the next several weeks. I became his submissive. He took me to his fetish parties and introduced me to people in the scene. I let him flog me while everyone watched. Alone the next day, I examined my bruises, fascinated and proud. One night, Sam asked me whether I would be willing to be tied down for a gang bang at one of his parties. I surprised myself by saying yes.

I've always been very sexual. I remember masturbating at four years old! By twenty-seven, I was a crazy mess of hormones. I even masturbated at work, at my desk or in the restroom. But there were other things going on besides hormones at the time I agreed to be the gang bang girl. The divorce was getting difficult, and I wanted a sexual outlet without all the emotional drama. See, I'm like a guy in that I am very good—or *was* very good then— at separating sex and emotion. At nineteen, I was raped in college by someone I knew, and the experience affected me deeply. During the rape, I remember feeling ashamed that I had no control over my body. At one point, I was in so much pain, emotional and physical, that I just went limp. But then, during that moment of surrender, something fantastic happened. Suddenly, I wasn't in my body anymore. The rest of my rape was like something happening on TV—I watched it happening but didn't feel any anything. After that experience, I learned how to switch off my feelings to protect the parts of me that could be hurt. There was a negative side to having this ability to shut down in that I had trouble connecting emotionally with men. But there was also a positive side—it was a liberating experience to be a young woman who could detach during sex and focus on the pure physicality of it. I was free to explore. In a strange way, that was a gift.

Though I had buried some of my desire for sexual adventure during my marriage, it was bubbling to the surface again

Then there was my relationship with Sam. I trusted him. He's very good at getting people to open up and feel safe. He seemed to know exactly what I needed. If he was with me, I could push myself further than I'd ever imagined.

My first gang bang was held in a warehouse where Sam staged underground fetish events. Some of his parties were held at nightclubs, but the more extreme events were held at private spots so that sex was allowed. People brought their own alcohol, and there were security guards stationed at the door. There was going to be a bukkake girl that night, too, and I would be tied between her legs. The guys would fuck me until they were ready, then they would cum on her. Being used by the men at the party would be an extension of being Sam's slave, a role I had been feeling more comfortable with after each experience.

I remember getting ready that night before the party. After spending years in an unhappy marriage, I was thankful to be in my own apartment even though there were dead roaches in every room. It was probably the most decrepit place I'd ever lived, but it was *mine*. In the tiny bathroom, with rotting tile and an iron-stained sink, I showered and did my hair. Then, while sitting on the floor because I had no furniture, I applied heavy Goth makeup. I put on black thigh-high boots, a sheer black dress, and a leather slave collar.

And then, just like that, I walked out of my apartment and into an adventure.

When I got into the elevator, a boy of about six years old got on with me. He looked up at me with a surprised look. "Are you from England?" he asked.

I laughed. "No, I'm from here," I said, smiling at him. I hoped he wouldn't notice that my dress was see-through.

"You're really pretty," he said.

I smiled again and bolted from the elevator when the doors slid open.

Feeling exposed, I quickly hailed a cab. The exact party location was difficult to find, and the driver eventually dropped me off a few blocks from the building. I began walking, wondering why Sam hadn't picked me up. Who lets a girl walk alone to a gang bang? I remember some of the people on the street looking at me as I passed. One girl chastised her boyfriend for staring at me. I could hear her yelling at him as I moved away. Finally, I saw a sign with the code word written on it and an arrow pointing down a long, deserted alley. This was the place.

My high-heeled boots clicked loudly on the uneven pavement. It was very dark and looked like a dead end. I continued on, and there was a turn, marked with another sign. I was relieved to see several men standing outside a door. One of the security guards recognized me from Sam's other parties. "No cover charge for her," he said.

There were only a few people in the room. Sam was at the bar. He hugged me and told me to take off my dress. He fastened a dog collar around my neck and attached a leash, which I found arousing. As he led me around the room, he sometimes allowed people to look at me or touch me. They always asked his permission first. At one point, I gave Sam a blow job while a young girl fingered me. "The party has started," I heard someone say.

More guests arrived. Finally, Sam led me upstairs. Some red velvet benches had been arranged to form a small bed in the center of the room. Other benches were spaced around the outer walls so that other people could play. There were mats on the floor, and the room was lit with candles.

Sam introduced me to the bukkake girl and then tied me between her legs in a kneeling position. He made sure we were both comfortable. There was a basket of condoms nearby. I asked Sam to blindfold me, too, because I didn't want to see the men.

The bukkake girl asked me, "Are you making them wear condoms?"

"Yes, of course."

"You'll dry out," she warned.

I felt a moment of apprehension. What had I gotten myself into? Was I going to be okay? I reminded myself that Sam wouldn't let me be hurt. I didn't have to do anything but have my experience.

Any remaining hesitation dissolved when the first fingers began exploring my pussy. I couldn't see anything, but I didn't need to.

What happened next? Two hours of constant orgasm.

While some men fucked me, others stuck their cocks in my mouth or felt my breasts. Someone fucked my ass, and I guessed it was Sam. When he was finished, another man tried to put his cock in my pussy. As I was getting sore, I pulled away from him instinctively, but I heard Sam say, "Don't let her get away with that." The man grabbed my hips and pulled me onto him. More men followed.

I was surprised at the intensity of my physical response. I'm loud when I orgasm, and the orgasms just kept coming. The young girl I'd been playing with at the beginning of the night joked with me to be quiet, but it was impossible. But the men were even more surprised. I could hear them talking sometimes. After he'd been with me, a man would say, "I think she liked it." You know—he heard me have an amazing orgasm! But then, he'd hang around the party and hear me continue to have orgasms with more and more men. It was obvious that one man couldn't have satisfied me, and I think I deflated a lot of egos that night.

But I wasn't interested in boosting their egos, anyway. One man fucked me roughly and kept asking me to call him by his name. "What's my name? What's my name?" Finally, I replied, with disdain, "I didn't come here to know your name." He shut up. I had slipped into my alter ego, a woman who could do any crazy sexual thing she wanted and say anything to men.

It was *my* party.

After two hours, Sam cut it off. I probably would have kept going.

He untied me, and I fell onto one of the mats on the floor. My hands were numb from being tied. I was overwhelmed.

After everyone left, Sam fucked me again, hard, in the bathroom. Then, I stumbled home alone like I was drunk, even though I hadn't even had any alcohol. My entire body tingled. I sat on the floor of my crappy apartment watching the sun rise over the city, a half-naked, roughed-up girl in smeared Goth makeup. My emotions were swirling. All at once, I was empty but fulfilled, desperate but hopeful, fearful but safe. Strangely, I also felt serene. I knew that even though my future was uncertain, I was moving forward from a place in my life that had become toxic to me. I might not be able to see what was at the end of the next dark alley, but I would be okay. I held the keys to my own future.

I e-mailed Sam the next day and asked how many men I had taken on. He told me he had counted twenty. *Twenty.* And to think the fantasy had started with five men.

After that night, everyone knew who I was in the scene. It was *my* name they remembered.

I continued doing parties for about two years. Sometimes, I would select the men from pictures they e-mailed to Sam. Sometimes, I let Sam choose. It was all sex, no emotion or attachment—except to Sam. But things slowly shifted. I began drinking. I hadn't needed to drink or do drugs at the beginning. My relationship with Sam was changing. I reached a point where I was no longer getting anything I wanted out of the parties. Not the intense relationship with him. Not the satisfaction of being indestructible. Not even the orgasms I wanted.

So I just stopped going. Everyone remembers me—still—but they respect that I've gone in a different direction.

My sex drive is still probably higher than most women's, but I've stopped having detached sex. I've stopped drinking completely. Part of my recovery requires understanding my motivations and learning how to connect with someone sexually *and* emotionally. I've learned that part of my desire to use men for my own pleasure and then discard them stemmed from a desire to hurt them.

But I have no regrets. The rape was awful, but the detachment that followed allowed me to have experiences that most women wouldn't be able to have. And being the gang bang girl—well, it's part of who I was and it made me who I am today. I've moved on, and you won't find me having those kinds of adventures anymore. I've learned a lot since then about myself.

But it's part of my story.

Confess that you have group sex regularly—or that you did a stint as the local gang bang girl but have now moved on—and you'll likely find yourself embroiled in pop-psychological conversations about your underlying motivations, relationship history, and level of self-esteem. Perhaps to avoid assumptions that one must be psychologically "damaged" or deficient to engage in transgressive sexual behavior, some participants focus on arousal or pleasure when queried about the appeal of group sex. As one man told me: "I'm not searching for some amazing high or spiritual awakening, just a little pleasure. Looking for the peak of Everest or the depths of the Marianas Trench makes one miss the land at sea level. Sex is fun. Sometimes a cigar is just a cigar. A lot of folks we know just like to have fun and think sex is fun. Sort of like eating a piece of chocolate because it tastes good."

But although group sex can, for some people, stir high levels of sexual arousal or satisfaction, it is never *just* about pleasure. Perhaps, someday, if sexual experimentation becomes a common occurrence—like trying new foods or sports—we might allow our explanations to rest there. Given the intensity of the boundary crossings discussed in chapter 4, however, it is unlikely. The tendency, unfortunately, is to concoct tidy explanations for— and judgments about—multilayered experiences.

A cigar *is* a cigar. But what makes a cigar appropriate after the birth of a son? Can a cigar aficionado detect a difference between a Montecristo and a San Cristobal? What happened to the days when velvet smoking jackets were donned after dinner so that the men could enjoy cigars while the "ladies" retired for a quick nap? (That nap sounds fantastic.) What does it mean when a woman smokes a cigar? What is at stake in debates over FDA regulation of cigars—or, when is a cigar more like a cigarette, a "tobacco product" that can be regulated in the name of public health? And what about the other uses to which cigars might be put, from live sex shows in Amsterdam to the oval office in DC?

As with the proverbial onion, there are many layers to peel.

THE "COOLIDGE EFFECT," SPERM COMPETITION, AND THE SHAKY BRIDGE

The Coolidge Effect

> [D]uring a visit to a large chicken farm, the president fell somewhat behind his wife. As the story goes: Mrs. Coolidge, observing the vigor with which one particularly prominent rooster covered hen after hen, asked the guide to make certain that the President take note of the rooster's behavior. When President Coolidge got to the hen yard, the rooster was pointed out and his exploits recounted by the guide, who added that Mrs. Coolidge had requested that the President be made aware of the rooster's prowess. The President reflected for a moment and replied, "Tell Mrs. Coolidge that there is more than one hen." [1]

Group sex fantasies, such as "gang bang," "sandwich filling," or "airtight" play on the idea of being overwhelmed by the experience—visual stimulation, tactile sensations, sounds, scents, possibilities, and pleasure (or power). Beyond the sensory aspects, there are other conscious and unconscious reasons that group sex is arousing, in fantasy or reality.

Habituation, or the "Coolidge effect," refers to the loss of sexual interest in individuals with whom one has previously engaged in sexual behavior. So don't feel bad if you're "too tired" for sex with your regular partner—it happens to rats, cats, rabbits, and goats. Even *Lymnaea stagnalis*, the hermaphroditic pond snail, is reluctant to mate as a male with any female more than once.[2]

Habituation in animals can be studied in the lab, and when it comes to sexual behavior, we know a lot about rats. There are important differences between rats and humans—for example, rats are limited lovers in terms of creativity, sticking to vaginal penetration and genital licking, and the males vigorously pursue novelty, free of guilt or economic constraints. But rats make good lab subjects because they like to mate and they are responsive to conditioning; that is, they can be convinced to mate preferentially with females through manipulations of sexual pleasure. Male rats have thus been copulating, ejaculating, and copulating again in the name of science for years, occasionally to the point of physical deterioration (exhaustion or death). They have been observed, timed, and videotaped. In the quest for sex, male rats have run mazes, sprinted across electrified grids, and climbed rickety towers. Novelty, researchers have found, grants many mammals a reward—a pleasurable dopamine dump in the brain. Repeated copulations with the same female result in less dopamine being released; the rat also takes longer to ejaculate each time. Familiarity thus breeds habituation, at least, if not contempt: even when male rats appear exhausted after mating, they are easily aroused again if presented with a new female.[3] Being confronted with a strange male rat—a competitor—can arouse a male again, as can copulating with a different female before returning to the original one.

Laboratory studies of habituation in humans are kinder—universities frown upon "physical deterioration" in human research subjects. Human studies are also more limited in design, as human females would never consent to the things that female rats must bear in silence. Still, both men and women exhibit habituation effects when exposed to the same segment of an erotic film, the same erotic image, or a repeated erotic fantasy.[4] Naturalistic studies—such as monogamous marriage—reveal similar trends toward habituation. Many people who have been in a long-term relationship, for example, can identify at least somewhat with stories of the "seven-year itch," and marriage counselors are besieged with couples seeking cures for a lack of sexual desire in one or both partners. What precisely this means varies, depending on who is complaining, but sexual frequency, sexual satisfaction, and sexual desire often wane for both men and women in relationships over time.[5]

Habituation plays a role in this decline. Human brains, after all, also reward novelty with dopamine releases. Both rats and humans display individual differences in how the reward centers of the brain are wired, however. Whether due to genetic, situational, or historical factors, some creatures seek these types of rewards more enthusiastically, have a stronger response to the chemicals released, or have more difficulty walking away when they *should*—be it a rat who should turn his back on the lever in his cage before he collapses in exhaustion but presses it again because doing so has produced a new female in the past, or a man who should check his watch, note that it is 5:00 a.m., and decide to forgo the cocaine on the nightstand and the hookers in his bed. The chemical underpinnings of a drive for novelty are well documented, although we cannot necessarily predict or explain behavior on this basis alone.

Some therapists believe habituation is also an emotional process whereby we cease to appreciate our partners as separate entities; the closeness of everyday life eventually hinders desire. If spouses increase their levels of "differentiation"[6] —developing individual interests or tackling their emotional weaknesses and unhealthy dependencies, for example—desire may spark again. A perusal of the self-help section of a bookstore might leave you thinking the situation can be remedied with better communication, frequent vacations, or a trip to Victoria's Secret. But although complicated physiological and psychological interactions make some individuals more likely to pursue the chemical cocktail produced by sex and novelty, one thing is relatively certain for *most* people: seeing one's long-term partner in a Miraculous Bra and thong, no matter how rare, might be more exciting than the usual flannel nightgown but will not be as electrifying as exploring sex with a new lover. Like rats, though, humans can become aroused by competition. For some couples, infidelity reignites passion even if it also causes emotional distress. Whether this is due to chemical surges, psychological distance, or a combination of factors is less important than the fact that nonmonogamy can produce both anxiety and arousal. Knowing that *someone else* saw that bra and panty set might be surprisingly provocative.

Group sex offers visual novelty and the possibility of competition, regardless of the extent of actual physical contact. "What do I enjoy?" an Australian gay man responded when asked about the large commercial sex events he attended. "Well, the sight of a hundred men naked, and having damn good sex. The energy, the camaraderie, and the pure visuals."[7] A circuit party attendee said that he feels "completely overwhelmed" at events: "My first party was like 'wow.' . . . This, to me, is my sexual revolution—to see all those guys doing those dirty things—that's exciting."[8] Other men prized the "voyeuristic aspects" of group sex, of "watching someone take it," or the exhibitionistic pleasure of being watched themselves. One man explained that group sex was "about fulfilling my little boy fantasy to be a porn star. . . . It's about playing the role, and maybe that's why it's about the numbers . . . its more sort of a performance act."[9] Group sex also offers physical novelty, as participants have access to multiple potential, possibly consecutive, partners. "Just the number of guys" available led some interviewees to claim that group sex was more adventurous, exciting, and "primitive" than dyadic sex.

In 1999 and 2000, sociologists Curtis Bergstrand and Jennifer Sinski studied more than a thousand self-identified swingers in the United States. They suggest that swinging "may be one creative solution to the problem of habituation—it provides sexual variety, adventure, and the opportunity to live out one's fantasies as a couple without secrecy and deceit."[10] Their respondents agreed: "It allows us to experience variety without cheating"; "Could we survive our marriage without variety, yes. It's a lot more fun this way though."[11] Many lifestyle couples derive pleasure from watching their spouse desiring and being desired by others in addition to their own experiences: "When your spouse sees others turned on by you and vice versa, they begin to see you once again in the light they once saw you. As a beautiful and desirable human being"; "I love to see her at her highest sexual arousal, it takes me there."[12] Another study found that twenty-six of thirty middle-aged lifestyle couples had sex at least twice a week; a 2010 study of the general population only found 16 to 26 percent doing so. The researchers suggest that the swinging rejuvenates marriages by activating "mild jealousies and related insecurities" in each partner that made the partners want to "sexually repossess" each other. As one woman said, "You see others wanting your man and you want him, too."[13]

Novelty can extend to routines and practices. One couple I interviewed, Candace and Claude, began swinging after more than thirty years of marriage. Candace claimed that her boredom with their sex life boiled over into a confrontation: "I said, if we ever have sex one more Friday night at 11 o'clock at night, and that Friday morning you say, 'Oh boy, guess what today is?' you're not going to get any more. *Ever.*" They began to experiment, attending lifestyle parties and visiting sex clubs. In the process, they discovered a renewed passion for each other—"If he comes home on a Friday night, I may not have on very many clothes. We may have lots of candles lit, music playing . . . we never did anything like that when we were monogamous." They became "more adventuresome" sexually because of experiences with outside partners, incorporating anal sex and light BDSM into their repertoire. While lifestyle couples might also take more adult vacations or buy more new underwear than "vanilla" couples, the erotic charge of potential new lovers—regardless of how far things actually progress in any given situation—contributes to a sense of adventure.

The Coolidge effect, however, is only one of the layers we need to explore. Despite their love of novelty, rats do *not* have group sex. Rats might copulate in front of each other—or, more likely, in front of overtired graduate students with stopwatches—but they do not "swing." And while hermaphroditic pond snails do indeed rack up more inseminations in groups than singly (and also when their aquariums are clean, for reasons we can't go into here), one couldn't exactly say they throw "sex parties." The appeal of group sex for humans is far more complex than a desire for novelty, then, even if this desire plays a supporting role.

Sperm Competition

Environmental stimuli can trigger unconscious and involuntary responses. Using a plethysmograph—a device that fits around the penis and measures the swelling or a probe inserted into the vagina to measure genital blood flow—psychologist Meredith Chivers has assessed arousal in both men and women. In one study, subjects watched short film clips—bonobos having sex, heterosexual sex, male and female homosexual sex, a man masturbating, a woman masturbating, a man walking naked, and a naked woman exercising—while their physiological responses were recorded. They also indicated how aroused they felt on a computer. Straight men reported subjective arousal during the sex scenes involving women, especially the lesbian sex scene. This matched their physiological measurements. Heterosexual women claimed to be most turned on during the heterosexual scene, even though, according to the vaginal probe, they responded genitally to *all* the scenes. This doesn't mean that women want to have sex with bonobos or get naked during spin class but that there is a split between subjective and physiological arousal for women.[14] Such a split could be related to the fact that women's genital cues are not as obvious as men's erections[15] or that women could have negative feelings about pornography that overrode their genital sensations in the experiment. There might also be evolutionary reasons for men and women's different response patterns. Women are believed to have higher reproductive costs (nine months of pregnancy, followed by nursing and child rearing). If women were highly aware of or motivated by sexual arousal, this might cloud mating decisions. Women's involuntary physiological responses to so many different sexual cues—from bonobos to naked joggers—could also prompt lubrication of the vaginal canal, which, in turn, may prevent injury should forced sex occur.[16]

Although men seem better at pinpointing when they are aroused in the laboratory, group sex provides an interesting example of how men also experience involuntary or unconscious physiological responses to environmental stimuli.

"Group sex" has advantages for some creatures reproducing through external fertilization. Horseshoe crabs, a journalist jokes, "host the longest-running beach party the world has ever known," ready to get "freak-nasty at a shore near you."[17] A single male crab can potentially fertilize all of the eggs laid by the female and attaches himself to her during the process. Due to intense competition, however, occasionally more than a dozen males cling to the female as she lays her eggs in the sand. According to paternity analyses, the initial male has the best shot at fertilization, but satellite males still manage to fertilize about 40 percent of the eggs.

But what about when fertilization occurs internally, as with humans? For years, the belief that women were naturally monogamous—and men were not—influenced theories about mating strategies and adaptations. Men's sexual jealousy and widespread attempts to control women's sexuality have been suggested as strategies to prevent their mate from being impregnated by another man. From a perspective that prioritizes men's need to win and guard their mates, why a man would find it arousing to see his partner with another lover or participate in a gang bang is somewhat of a mystery. But what if women in ancestral environments were also nonmonogamous? Multiple matings, some researchers suggest, could increase a woman's chances of viable offspring by providing more opportunities to access resources controlled by males and potentially diversify the paternal care her offspring obtain. Sperm competition suggests an element of postcopulatory struggle in mating—the possibility that sperm from more than one male compete internally in the female's reproductive tract for egg fertilizations.

Some researchers believe that existing evidence supports theories of sperm competition in humans. Although sperm competition looks different across species, anatomical, physiological, and psychological adaptations to sperm competition in humans have been proposed.[18] In species with more intense sperm competition, for example, males have larger testes. Human testis size falls between that of gorillas, where female "promiscuity" is rare, and chimpanzees, where females engage in multiple matings, suggesting intermediate levels of promiscuity in our evolutionary past. ("Promiscuity" in the context of this literature should not be taken to have the same negative implications as in everyday usage.) The length and shape of the human penis could be related to the need to displace rival sperm in a woman's vagina, and some researchers even suggest that a man's rapid loss of erection after copulation prevents him from inadvertently removing his own semen. The intensity of male sexual jealousy can serve as evidence not just of an evolutionary history of female infidelity but also of sperm competition. Despite jealousy, many men experience acute sexual arousal in situations of potential sperm competition and report stronger orgasms—this increased arousal could have an adaptive quality if it motivated men to copulate and displace rival sperm. Some evidence also suggests that males unconsciously adjust the number of sperm or the quality of sperm ejaculated depending on how much risk there is that their partner has recently had another lover.[19] In a 2005 study, men viewed a randomly allocated set of sexually explicit images—images of either three females or two males and a female—and provided semen samples. Subjects who viewed the images of sperm competition (two males and a female) had higher proportions of motile sperm in their ejaculates.[20]

If theories of sperm competition are accurate, they point to a partial ultimate-level explanation for why humans engage in multiple matings, of which group sex would be one example. If unconsciously sensing a competitor affects the composition of a man's ejaculate, it makes sense that actually observing a competitor in the act would also have an impact. (If mice, owls, beetles, horseshoe crabs, and stickleback fish engage in sperm competition, why shouldn't we?)[21]

"Hotwife" enthusiasts, men who enjoy vicariously experiencing or watching a female partner with other male lovers, report high levels of arousal from their experiences. David Ley, a clinical psychologist who began studying the "hotwife lifestyle" in 2005, argues that, as with most instances of nontraditional sexualities, therapists tend to see people in such relationships as "inherently dysfunctional" and their desires as "emerging from deep-seated psychopathology and personality disturbance."[22] But this is not necessarily the most productive way of understanding this behavior, according to Ley. Hotwife couples are creating fantasies—the wives are *not* actually cheating, and sometimes cuckoldry isn't even part of the game. The sexual encounters take a variety of forms, from the man only hearing about his partner's adventures, to watching either openly or secretly, to participating in the scene. Many of Ley's interviewees sought extramarital encounters independently of each other; group encounters were not mandatory. Yet an interest in these outside activities is central to the erotics of the relationship. One man kept a diary of his wife's exploits and how many men she'd been with, for example.[23] Such couples, Ley writes, may be "co-opting" sperm competition to fan the flames of relationships "long past the time when they might have normally subsided into a comfortable, quiet love where sex is nice, but not necessary."[24]

Evolutionary theories are difficult to prove (though psychoanalytic theories are equally tough to substantiate), and despite a growing number of studies exploring sperm competition in humans, many researchers still consider the idea speculative. It is tough to design scientific studies to answer questions that are overdetermined in so many ways, and experimental designs are limited when you can't actually ask people to have sex in the lab while you watch or take notes. Asking people to explain *why* they became aroused in a particular situation or by a specific cue is possible, but the problem is that people don't always know. Sometimes they do not even know they are aroused, as we saw in Chivers's study, or the arousal surfaces later in another encounter or fantasy. Historical examples might be provocative but are ultimately incomplete. The Marind-anim practice of *otiv-bombari*— where multiple men had sex with a woman in quick succession—has been offered as an example of sperm competition in humans. Marind-anim even believed that *otiv-bombari* was necessary for enhancing women's fertility and should be repeated throughout a woman's life. Because Dutch colonial officers suppressed the practice more than a hundred years ago, researchers missed their opportunity to ask Marind-anim men to ejaculate into a cup so that their motile sperm could be measured. The fact that *otiv-bombari* might have actually contributed to sterility in the women does not invalidate sperm competition as an underlying evolutionary impetus for the practice. Still, questions arise—why were situations involving sperm competition elevated in some cultures and denigrated in others? Even among the Marind-anim, why was *otiv-bombari* celebrated but female infidelity punishable by death? Clearly, many other factors intervened.

Turning to the Internet as a naturalistic study of sexual preferences presents problems as well. Writers Ogas and Gaddam point out an asymmetry in the sex of participants in gang bang pornography, for example—there are far more depictions of multiple males having sex with a single female than vice versa. About the website PornHub, they write:

> There are dozens of "mega-gang bang" videos featuring more than one hundred guys having sex with a single woman. In contrast, there are no videos featuring a guy having sex with more than a dozen women. . . . (Of course, this might also say something about how much easier it is to round up one hundred guys to be in porn than it is to find one hundred willing girls, especially considering that the guys would be willing to do it for free. But if you're a straight male, ask yourself—would you pay to see one guy have sex with a hundred women?)[25]

Ogas and Gaddam also suggest that the significance of black men in gay and straight porn is related to their association with dominance and that sperm competition also hypothetically fuels viewer pleasure in gay male gang bang films. The more dominant a potential rival, they argue, "the stronger the sperm competition cue and the more intense the arousal, perhaps because dominant males tend to ejaculate more vigorously than submissive males."[26] But does the proliferation of porn websites such as "Gang Bang Arena," "Orgy World Girls," and "Russian Orgy" support the idea that sperm competition underlies the appeal of group sex, as they suggest?[27] Or might the explosion in such sites be driven as much by the fact that few people want to actually own a copy of *10 Man Cum Slam* and display it in their DVD rack or are more likely to pay for scenarios they don't experience in everyday life?

Despite unanswered questions, sperm competition has spread as a folk explanation for nonmonogamous and stigmatized forms of sexuality. Advice columnist Dan Savage, for example, takes a turn at therapeutic evolutionary psychology, suggesting that a wife whose husband shows no sexual interest in her might open her relationship: "Maybe knowing that you're having sex with other dudes—or just knowing that you can have sex with other dudes—will cause your husband to develop a bad case of sperm-competition syndrome (Google it), and the husband will be inspired, fucking you three times a week instead of his fist."[28] In *The Lifestyle* (1999), journalist Terry Gould uses sperm competition to explain why lifestyle couples report increased sexual desire for each other as a consequence of swinging. He writes: "If we look at all lifestylers in this biological way—from the inside out—we can at least begin to comprehend why they do what they do and the reasons they say it gives them pleasure." Instead of declaring the lifestyle "abnormal," he proposes that swinging creatively combines

> the programmed urge of both males and females to promote or fight sperm wars in females, the casual female bisexuality and group sex so prevalent in our close relatives the bonobos, and the voyeuristic pleasures of males who—as assured of their partner's emotional fidelity as their partner is of theirs—know how to enjoy the reaction of their bodies to spousal "infidelity."[29]

Gould coined the phrase "sperm competition syndrome" to explain the intense orgasms experienced by male swingers.[30]

Discussions of sperm competition appear regularly in lifestyle forums, often similarly to defend men's participation (although commonly appearing alongside spurious statistics and explanations stretched a bit thin): "If sperm competition syndrome has been triggered, the man will have an orgasm 3 times stronger than usual, his pelvic thrusts will be 3 times as hard when he next has sex with his partner. And he will want to immediately. . . . The desire has nothing to do with a man's masculinity, sexuality, or psychology. It is primal, plain and simple."[31] Sperm competition appears as an explanation for sexual behavior in hotwife forums as well. As a man expresses it in more mainstream verbiage:

> Men cum and need a rest. Women cum, and they're ready for more! It's because men compete to fuck women, women fuck as many guys as possible to get the best chance of getting good sperm. Group sex is hard-wired into humans. Guys have a refractory period, a time to recover, from orgasms. While they rest, another guy takes his turn. This also stimulates the resting man to want to get back into the action again. It also produces more intense orgasms for the guys. His balls want to pump cum into the woman's cum-filled vagina. Isn't Nature wonderful?[32]

A woman similarly asserts:

> In the cuckold relationship you openly become involved with another man, and [your husband] knows it! His primal sperm competition reaction will kick-in, resulting in a sex drive in overdrive, and increased sperm and testosterone production as soon as he is back in your presence. He will pursue you and even dote over you obsessively upon your return. That's why husbands in the cuckold lifestyle are more attentive to their wives than men in traditional marriages.[33]

As another blogger "scientifically" describes hotwifing:

> The two of you (you and your wife) become sub-serviant to him. What a stud he is! The fact that you have been conquered by this superior male makes your wife want him all the more. He has now come between the two of you and has stolen your mate. He's also made you like it! Watching or listening to them make love or smelling and tasting the aftermath of their sexual encounters causes your sperm competition reaction to make loads of sperm, and starts to demand a quick release, and that's what gives you guys "the thrill" of being cuckolded. Of course all of this is chemical-biological, and has no effect on intellect.[34]

For individuals whose erotics clash with the classic story of "natural" human sexuality, the theory of sperm competition provides a measure of reassurance.

Sperm competition, though, even if it plays an underlying role in any of these practices, can't be the whole story. After all, if sperm competition is such a significant source of arousal, why don't more people avail themselves of the pleasures it promises? Why do some men, in some places, pursue sperm competition scenarios while others avoid them at all costs? And for those who do find sperm competition arousing, why would one man prefer the egalitarianism of swinging while another eroticizes a hotwife scenario, sitting on the sidelines watching his partner's sexual encounters, occasionally humiliated or temporarily frustrated?

TAXI CAB CONFESSIONS (INTERVIEW, MADELINE)

My boyfriend was married and high profile. We would sneak away sometimes, for a few nights, although we never had enough time together and the time we did have could be stressful logistically. We were always worried about getting caught, so we spent a lot of time sequestered in nice hotels, ordering room service, and having as much sex as we could, just the two of us. Even when we did venture out, we were careful to pick the right restaurants and make sure he wasn't recognized.

One night we started fooling around in the cab on the way to one of our clandestine dinner dates. I was wearing a loose, sexy dress. At one point, my lover lifted my dress to reveal my breasts, and said to the driver, "Hey, isn't she hot?" The driver glanced back, first turning his head and then again using the rearview mirror. He seemed unsure of how to react, but nodded. My lover pressed the issue. "Really . . . Look at her breasts. She's so beautiful. Don't you want to touch them?" Then, a minute or two later, he offered again, "You should touch them. Here. Give me your hand."

The cabbie finally reached back, and my lover guided his hand to my nipples. "Pinch them," he instructed. "I pinch them, bite them, treat them like they are mine. That's how she likes it." The man did as my lover suggested and pinched my nipples roughly. The two of them touched my breasts together, while my lover also kissed me and put his fingers between my legs. He dropped us at the restaurant, but we were so turned on we barely made it through dinner. All we wanted to do was go back to our hotel and fuck.

It became part of our routine to involve our driver, even though it meant that we couldn't use the nicest car companies—we were sure the drivers gossiped about us and didn't want to risk it. I would wear clothes that were easy to take off, lift up, or pull aside. "Look at her body," my boyfriend would say, undressing me during the ride. "She's beautiful and I know you want to touch her. She wants you to, so it's okay."

One night, my boyfriend stripped off my clothes and the three of us made a scene on the drive. At each stoplight, I could see people staring at us from their cars. The windows steamed up, but it wasn't hard to tell what was going on. It was a long ride back to our hotel. We made out for a while, and then we had sex while the driver watched us, sometimes reaching back to touch me. My boyfriend pulled my hair while the driver played with my breasts. Afterwards, the driver dropped my lover off at the hotel first—we couldn't risk walking in together. Then he circled the block while I picked my clothing up off the dirty floor of the car and got dressed alone. We were silent.

When I got up to the hotel room where my lover was waiting, we had crazy sex.

If I were alone, thinking about a random cab driver touching me would freak me out. But with my lover there, it became the hottest experience I've ever had. I knew I was his, and it was his decision to share me. He got off on having these strangers want what he had. I was proud that he thought of me that way. But for me, the driver was also a source of reassurance. I'd been in love before, though never as in love as I was with this man. But while my friends could fall in love, post pictures on Facebook, talk about their boyfriends, and go to parties with their guys, my whole relationship was a secret. Here I was, in the most intense relationship of my life, and it was a fucking secret. Of course, I wanted the whole world to know. But I was willing to settle for the cab drivers. One after another.

Once, we had sex during a theatrical production of Macbeth. It was the kind of performance where the audience moves around and interacts with the actors, following them through the different rooms. The staff sometimes separated you from the people you arrived with to make the experience more intense, and that was what happened to my boyfriend and me. They sent me out first into a spooky five-story building with dozens of rooms. I remember my high heels sticking in the floorboards of the old house as I wandered around, always looking for him. I was uneasy and couldn't concentrate.

Finally, I found him and he took my hand. We saw more of the performance, moving through a bedroom scene, a hotel room, and an insane asylum. In that area of the building, I noticed a padded cell. When the actors and audience members moved on, my lover and I slipped into the cell and locked the door. There was a small slit in the door and he opened it. Then, he pushed me up against the wall and started kissing me. He lifted up my dress. I was wearing thigh-high stockings because I'd gotten used to dressing for our public performances. I undid his pants and pulled out his cock. Just before he entered me, he said, "Someone's watching."

My heart started beating faster. We had our audience. I couldn't see much of the man watching us, just his eyes and a bit of his face. He looked young, maybe in his twenties, with a bit of stubble. As we had sex, I kept looking over at the man outside the door. He kept watching. Finally, my lover came inside of me, pulling out slowly so that his cum ran down my leg.

We waited until the man outside left, but it wasn't more than a moment; he seemed to know our show was over. Then we opened the latch and snuck back out to the real performance, still in progress. I wondered if I would recognize the man who had watched us. Every male face had potential—was that *him*? I know my boyfriend was more turned on by flaunting me, but I loved having an audience, even of one, to validate our passion, our relationship.

The Shaky Bridge, Sensation Seeking, and Sexual Adventurers

In the fourteenth season of *The Bachelor*—a "reality show" where a man dates twenty-five preselected women, hoping to propose marriage to one at the end—bachelor Jake Pavelka chose a tall blonde named Vienna for his first "one-on-one date." Their helicopter ride through the San Gabriel Mountains included a landing on a bridge, where the two acrophobes would bungee jump in tandem. Even though Jake planned the date as a test—"I need to know that I have somebody there that I can rely on and draw strength from if needed"—he had second thoughts about jumping as he peered down at the river below. Vienna, also pale and scared at first, soon comforted Jake and helped him stand up on the ledge. "Don't look," she warned. After taking a 120-foot plunge (screaming all the way), the two clung together in their harnesses, upside down and swaying over the river. Still "terrified," Jake kissed her and was stunned by the intensity. "My first kiss with Vienna is unlike any kiss I've ever had in thirty-one years," he said afterward. Vienna gushed that kissing Jake was "amazing," that the "whole world stopped," and that the jump was "a memory that the two of us will share forever."

Vienna was the last girl standing that season, receiving both the final rose and Jake's marriage proposal. Although the couple split a few months later, they undoubtedly do still share the memory of that fateful bungee jump.

Producers didn't wait until season fourteen to pull this trick out of their hats—previous contestants zip-lined, rock climbed, and dived with sharks. Sexual arousal, after all, can be heightened by risky situations. Under stressful or anxiety-provoking conditions, the adrenal glands produce cortisol, epinephrine, an amphetamine-like stimulant, and norepinephrine, which elevates blood pressure and speeds up the heart rate. After even a "moderate biochemical emergency," people may experience amplified "feelings of physical prowess and personal competence, often associated with strong sensations of pleasure."[35] This "stress drunkenness" may also be accompanied by lightheadedness and a loss of inhibitions. Even more importantly, people experiencing these effects can misattribute their true cause. In the mid-1970s, a pair of social psychologists designed the now famous "shaky bridge" study. An attractive woman—a confederate who was part of the project—approached a male subject as he walked alone over either a low, stable bridge or a shaky suspension bridge. She asked each man to take a TAT, or thematic apperception test, and then gave him her phone number to call if he had questions about the study. The TAT is similar to the Rorschach test, requiring subjects to write a narrative about an ambiguous picture, which is then analyzed for each subject's projections. Men who had been approached by the woman on the shaky bridge wrote more sexual or romantic narratives than those who met her on the stable bridge. They were also more likely to call her.[36] Subjects believed their emotions were triggered by attraction to the woman rather than their fear of heights or the unstable bridge. Similar misattributions have been reported when arousal was created in male research subjects through exercise or hearing a violent description of a murder. Even when long-term partners participated in arousal-generating activities, they reported increased love and satisfaction.[37]

As reality TV producers understand so well, when we feel stress-drunk, we may not distinguish between the person we're looking at and the fact that we just jumped out of an airplane into a crocodile-infested lagoon. And if we've already peed our pants in fear that day—or feared we were going to—we might be more willing to strip naked and have sex with a stranger. On television. (There are limits, of course. While there may be a "baby boom" nine months after a disaster strikes, it will likely be the result of traditional couplings rather than the spontaneous, indiscriminate orgies of literature or film.)

But there is more to the equation: if we initially risked becoming a crocodile snack out of fear that twenty-four other women are being kissed more ardently than we are, we might believe we are passionately in love—and even say "yes" to the bachelor's proposal at the end of the season—only to realize that our attraction to him falls flat without the rivalry.

People handle stress differently, of course, responding to situations with varying levels of arousal. Some individuals do consistently seek more stimulation than others, and some are more likely to seek that stimulation through sexuality. Sensation seeking is a personality trait "defined by the seeking of varied, novel, complex, and intense sensations and experiences, and the willingness to take physical, social, legal, and financial risks for the sake of such experience." High and low sensation seekers, some researchers believe, may actually be equipped with "different evolved biological strategies for processing novel or intense stimulation."[38] Preliminary findings suggest that genetic influences on the dopamine system, which is involved in reward and motivation, impact novelty and sensation seeking. Variation in the dopamine receptors D2 and D4, especially the minor alleles, appears related to differential human reproductive and sexual behavior. The presence of the 7-repeat allele (7R+) in the dopamine receptor D4 gene, for example, makes individuals exhibit a higher reactivity to dopaminergic rewards and is associated with higher propensities for risk taking of various sorts, from gambling to substance abuse. Some scientists believe that this polymorphism might have been positively selected for between forty and fifty thousand years ago, as it is found at higher frequencies in populations that have migrated farther—an orientation toward novelty and sensation seeking would have been adaptive in dynamic social environments or changing ecological landscapes.[39]

Other biological correlates—neurotransmitters, enzymes, and hormones—also play complex roles in this process; testosterone levels have been correlated with susceptibility to boredom in young men, for example. Individuals may thus not only desire higher levels of stimulation but actually perceive risk differently: high sensation seekers, for example, "have differing responses of the sympathetic nervous system, which affects the behavioral-inhibition system leading to less fear, anxiety, and stress." Because "high sensation seekers do not view the environment as threatening and leading to negative consequences," they tend to engage in activities that others view as dangerous and seek out peer groups with similar outlooks on the world.[40]

Not surprisingly, men tend to score higher on sensation-seeking scales than women; younger people usually score higher than older people. But while sensation seekers desire to increase their stimulation, they do not necessarily court physical danger. The four subcomponents of sensation seeking—thrill and adventure seeking, experience seeking, disinhibition, and boredom susceptibility—illustrate this diversity.[41] Sensation seekers can choose activities that are risky, such as drug use, gambling, or "varying sexual experiences." They can also choose nonrisky outlets, "such as occupations, music, travel, art, media, and sports." Firefighters, race car drivers, and

US Navy divers, for example, are often sensation seekers with an elevated desire for thrill and adventure and an acceptance of risk. Other occupations are stimulating enough to draw high sensation seekers without being risky, such as rape crisis counseling, journalism, or surgery. [42] "Sex, drugs, and rock 'n' roll" is more than a cliché among high sensation seekers, who have been found to choose more "arousing" music (rock over classical), be prone to using drugs or alcohol, have more sexual partners, hold more permissive sexual attitudes, and engage in riskier sexual behavior than low sensation seekers. [43]

Had you volunteered for a study on sensation seeking in 1974, you would have been asked to rank how true statements like the following were for you: "I enjoy the company of real swingers" or "I would like to make friends in some of the 'far-out' groups like artists or 'hippies.'" Twenty years later, researchers updated the scale—revising the statement about "swingers," for example, to "I like wild and uninhibited parties"—and focused sections of it more specifically on sexual behavior. This newer Sexual Sensation Seeking Scale has been found to predict HIV-risk behavior in gay men and sexual permissiveness in college students.

Sexual adventurism is a concept derived from sensation seeking more generally and refers to a tendency toward a high number of partners, high sexual frequency and duration, unprotected anal intercourse (UAI), group sex, "esoteric" sex practices (BDSM, fisting, anal fingering or rimming, the use of sex toys, etc.), membership in particular groups (or "subcultures"), and the use of sex clubs. Sexual adventurism is usually used in reference to urban gay male subcultures, but there are other sexual enclaves that attract an edgy, experimental, sensation-seeking crowd, some of which are discussed in this book. Sexually adventurous "subcultures" are "geared to the maximization of sexual pleasure," often "having as much to do with modes of socializing and 'partying' (such as frequently attending dance parties) as with sexual behavior." [44] "Intensive sex partying," or ISP, is another way to refer to linked behaviors—frequent partying and unsafe sex, multiple partners, specific drug combinations, and sexual experimentation—that does not rely on assumptions that people do these things only within "subcultures" or at public venues rather than in domestic spaces. Neither does ISP assume or imply that everyone who goes to circuit parties or uses bathhouses engages in sexual adventurism. [45] Not all gay men, lifestylers, or others who seek group sex in combination with other types of stimulation do so "frequently" or fit the definition of "intensive sex partying." "Most gay men," researchers stress, "probably live far more mundane lives than might be suggested by the literature." [46]

Sensation seeking, sexual adventurism, and ISP are frequently viewed as negative tendencies that increase people's risk of addiction, illness, or death. Unfortunately, studies meant to be value-neutral can reflect the assumptions of researchers. Take the category of "esoteric" sexual practices. As Australian researchers Jonathan Bollen and David McInnes point out, "It may only be from the perspective of the ordinary, the normal, or the regular that fisting is regarded as 'adventurous,' 'heavy,' or 'extreme.'" Their informants, gay men who self-identified as being "into adventurous sex," were motivated "by an erotics of unpredictability," an openness to exploration, experimentation, and improvisation. As these men understood it, sexual adventurism was a way of describing their overall approach to sexual activity rather than a way to categorize or hierarchically rank sexual activities. One man, for example, described fisting as "the most boring experience on earth."[47]

A focus on negative consequences has often overshadowed the positive aspects of seeking sensation, novelty, or adventure in a modern world. Sensation seeking may play a role in keeping people happy and healthy over their life span, researchers argue.[48] Many wealthy and powerful individuals have been exposed over the years as being involved in sexually "adventurous" activities. While they might have a stronger drive for novelty or sensation seeking (and perhaps this is part of what helps them become wealthy or powerful), it could also be that power and money provides opportunities to indulge in activities many others would find desirable if they had the resources. Given entrenched notions of sexual risk in Western culture, it is often difficult to accept that sex can be a realm of positive exploration. On the other hand, sexual excitement draws on unconscious sources of inspiration and gains steam from prohibitions and emotional ambivalence. Distinctions between positive and negative may thus be too simplistic.

ADVENTURES IN COSMIC ECSTASY

Group sex can be a route to experiencing a transcendent state, sometimes termed a "high" and sometimes pronounced as spiritual or sacred. Psychologist Abraham Maslow analyzes peak experiences as "moments of highest happiness and fulfillment" potentially including love, "parental experience, the mystic, oceanic or nature experience, the aesthetic perception, the creative moment, the therapeutic or intellectual insight, the orgasmic experience, certain forms of athletic fulfillment, etc."[49] These experiences are self-justifying and self-validating; even pain becomes worthwhile in the quest to attain such states, which may also be characterized by "complete, though momentary, loss of fear, anxiety, inhibition, defense and control, a giving up of renunciation, delay and restraint."[50] Peak experiences can also involve feelings of both separateness and belonging: "the greatest attainment of identity, autonomy, or selfhood is itself simultaneously a transcending of itself, a going beyond and above selfhood. The person can then become relatively egoless."[51] Many writers in psychology, aesthetics, and religion suggest that peak experiences are intrinsically valuable, "so valuable," in fact, "that they make life worth while by their occasional occurrence."[52]

Some individuals and religions refuse the pleasures of the body or sexuality as a poor substitute for the ecstasy of the divine, or they go further to deem sex sinful. Still other traditions locate religious elements within particular bodily experiences, believing in the promise, or hope, that sex can deliver more than temporary pleasure. Certain unions are blessed as sacred. Lovers might be seen as mirroring godly wholeness or as embracing the divine in each other. Sexual desire and pleasure can be pathways to accessing "the Source." Like trance and death, sex is a physiological experience that takes on complex meanings and cultural forms. Trance is sometimes referred to as "'half death' or 'little death'" and can involve actual orgasm;[53] "near-death experiences" have reportedly been triggered by orgasm. Words such as "bliss," "passion," and "ecstasy" are used to describe both sex and spirituality in various languages. The French phrase *la petite mort* can refer to orgasm, spiritual experiences of transcendence, or inner feelings of loss. Some individuals describe sex as spiritual, although the descriptions vary by tradition: to varying degrees and frequency, people recount "feelings of oneness with the universe during orgasm"; out-of-body experiences; weeping with joy; feeling "enveloped with a loving light," "touching souls," and encountering "universal healing energy."

Mythical orgies—and occasionally real ones—are viewed as potentially amplifying these experiences. Powerfully transcendent experiences, some theorists believe, can also potentially lead to orgiastic expression, as the "intensity of religious sentiment" becomes an "expression of collective desire." According to French sociologist Michael Maffesoli, an orgy is not reducible to sexual activity: "Eros cements and structures sociality; it leads the individual to transcend itself and to lose itself in an ensemble more vast."[54] Maffesoli's argument is reminiscent of Eliade's, where the breakdown of social order into chaos during the orgy and the loss of individual selves into the multitude are regenerative of civilization. Not surprisingly, many of Maffesoli's examples of orgies are drawn from Eliade, who drew from Frazer, and so on. As discussed throughout this book, many such reports of sexualized worship are historically unsubstantiated, exaggerated, or possibly fallacious. Nevertheless, links between spiritual experience and group erotics persist across time and place.

Painful experiences and rituals can also induce altered forms of consciousness, which sometimes generate experiences of spiritual communion. Once an individual has gone through a period of pain, endorphins—"natural opiates"—are released in the brain. Athletes have long chased endorphin highs; BDSM players do similarly. Altered states of consciousness vary in intensity, and experiences are given different meanings across contexts ("runner's high," "subspace," "oneness," etc.), but people attaining such states report similar effects, such as the disappearance of pain, a loss of sense of self, and feelings of deep connection. Anthropologist Harvey Whitehouse argues that "traumatic ritual ordeals feature in all the world's religions, at least as locally or regionally distinctive traditions rather than universal features."[55] From the Native American sun dance, where dancers pierced their chests with hooks, attached ropes, and then suspended themselves until the skin ripped away, to the self-flagellation of monks, and from religious fasting to firewalking, people have pursued transcendent experiences through physical trials. Some initiation ceremonies cause extreme pain or instill extreme fear in participants through severe deprivation, violence, genital cutting or other bodily modifications (circumcision in men or women, penile subincision where the uretha is slit lengthwise, "penis bleeding"), and so on.

Peter Allison Larkin spent more than a decade immersed in the Roman Catholic Church; he also earned a master's degree in theology. After he retired from religious life, he changed his name to Christopher Larkin, made a film about being gay, traveled the world, and began exploring tantric sexuality. He renamed himself yet again as Purusha Androgyne Larkin and in 1981 published a book called *The Divine Androgyne according to Purusha.* Although detractors of the work termed it an "extended, egotistical essay on fist-fucking," Purusha preferred to think of it as a description of his "adventures in cosmic erotic ecstasy and androgyne body consciousness."[56] Purusha described pouring his early homoerotic desires into the church—"I fell in love with this man Jesus and that a man could live on the earth like he did." Eventually, he grew restless with trying to sublimate his erotic energy, left the church, and developed a new theology based on the body, sexuality, and love. Androgynes, he alleged, were beings that had reconciled dualities in their own bodies, achieving an inner equilibrium and sense of wholeness; this could be accomplished through certain erotic practices. Believing that "ninety-nine percent of all the people in this country are not only touch-starved, they're ecstasy-starved," Purusha proposed that every man and woman should have "one full, intense orgasm per day by sexually love worshiping themselves, and others, without guilt." Doing so would "transform our species and change the course of evolution," leading to a deeper fulfillment of human potential. "Awe" and ecstasy were meant to be experienced daily.[57] "Fist-fucking" and piercing, for Purusha, were advanced forms of practice, producing transcendent experiences. Fisting is described as beautiful, profound, "mind-blowing," and like "being fucked by the whole universe." "The extreme sensations of pleasure or pain, or especially the combination of both together," Purusha claimed, concentrates the mind and "*unifies* the consciousness in a way that leads in the direction of what is called the mystical state, or ecstatic states of consciousness." These states, he argued, are called by different terms even if they are ultimately similar—*satori* in Zen, *samadhi* in tantric Indian traditions, or Maslow's "peak experiences." The pain sometimes involved in achieving these mystical states could be distinguished from the "hurting, degrading, and abusing" that could occur when people approached BDSM without first clearing their "negative conditioning."[58]

"Sacred kink" and "spiritual BDSM" take various forms today, using different language and practices ranging from a focus on appropriating primal or tribal characteristics to the recovery of suppressed religious doctrines. Entering, or producing, a space of altered consciousness is for BDSM players what orgasm is to "vanillas"—that is, an experience that is valued, sought, and remembered though not always attained. Players claim that their intense physical and emotional ordeals produce a "natural high." Throughout the literature on BDSM, players report experiences of euphoria, hyperreality, dissociation (out-of-body-experiences), spiritual transcendence, emotional release, "flow," and energetic connection with others in the scene. During the high phase, sometimes referred to as "subspace" or "headspace,"[59] players may no longer experience pain or be aware of their surroundings. After coming down, however, some players may feel confused, disoriented, and disconnected; occasionally, they may be unable to communicate or even feel temporarily paralyzed.

Explicitly connecting this kind of BDSM experience to transcendence is extremely important in some enclaves and negligible in others. Pat Califia argues:

> The impulse to get tied to a bench and flogged for two hours until you are flying out there with adrenaline and endorphins is no different than the impulse to snort a line of coke, or swallow a hit of MDA, and be someplace else. It's about looking for transcendence, it's about getting past fear, it's about being able to make a deep heart connection with other people that is not cluttered by all of this critical self-talk and self-consciousness that normally pollutes our experience of the world.[60]

In *Leatherfolk*, an edited collection focusing on the spiritual elements of BDSM, several practitioners recall early quests for transcendence, often sounding a lot like sensation seekers who had not yet settled on an outlet: "I craved the excitement of life. I was searching. Searching for something—the highest highs, the biggest thrills—yet never finding it"; "I was always restless. . . . I started the long journey toward what we're all looking for, which is liberation."[61] They found their answers, at least temporarily, in "cosmic" or spiritual ecstasy, although we cannot overlook the importance of context in this process—it is not an accident that mid-twentieth-century San Francisco figures prominently in their journeys (this is discussed in more depth later in the book).

BDSM play thus makes use of timeless human capacities—both physiological and psychological—but in a manner that is resolutely cultural and historical. As Gayle Rubin writes:

I do not see how one can talk about fetishism, or sadomasochism, without thinking about the production of rubber, the techniques and gear used for controlling and riding horses, the high polished gleam of military footwear, the history of silk stockings, the cold authoritative qualities of medical equipment, or the allure of motorcycles and the elusive liberties of leaving the city for the open road. For that matter, how can we think of fetishism without the impact of cities, of certain streets and parks, of red-light districts and "cheap amusements," or the seductions of department store counters, piled high with desirable and glamorous goods . . . ? To me, fetishism raises all sorts of issues concerning shifts in the manufacture of objects, the historical and social specificities of control and skin and etiquette, or ambiguously experienced body invasions and minutely graduated hierarchies.[62]

Simple comparisons of modern Western practices to tribal rites, then, are problematic. The processes involved in producing the experiences are real; the explanations given for such practices by rooting them in particular histories are sometimes mythical. Experiences are interpreted in light of historical data, fantasy, and contemporary discourses of sexuality and spirituality. Contemporary "suspension" enthusiasts, for example, sometimes recreate the sun dance ceremony but have elaborated on the idea through group "pulling" sessions, where people pierce their flesh with hooks, attach ropes, and then fasten the ropes to other individuals or objects, using each other's weight as resistance to collectively intensify their experience. Further, during altered states produced by trance or ritual, on drugs, or when having sex, people usually do what they've learned to do and what other people around them do. Dancers become "possessed" by the appropriate spirits. Modern college coeds trip and watch television; Timothy Leary's followers tripped and spoke to God. American lifestylers generally do not profess love to their outside partners before sex; tantric practitioners remind each other of love and divine connection as the basis of sexual union. What people consciously *believe* they are doing is also important—those undergoing physical trials to attain a spiritual experience might not like the thought that what they are doing is no different from people who want to "get tied to a bench and flogged for two hours," as Califia suggests. Supposedly, some members of the controversial Roman Catholic sect Opus Dei engage in "corporal mortification." But is wearing a cilice (a spiked bracelet around the thigh) or engaging in "the discipline" (self-flagellation, occasionally with razors or pins in the whip) best understood as sexual or religious? Could it possibly be both or perhaps depend on the occasion, person, or level of analysis? Justifying an activity as spiritual rather than sexual can elevate it in the eyes of nonparticipants, who might be primed to interpret it as deviant or hedonistic. But even the same activity can mean multiple things on different occasions. Andy, a participant in "flesh-pulling" rituals, explains: "For some people, it's a spiritual thing, for some people it's for shits and giggles." Some events were sexual for

Andy—"It's great to come [orgasm] with the hooks in"—but others could be "very mellow and spiritual . . . it all depends on the participants."[63]

Sex remains sacred for some Western tantric practitioners, who use sexual practices to heighten spiritual experience and divine connection. At the mention of tantra, many people think of Sting, the rock musician who supposedly claimed that his mastery of tantric sex meant that he could perform sexually for seven hours straight. Or five hours, or twenty-four hours, depending on the article one reads. His wife, Trudie Styler, has attempted to bust the myth, but given its persistence for more than twenty years, Sting is unlikely to be dethroned anytime soon. (Of course, there are worse reputations to have.)

Religious scholar Hugh Urban suggests that tantra serves as a "Rorschach test or psychological mirror of the changing moral and sexual attitudes of the last two hundred years."[64] Tantra has a quasi-mythical history, traced back either to the Indus Valley's ancient matriarchal civilization that practiced goddess worship and fertility cults or to an inner core of Vedic teachings that were suppressed in modern contexts.[65] Early European missionary accounts referred to "the so-called Tantra religion," where "nudity is worshipped in Bacchanalian orgies which cannot be described." *Sound familiar?* While scandalous representations of tantra appeared in both Victorian novels and Indian popular literature, other Western and Indian authors attempted to squelch such sexualized images, presenting tantra as a "noble and orthodox tradition."[66] More recently, Urban argues, Western cultures have seen a neo-romantic celebration of tantra, imagining it as an "engine of political change," a path of "social defiance" to society's religious restrictions, and a symbol of "sexual pleasure, sexual liberation, and political freedom."[67] Pop tantra, or what some scholars somewhat condescendingly term "California tantra," doesn't usually focus on a guru, involve extensive meditative practice, or prescribe traditional rules of conduct. But it does emphasize female equality and the physical and spiritual benefits of sexual pleasure, features which have made it attractive to people beyond those considered "new age."

Issues of historical authenticity aside, tantra classes and workshops have sprung up around the United States and elsewhere. Not every tantra class involves nudity or sex. Some practitioners would dislike tantra's inclusion in a book about group sex, preferring a focus on other facets of their spiritual traditions—asanas or yoga techniques, mantras, mandalas, meditation, and other practices. But in some teachings on sacred sexuality, solo or group sexual practices have an educational purpose. Students are given instruction on how to generate, balance, and harness sexual energy in their body and interactions. Some practitioners focus primarily on techniques such as breathing, yoni massage, or the prevention of ejaculation, while others more systematically link those techniques to spirituality. My experience with tantra is limited, and in the few workshops I attended, we merely paired off in dyads, gazed into each other's eyes, practiced breathing, and occasionally massaged a stranger (while clothed). Trying to experience the humanity in each individual, respect the person's unique gifts and wounds, and respond with love was a worthwhile exercise, however; attempting to be comfortable both giving and receiving pleasure from a stranger—even the PG-rated kind—is actually quite difficult for many people.

Sasha and Janet Kira Lessin run Club Tantra in Hawaii, an event that blends the instructional aspects of coached tantra with the erotic environment of a play party. The teachers at Club Tantra focus on honesty, respect, and the process of setting and honoring boundaries. Through control of one's sexual energy, expansive feelings of love, and the mastery of special techniques, the limits of the individual body are ideally transcended in favor of ecstatic merging. People of all sexual orientations and relationship types are welcomed, making it more inclusive than many venues, and the opportunity to immediately practice their skills probably appeals to students who have been shelling out thousands of dollars for instruction at the School of Tantra, also run by the Lessins.[68]

Like other cosmic orgiasts, Janet Kira Lessin links particular sexual practices to the possible achievement of *satori*, or divine understanding. Double penetration, for example, can allow a practitioner to

open your inner stargate, touch the face of God and remember your source. As you embrace two or even three magic wands, the *lingams* (as we call penises) with your most sensitive inner sensual shrines, you feel ecstasy, get total personal and transpersonal recall. You drop concepts of physics, science and religion and instead zoom, as your multidimensional self, through space and time. You and the beloveds entering you merge with divinity, source of all inchoate forms. Home, you experience everything everyone told you as illusion and, at the same time, truth.[69]

For Lessin, "group synergy, tantric lovemaking, polyamorous merging and multiple penetration" can all be used to achieve altered—higher—states of consciousness that can fundamentally change the world: "Together we stop war, pollution, overpopulation, disease and hunger."[70]

Physical experiences, especially those that are highly stimulating, can produce altered states of consciousness. Whether such states are interpreted as sacred or mundane, however, depends on many factors, and privileging specific practices—whether fisting, flesh pulling, or double penetration—with an essential role in achieving these states is problematic. After all, Purusha might experience fisting as "mind blowing," but what does it mean when someone else regards it as "the most boring experience on earth"?

"I'M CAUTIOUS NOW . . ." (INTERVIEW, MICHELLE)

Stan and I picked out the man who would join us in bed. I liked that Jack was bisexual, because Stan will sometimes be with a man also. We got together three times, and each time I was more turned on. I had a no kissing rule, and Jack was respectful of my boundaries.

The first night, we were all in front of the fireplace and Stan intentionally left the room. Jack massaged my back, and it started feeling sexual. After we started fooling around, Stan came back and joined us. The second time was playful. I was reading *The Guide to Getting It On*, so I'd try the hand job techniques on both of them at once. They would tell me which moves they liked best.

The third time was when I sat on top of Jack having sex. I remember that because I hadn't done that before with him. Stan remembers working with compersion[71] while he watched from the couch. I never had an orgasm, but was turned on. Then Jack and Stan played with the BDSM equipment and I participated a little, tickling Jack's penis with my hair. I was a gentle addition. Following that, still in the dungeon, Jack had intercourse with me and ejaculated. Stan said, "I like sloppy seconds." I use condoms with them both, so it wasn't really "sloppy," but Stan liked the idea. I was on my back and Stan got on top. I was less into it at that point but knew I could say yes or no. I didn't say no. So we had sex. While Stan was inside me, Jack manipulated my clit. I remember saying they were turning me on. Then it ended.

Later that evening, I went to shower before bed. In the shower, I had this sudden feeling of wanting to wash Jack's touch off me. I remember scrubbing my neck—he had kissed me on the neck—and then I got this image in my mind of a raped woman washing herself off in the shower. I thought, this is what a raped woman looks like. I detached, seeing myself as a woman who wanted to be washed clean. But why? Was I someone who had done things she didn't want to do? I hadn't said no and was mostly turned on. But at that moment I realized something happened to me that I didn't feel good about, even if I hadn't been hurt or violated. I said, I'm not doing this anymore until I figure it out.

I talked with Stan about my feelings but didn't tell Jack right away. He wasn't a close friend. Eventually, I just told him I didn't want to experiment again.

I'm still confused about my reaction. Maybe it was cognitive dissonance. "Michelle doesn't do those things"—have sex with two men—but there I was, getting turned on. Maybe I was afraid of becoming someone I don't think of myself as. If I define myself as monogamous, how do I feel if someone is turning me on and it's not Stan? I also don't like the image of myself lying on my back and having two people over me. I was married for twenty years, and the last ten years were platonic. One day I had intercourse with my husband, and I remember it was an effort. I still have this image of him on top of me, with me knowing I'm not turned on, feeling like I'm giving my body away. Maybe I overreact when I'm not turned on now, or maybe it's that image of having someone above me. It wasn't like sex wasn't good with my husband. I usually had orgasms during intercourse and didn't even know that was unusual for many women. But I've never forgotten that experience, and it was the last time we had sex.

Stan really likes threesomes, but I'm cautious now. I didn't like how threesomes all revolved around me. We had a threesome with a woman who was bisexual, but things went too quickly for me. When that happens, I shut down but feel pressure because it's my fault everything stops. After each experience we had, I thought, "I don't need to do that again." Not, "I need to do that differently." Just, "Okay, that's it." We've gone to swing parties and I can have sex with just Stan in a group situation. I have a mild exhibitionist side. But if he's going to have sex with someone else, it's better for him to leave me at home. When he had his orgy party a few months ago, I was uncomfortable. It's easier for me to think of him fucking someone else than to see him having a connection.

But strangely, threesomes come up in my fantasies when I masturbate. There are two frequent scenes that I visualize. One is a scene with two Russian brothers. I have a connection with one but the other has never been with a woman. So the first asks me, "Do you mind if my brother watches?" I let him watch and then the brother fucks me. There's another version of this where one has a finger in me and I'm giving the other one a blow job. The other fantasy is based on an experience I had watching a woman at a party who was with two men. She was lying on her stomach. One man was having sex with her from behind and the other guy was in her mouth. They moved her back and forth. It's not like I picture myself in there between the men. It's *her*. But I use the memory to get off.

Psychotherapist Jack Morin surveyed 351 people about their most memorable erotic encounters and favorite sexual fantasies. Expanding on Maslow's theory of peak experiences—intensely joyful or exciting moments in an individual's life—Morin used the narratives he collected to delve into the erotic mind, which he believed was key to understanding human needs and potentials. Unlike other peak experiences, however, he found that "in peak sex the erotic impulse frequently strays far from our ideals," revealing "our idiosyncrasies, conflicts, and unresolved emotional wounds."[72] Morin's "erotic equation" is relatively straightforward: attraction + obstacles = excitement.

"Although sexual desire and arousal can be stimulated by all sorts of people and situations," he writes, "your most passionate responses spring from the interaction of competing forces."[73] The obstacles could be a partner's unavailability or inappropriateness, distance (physical, emotional, or geographic), uncertainty about the future, or taboos. Secret sexual encounters are notoriously exciting, for example, and specific sexual acts may be more or less acceptable across time and place—and correspondingly more or less exciting.

Because each individual's history is unique, different obstacles heighten arousal for each of us—at least up to a point. Morin argues that there are "four cornerstones of eroticism," or existential sources of obstacles: longing and anticipation, violating prohibitions, searching for power, and overcoming ambivalence. While a peak erotic experience does not require that these cornerstones be present, many such encounters will include at least one, and sometimes more, because they are "extremely effective arousal intensifiers."[74]

People tend to be aware of the positive emotions "energizing" their peak sexual experiences—love, tenderness, or affection. But the "unexpected aphrodisiacs"—anxiety or fear, guilt, shame, hostility, anger, and vulnerability—also intensify arousal, though most successfully in low doses or controlled situations.[75] The best time to flirt with someone, for example, according to "pick-up artists," is when the person is feeling slightly insecure. *The Art of Seduction* suggests techniques drawing on the sexually arousing nature of anxiety: for example, send "mixed signals" to confuse the "victim," create "triangles" so that the victim must compete for you, stir up feelings of inadequacy in the victim, generate suspense about what you will do next, and mix kindness and cruelty to heighten the erotic charge ("The lower the lows you create, the greater the highs").[76] Potential lovers who make us work for their attention often seem more exciting than those who throw themselves at our feet (or even those who are just nice to us). While we may not all want to scheme to such an extent, it is wise to keep in mind why our hearts beat faster in some scenarios than in others.

Arousal depends, in part, on an intricate psychological dance between safety and danger. While actually being caught licking someone's genitals might be too shameful to bear, *almost* being caught could be wildly exciting. For someone like Millet, being witnessed, either literally or figuratively through narrative, is a source of pleasure or arousal. Until it isn't. As a memory, a story told to others, or a scene revisited under controlled conditions, a sexual experience can transform over time from traumatic to arousing or vice versa. This does not necessarily mean that anyone who was raped will be "healed" by organizing her own gang bangs. But it does point to the complexity of emotional experience involved in erotics. We may not all have dramatic events in our history that directly impact our sexuality, but we can be fairly certain that our idiosyncrasies, conflicts, and unresolved emotional wounds will eventually turn up in our erotic life. As Brianna's story illustrates, group sex can also be physically challenging or overwhelming. To truly understand any particular individual's motivations requires traversing a vast territory of fluid meaning.

Morin found fantasies involving multiple partners to be the most frequent scenarios reported by his respondents; fantasies about anonymous partners ranked second.[77] Given social prohibitions on nudity and multiperson sex, the intricate negotiations required, and preexisting folklore highlighting the explosive potential of orgies, group sex easily rests on the "cornerstones" that Morin discusses. When we add in potential emotional experiences that generate ambivalence, we have enough obstacles for a four-hundred-meter hurdle course. It is not surprising that swingers are more likely to describe their lives as "exciting" than the general population.[78] One woman described her first orgy as "a fantastic adventure."[79] Hotwife scenarios, dogging, and other sexual adventures, can generate arousal for the individuals who crave them on numerous levels—whether through the experience of novelty, social and interpersonal risk, the emotional stress of competition, jealousy, shame, overcoming prohibitions, or all of the above, depending on the person.

But what makes someone choose an orgy over a safari?

And how do they decide which kind of orgy to go to?

Chapter Six

Games People Play

Group Sex as Experimentation, Adventure, and Play

THE ORGY DOME (INTERVIEW, ZACH)

One of Burning Man's most valued concepts is "gifting," the giving of things to others just because one can and with no expectation of receiving something in return. The "orgy dome" was intended to be our "gift" to other Burners—a safe space for people who were already in the lifestyle, or into swinging, to play. Somewhere along the way, our camp also decided it would be great to introduce interested newbies to open sexuality—safely and without judgment—what we call being "sexually social." Now, the "orgy dome" is open to experienced lifestyle couples, curious couples, and even some who are sharing camping space and just don't have anywhere else to go. We are mostly visited by heterosexual couples, but we do get gay and lesbian couples occasionally (and combined groups we call "moresomes"). They are welcome, although there are other camps dedicated to those groups. One year, a girl wanted to celebrate her birthday with a gang bang—we were going to allow single men that day, but it didn't end up happening. Singles aren't usually allowed, but they still try to get in. We've even had obviously straight guys try to get in by pretending they are a gay couple. "Okay, kiss each other," I'll say, and that's usually the end of that.

Campmates share "greeter" duties, where we go over the rules with visitors or watch the door to make sure that only couples or moresomes enter and leave together. We answer questions and warn people who break the rules. Unfortunately, sometimes we have to eject them. So what are the

167

rules? No shoes inside. Leave your dusty backpacks or coats in the cubbies. Couples enter and leave together, and no gawkers (unless specifically asked to watch—we do have exhibitionists). The most important rule is to ask before you touch anyone, and if they don't actually say "yes," they don't mean "yes." Use a towel when you have sex, and clean up after yourselves. We provide towels, condoms, and lube. It's tough enough to keep things clean in the desert, but we change the sheets, empty the trash, and stock clean towels. It takes a lot of work to keep everything going, and people are very thankful. I've received some very special playa gifts over the years.

After people listen to the orientation, they can go inside. It's a double zip-door both for privacy and to keep out the dust, so we request that they unzip the first door of the tent, step inside, zip it back up, and then unzip the second door. Inside, we have seven air conditioners. There is at least one massage table (sometimes more) and a small room with a sex swing that gets used quite a bit. There is a larger room for group play.

Occasionally, a couple will go inside and be back out in just a few minutes. There's a bit of a "sensory overload" issue sometimes—they need to think about it, or they aren't sure if an orgy or public play is right for them. That's fine. It might *not* be right for them. But I love it when a new couple comes just to check it out, and then disappear inside for an hour or more. They come out flushed, exhilarated, dazed, and very, very happy.

A few years ago, I had a small group of cocky drunken frat boys who stopped by. I couldn't let them in, of course, but it was very dusty, so they were hanging out in the overflow area, trying to decide where they were going to go next. Well, about twenty minutes before they arrived, a gorgeous young girl had gone inside the dome with her boyfriend. She was very enthusiastic and we could all hear her enjoying herself. The guys could only imagine what was going on inside—they hadn't been inside the tent, and they hadn't seen the girl.

All of a sudden, the tent unzips and she steps out, naked. *Beautiful.*

"I need another cock," she said. She looked around, noticed one of the frat boys, pointed, and said, "How about you?"

He looked like he was going to pass out. "Uh, I can't," he stammered. She asked a few more of them. None had the nerve to take her up on the offer. All of their bravado was gone. Eventually, she just shook her head and stepped back inside, zipping the tent behind her.

I laughed. "In twenty years," I told them, "you're going to look back on this moment and really regret it."

But at Burning Man, a lot of people are out of their comfort zone. They're suddenly in an environment of "radical self-expression" and it's intense. Long-term Burners are there with their peer groups, so it's easy to forget what it was like their first time. Newcomers are often overwhelmed. They might sit next to a swinger at work every day and have no idea. But at

Burning Man, people are free to be themselves. Suddenly, newcomers see things they've only heard or fantasized about. The first day or two, some people end up sitting in their tent saying, "Holy shit. I don't think I can go out there again." But by the third or fourth day, they're feeling more comfortable. Obviously, being out there in the desert is not *just* about sex, although sex makes a lot of people uncomfortable, so there's sex to grapple with. Being out there is about a lot of things we aren't supposed to do or be in the everyday world.

BURNING MAN: A MOVABLE FEAST FOR THE SEXUAL TRAVELER

Sexiled? Need a place away from your campmates to get it on with your new playa friends? Can't find a place to safe-sex it up on playa? . . . We have a fully equipped, environmentally sealed, safe-sex space ready for you and up to a dozen of your friends to use anytime, day or night! With massage table, mattresses, sheets, supplies, and surprises you can share. *** Open to all genders and preferences—closed to the creepy.
—Advertisement for the Orgy Dome

"In all known cultures and civilizations," anthropologist I. M. Lewis argues,

we find essentially two, at first sight contradictory processes which induce trance. One involves sensory deprivation—trauma, stress, illness, isolation, fasting, and deliberate physical mortification as in many mystical religious traditions. The other equally common stimulus involves sensory overloading—with musical and other sonic bombardment (especially monotonous drumming), strobe lighting effects, the ingestion of hallucinogenic drugs, and more mundane procedures like over-breathing and even strenuous exercise such as jogging (which has been shown experimentally to increase endorphin levels).[1]

Trance, for Lewis, is a term referring to altered states of consciousness ranging from dissociation to religious ecstasy, meditation to peak experiences.

At the Burning Man festival, which takes place in a high-altitude desert basin too bleak to support natural plant or animal life, both of these trance-inducing processes occur simultaneously. The harsh physical environment—hot during the day and cold at night; frequent dust storms; a lack of physical features other than the distant mountains and the desert floor; and the inability to access everyday comforts—becomes the setting for a new landscape created to indulge and engulf the senses. Loud, continuous electronic music, elaborate costuming or nudity, performance art and installation art, and a novel set of cultural expectations (embraced to different extents by participants) appear within a new arrangement of time and space. Somehow, it becomes almost impossible to arrive somewhere "on time," although time also gains new meaning with a twenty-four-hour clock. Some people find it easier to sleep during the heat of the day and venture out at night. Others find it impossible to sleep at all. Navigating through the dusty city becomes easier with experience, although it is challenging for newcomers. "The Man," in the center of the playa, becomes the primary reference point; the streets that encircle him form a wheel, marked around the circumference by the numbers on a clock (2:00, 2:30, 3:00, etc.) and outward by the letters of the alphabet, with "A" being closer to "the Man" than "L." Transportation is limited to bikes or feet, or an occasional art car. (The problem with art cars, however, is that you're quite literally "along for the ride" and might end up miles from your camp.) Contact with the outside world is difficult—the drive from Reno is about three hours, and with traffic on the two-lane country roads and lengthy backups at the front gates, it is rare for someone to leave the festival and return. Many years, cell phones do not work, making communication difficult. Being on the playa is described as similar to being on Mars, the moon, or "another planet." Substances are not necessary in order to experience an altered state of consciousness in such an environment, although some participants add drugs into the mix.

Burning Man had its origins in San Francisco, and a hippie ethos filters through even its more mainstream contingencies. The event is quintessentially American in principle and practice, although participants hail from around the world. As Matt Wray writes:

> There are all sorts here, a living breathin' encyclopedia of subcultures: Desert survivalists, urban primitives, artists, rocketeers, hippies, Deadheads, queers, pyromaniacs, cybernauts, musicians, ranters, eco-freaks, acidheads, breeders, punks, gun lovers, dancers, S/M and bondage enthusiasts, nudists, refugees from the men's movement, anarchists, ravers, transgender types, and New Age spiritualists.[2]

The emphasis on radical self-expression occasionally becomes another source of conformity: most participants respect the informal ban on visible corporate logos on their clothing or gear, but it is impossible to bike a block without seeing colorful tutus, Native American headdresses, or men wearing utility kilts, for example. Still, for most people, such adornment is far from everyday attire, and you might also encounter naked people painted head to toe in metallic colors, hundreds of partiers wearing bunny ears (probably participating in the "Million Bunny March"), or a guy wearing a disco ball that fits over his entire head. After a few days, you'll barely glance at the topless girl dancing along the Esplanade with a parasol, but a guy in a Tommy Bahama Hawaiian shirt will stop you in your tracks: Why is he wearing *that*? What does it *mean*?

Another treasured value of the event is a focus on individual and community meaning-making. Rather than proclaiming what the event itself or any particular work of art stands for, the organizers and contributors have long privileged the possibility of diverse and even contradictory interpretations. Even the meaning of "the Man" himself is left up to individual participants to discern. For some, the ritual burning of "the Man" is a somber event; for others, it is celebratory. Participants are *expected* to make meaning out of their experience, and they usually do. Ideally, participants also remain free to "have their experience" without the imposition of others' judgments, rules, or expectations. Each year a temple is constructed on the playa, to be burned on Sunday night. The temple is a nondenominational and participatory space—people pray, write on the walls, contribute items for the bonfire, do yoga inside, and even spend the night there. One of my most vivid memories is of watching the sun rise over the desert with people who had gathered on top of the temple. Except for the mourners, some of whom were being embraced by their companions, everyone was nearly silent and still. Some people meditated; others slept or were lost in their thoughts. A couple cuddled next to me, sharing a heavy jacket. As the sun peeked over the horizon, we rose as a group. We were teary-eyed, tired, and chilled. People began solemnly hugging their neighbors; some raised their arms to the warming sun. Someone began to sing "Amazing Grace." At that moment, a giant boat floated past the temple, blaring music so loud that it completely drowned out the singing. Ravers danced on the roof of the vehicle and people sprawled across every surface, hanging off the railings and dangling their legs over the wheel hubs.

They waved.

We waved.

Opinions on what actually happens "out there in the desert" range from condemnation to glorification. Critics have described it as "a 192-hour drug orgy," "a dance orgy," an "aural orgy," and even "a 24/7 bacchanal of booze, drugs, nudity, S&M, public sex, and bad art."[3] One man told the press that Burning Man wasn't about art at all, but "really about sex, drugs and rock 'n' roll—a lot of sex."[4] (I'm still wondering where he heard the "rock 'n' roll.") Supporters champion the possibility of personal growth and social transformation as the experiences and values of Burning Man trickle back into the everyday lives of participants. As an academic writer claims: "Burning Man does more than merely offer a means of escape—it offers the means to perform alternatives, and to enact a different social reality that may have practical implications."[5] Participants do not necessarily have a unified vision of that alternative social reality, however. Over the years, the more radical factions at Burning Man have warred with the "ravers" over the focus on partying rather than community or political change. Contradictions flourish. For every person extolling the virtues of desert tribal ritual, someone is fixated on global cyberculture. The "barter" and "gift" economy is fascinating to people used to whipping out their credit cards at every turn, and the media often underscores the fact that money only exchanges hands during the event for the purchase of ice or coffee at Center Camp. On the other hand, a *lot* of money goes into preparations for Burning Man, from renting RVs to purchasing tickets, tents, supplies, and enough fresh water to survive a week in the desert. Some of the more extravagant camps—which "gift" everything from meals to art cars to TEDx talks to mainstream DJs spinning on high-quality sound systems—are funded by entrepreneurs, bankers, and CEOs.

But what about the sex?

In addition to the "orgy dome," there are other opportunities for sexual experimentation, many of which transgress norms of privacy and decorum. The "safer sex" camp offers free lube and condoms, and the Bureau of Erotic Discourse (BED) holds discussions on sexual negotiation. One camp sponsors a "human carcass wash," where visitors are bathed and felt up at the same time by their launderers—*after* agreeing on boundaries. (Even individuals who aren't into group gropes may find themselves tempted to trade suds for fondling after a few days in the dust.) Several camps provide dungeons and BDSM equipment. You can find erotic rope bondage, pony play, and discreet places for men who are closeted or curious to play with other men. You might happen upon a game of naked Twister, a game of naked *wet* Twister, a topless disco, or a "petting zoo." Many workshops and demonstrations are sexually themed—rather than being sequestered away from passersby, these can occur right along the main streets. A friend of mine, biking through Black Rock City one afternoon, noticed a large group of people gathered at a camp. When he investigated, he saw a woman penetrating a man using a strap-on while the man explained his sensations and answered questions. In 2012, workshops were offered on double penetration, cunnilingus, and fellatio. If you're interested in sex toys, you can try out the Orgasmatron, Orgasamator, or the Spank-O-Matic, or even sit on the vibrating handles of my friend Kevin's Daiquiri Wacker, a blender mounted on a golf cart and driven by a gas-powered motor. (At the very least, you'll end up with a margarita, which is nothing to complain about in hundred-degree heat.)

Not all erotic activity is organized. Some art installations are strictly off-limits for sexual activity; others seem designed to invite it. In the wee hours of the morning, the many "chill domes" provided by camps—usually carpeted and furnished with pillows or mattresses—occasionally shelter couples having sex, "cuddle puddles," and smaller, impromptu group sex scenes. But given that public sex is illegal, and the law is enforced by the Bureau of Land Management and Nevada police, larger sex parties follow norms of spatial segmentation and interaction as you'd find at other public sex venues, where entry is controlled, rules are posted or explained, and the explicit nature of activities is progressive rather than "in your face."

Despite the variety of erotic entertainments, many regulars see the focus on sex in media accounts as misguided. Not everyone is there for sex, and the conditions aren't ideal—unless you eroticize dust, the taste and smell of baby wipes, or performing in front of a crowd. Continually asking for directions to an "orgy camp" marks one as a newbie quicker than wearing Nike sneakers. As a blog writer points out: "Tourists at Burning Man can all be recognized by their distinct, annoying, and fucktard behavior; generally they tend to be males (of any age but most often 19–22 year old frat boys or 50–60 year old men in $500,000 RVs) who come to Burning Man expecting an orgy of hot chicks undulating naked and ready to fuck on a moment's notice. If this is your reason for attending Burning Man, do yourself a favor and go to Lake Havasu instead."[6] Blogger Jay Michaelson writes that although there are some "naked people running around on drugs," the event is far more diverse than the media representations of it: "For every NPRAOD, I'd guess there are two people wishing they had the courage to do so, one person playing the violin on a sofabed in the middle of a desert, two people cooking pumpkin ravioli, and another person writing the name of her beloved on the wooden walls of the Temple." "If it's just a big party," Michaelson asks, "why is there a temple in the middle of it?"

For many of those devoted to Burning Man, sex and erotic experience simply plays a supporting role in a week that is really about a more ineffable experience—"a lot of something that can't be grasped," like trying "to describe color to a blind person." The event produces altered states of consciousness and feelings of liberation, freedom, and authenticity; sex is associated with these same experiences in American culture. For some participants, the experience is one of spiritual transcendence. As Michaelson suggests, "peak experiences such as those encouraged at Burning Man give a glimpse of the ultimate, the infinite." Although Burning Man doesn't provide this for everyone, it does so for enough people to attract fifty to sixty thousand each year and to have persisted for over twenty years, serving as an annual pilgrimage for many participants.

As with other liminal spaces or "temporary zones of altered reality," such a setting is conducive to sexual experimentation, even if not every participant chooses to do so. Unlike everyday life, commitment is not required for experimentation in such an environment—temporary, relatively anonymous, removed from everyday roles, norms, expectations, and comforts, and shaped within a set of cultural values supporting individual exploration and expression. A focus *just* on the sex, however, misses a great deal of how, and why, adults play.

Let's look at another experimentation zone—the world of the Internet.

GROUP SEX AND THE SINGLE AVATAR

Second Life is a virtual three-dimensional world where human users interact as avatars, both visually onscreen and through chat, instant message, and voice technologies. Second Life has had up to twenty-nine million sign ups since its inception in 2003; around five hundred thousand users log in each week. Although Linden Labs created the platform for Second Life, the world is actually driven by user-created content, which means that individual users can build objects or produce animations, retaining their copyrights. [7]

As with other Internet forums where control over content is ceded to the masses—say, Craigslist or YouTube—sex was inevitable. Philip Rosedale, the head of Linden Labs, allowed users to create sexual content in Second Life, even though other virtual worlds at the time restricted it: "We believed that freedom was fundamental to the environment and freedom is not something you can split hairs on. Second Life, like the Internet, is open to all, and what people want to do there is their own decision." [8] Controversy was also inevitable. During its peak years, Second Life sparked concerns: Would people begin spending all of their time at their computers and cease pursuing real relationships? And would the accessibility, anonymity, and instant gratification available online spur users to ever-greater sexual depravity? In the mid 2000s, Linden Labs created adult areas requiring age verification for admittance and banned certain activities, such as "ageplay," or sex where an avatar appears as a child. Since then, a decade has passed; panics have arisen around the sexualized use of other technologies (sexting, anyone?). Some gamers dismiss Second Life as a relic. Other virtual worlds have since sprung into existence, some of which are more exclusively focused on sex. Red Light Center, for example, is an adults only, "multiuser reality" site. In addition to experimenting with sexuality, Red Light Center users can smoke marijuana or take magic mushrooms—the game is modeled after the red-light district in Amsterdam—and visual changes associated with each substance appear onscreen.

Still, Second Life remains the prototype for virtual sociality and provides an interesting environment in which to study sexual fantasy and adventure. In many ways, Second Life has become a lot like "Real Life" (referred to by users as SL and RL). Because users sell the content they create, SL revolves around the marketplace. The local currency, the "linden," has a fluctuating exchange rate, hovering around $300L to $1 USD in 2011. But lindens add up: SL profits have reportedly made some RL millionaires. [9] And similar to RL, how an avatar looks and what it owns—from sneakers to real estate— becomes a way of claiming identity, displaying status, and making connections. Users initially choose their avatars from eleven standard models. Rather quickly, however, new "residents" usually refine their look by purchasing clothes, changing hairstyles, and customizing their bodies with everything from realistic "skins" to elaborate wings, horns, or tails. Supporting a shopping habit requires lindens, so residents go to work. They earn, save, and spend. They make friends, fall in love, get married, have children, cheat, and get divorced. And, of course, they have sex (usually after buying genitals, which aren't included with the basic model).

Given the creativity of erotic entrepreneurs, SL users can experiment with BDSM, sex work, orgies, and anonymous hookups in dark alleys. Some residents have sex at home; others retire to relatively private areas such as "skyboxes," tall objects where other avatars can't easily view what's happening at the top. Purchasing a "full sim," or a large chunk of land, allows one to hide one's virtual erotic activities more completely—it won't even show up on the map to those who aren't invited in—but can cost about $1,200 to create and around $200 a month in upkeep.[10] Some residents form private clubs, using membership dues to support these expenses. Many users, however, want public sex. After all, you can hide away in your own bedroom in RL, shades drawn and lights out, so why not try something different online?

Misty Crimsonlay is an avatar that has parlayed her erotic exploits into a series of self-help books and memoirs available for purchase with "real" USD, such as *A Slutty Day in Second Life, Second Life: How to Get Laid—Fast!* and *Second Life: Dirty Lesbian Sex.* She even publishes *Second Life—Sex Guide 2011* and, of course, *Second Life—Hot Orgies.*[11] "Sometimes I like to watch," she writes in *Hot Orgies,* "sometimes I join in." The following threesome scene, presented as it might look in Second Life chat, involves Misty, a shemale named Julia, and a lesbian named Alice:

SecondLifeNowPlaying:

Dip It Low

Christina Milian

Misty: oh yes with your pussy in my face

Misty: hmmmmm.

Alice: lick it baby

Misty: and Julia's fingers exploring

Misty: hmmmm

Alice: looks lovely

Misty: oh god yes

Misty: push down on me honey

Misty: smother my face

Misty: smother me with your pussy and rub it over me

Alice: your glasses are a bit sharp sweety

Alice: lol.[12]

An ethnographer at heart, I wasn't satisfied with reading *Hot Orgies*. I had questions: What were people looking for in Second Life, and how did they find it? What does virtual sex actually look like?

There was one good way to find out. I signed up, chose my avatar—a blonde woman in a red tartan skirt and turtleneck—and headed straight for the adult territories. Teleporting and flying, which is the best way to explore SL, were easy. I'm a natural, I thought. I had high hopes for my expedition.

But after thirty minutes of teleporting to deserted islands, I felt more like an archaeologist wandering the ruins of Pompeii than Margaret Cyber-Mead. I understood why some residents sought advice from Misty. *Where was everyone? How was I going to get laid—fast?* Just as in RL, you need a partner (or three) for group sex.

Finally, I found a crowded club called the "Dirty Bar." Residents sprawled across couches and chairs; some chatted in groups. Many were already in various stages of undress. A few female residents gave lap dances, while others whirled around poles. I approached a brunette woman in a purple raver outfit, thinking I'd ask her where she bought her leg warmers and maybe seduce her in the process. For some reason, choosing a woman for my first online sexual experience felt safer, even though I reminded myself that she might not really be a woman. But it didn't matter, anyway. Raver Girl had clearly come to the Dirty Bar for something or someone specific, and it wasn't me. She teleported. Perhaps she knew I was an SL virgin by my outfit. Also, like a typical newbie, I was making mistakes. Flying over vast waterways and uninhabited islands might have been effortless, but maneuvering around other avatars was more challenging. I bumped into walls and spun in circles. I peed on the floor. *How was I supposed to know that would happen if I clicked on the rug?* When I tried to sit down in a chair, my schoolgirl avatar instead mounted a mechanical sheep from behind. (Whoever created the animal, in addition to a warped sense of humor, had the foresight to design it to look as if it were constructed with nuts and bolts. Bestiality is scandalous even in SL.)

The sheep began bleating and circling the club, picking up speed. Panicked, I frantically searched for a way to disengage. In the main chat box, unfolding on the left side of my screen, residents mocked me:

Xxxx: it's okay everyone humps the sheep at some point

Yyyy: she should borrow my strap on . . . or buy one

Zzzz: second day in second life, wait until tomorrow

Yyyy: *baaaaaaaaa*

I tried to ignore them. Finally, I noticed a button on my control box that read, "STAND." I clicked it. My avatar, thankfully, returned to her upright position, and the mechanical sheep resumed a grazing posture.

How embarrassing.

Who cares? I'm a blonde standard model here. Nobody knows me.

Still, I teleported—*fast.* Perhaps it would be best to spread myself thin until I learned the ropes.

As I quickly figured out, one needs to pay close attention to the cursor. The round objects appearing on the computer screen are "poseballs." When clicked with the mouse, poseballs can make your avatar sit in a chair, kiss, or lie down on a pool table with her legs spread. You can become a "Waiting Prostitute" or position yourself for "Public Use." In BDSM clubs, poseballs were politely balanced: "Dom" or "Sub," "Give" or "Get," "Rape" or "Get Raped," "Pee" or "Get Peed On." Sometimes, though, poseballs are clustered so close together that it is hard to tell exactly what will happen—just like that, you end up humping a sheep. Residents can also purchase furniture, such as a bed or table, with built-in scripts for more complex options, although I wouldn't say they create a seamless fantasy.

Along my high-tech trek, I found places to congregate for Goreans, who practice master/slave relationships based on a series of science-fiction novels, and special islands for "furries," who anthropomorphize animals (only some of whom extend this interest into sex). I visited gay and lesbian communities, dungeons, orgy rooms, and sex clubs with names such as "Bukkake Bliss" or "Orgy in the Forest." Destinations such as "Public Disgrace" cater to residents interested in more extreme activities such as "rough sex, forced sex, swingers, prey, bukkake, slut, rape." (I found the appearance of "swingers" in the description to be curious and didn't run across any avatar couples on my visits.) On Orgy Island, couples had sex in a sandbox in every conceivable position; one man was break-dancing over a woman lying flat on her back. In Bukkake Bliss, a group of men stroked their penises while a naked woman did yoga poses in a bathtub, rhythmically opening and closing her mouth. A few female avatars gave blow jobs, and dozens of strippers whirled around poles. In fact, I saw so many strippers that I wondered whether more people came to SL to strip than to have sex.

Some of the more exclusive sex areas, I learned, can cost a pretty linden to enter, as can the costumes and equipment that mark you as a "real player." As in RL, garnering attention is part of the game when you're seeking sex. And when it comes to genitals, you get what you pay for—so unless you're satisfied with looking like a Ken doll or with the "free penis" sometimes offered as an incentive to visit a less trafficked sex club, you should invest wisely.

Hours passed. I was still a virgin. Just like in RL, everyone seemed to be waiting for someone else to make the first move. It was going to have to be me.

Am I really nervous about having sex as a computer graphic?

I teleported back to the Dirty Bar—*hey, they know me there*—and strode in confidently, avoiding my ovine friend. *No chickening out.* Catching sight of a muscled blonde resident who had obviously spent big bucks on his penis, I approached him and clicked the poseball that read, "Suck." My avatar dropped to her knees. After a few seconds, I clicked "Stand" and wandered off. *Well, that was easy.* Next up—threesome. I clicked on another poseball, and my avatar sprawled on the ground. Within minutes, a naked man with a long demon tail and tattoos on his arms positioned himself above me. Another naked man soon joined us, but as he hadn't claimed even a free penis, his humping movements above my head looked bizarre. I decided it counted anyway.

But how long should one have avatar sex? How does an encounter culminate without any physical cues? Pondering this issue, I waited about two minutes before moving on. Another mistake, as my tattooed partner twice turned his back on me when he saw me again in the club that evening. Later, I realized I had inadvertently ignored his attempts to chat privately with me: "nice ass, fuck, this is so good." Unsure of how I would have responded, I still grasped how rude my behavior had been. *Communication. That's how you know what to do next.* And, of course, that's where newbies make the most mistakes.

Eventually, two male avatars took me under their wing, demonstrating how the scripts worked on one of the beds. They contorted my avatar into a rapid string of sex positions that made me once again wonder if computer programmers have a fetish for Ashtanga yoga. And once again, I found, SL starts to look rather like RL. Sure, an RL man can become a busty redhead with a skunk tail, elf ears, and latex gloves in SL. But the overall menu is fairly familiar. I rarely saw an overweight avatar. No one buys a small penis. Residents have oral, anal, and vaginal sex. They flip-flop top to bottom and have sex standing, sitting, and lying down. They masturbate, sometimes as a way to get attention in sex clubs. They tie each other up on pool tables and get kinky with whips and chains. But I didn't come across anything unexpected, and even the "alien captors" I encountered aimed their lasers and examination probes at predictable bodily regions on their hostages. (Sure, some residents had sex with unicorns, or *as* unicorns, but somehow that didn't seem like bestiality.) More residents seek "tops" than are interested in topping others, judging by the number of slaves tied patiently at "Public Use" stations or wandering around with signs reading "waiting for master." Violence makes an appearance even though users can be banned from areas if they do not respect the rules. Communities form, developing their own norms and expectations, and there is no escaping social hierarchy. In the crowded sex clubs, a few users dominated the public chat, usually those with the best outfits or the most knowledge about SL (some of whom would call out other residents for mistakes). In both talk and appearance, there was jostling for attention and status.

Avatars may be infinitely flexible, but players are only willing to stretch so far.

SL sex carries fewer risks than RL sex, as there are no STDs, pregnancies, stigmas, or physical dangers. You can hire an escort without worrying about your picture showing up on the evening news. Other barriers to sexual experimentation are also lowered: disgust rules don't hold as powerfully when it comes to computer graphics, and shame organizes social interaction to a lesser degree. In an uncomfortable situation, one simply teleports, never to return again—or to return as a giant, fire-breathing demon. On the other hand, SL sex occupies an intriguing borderland between real and virtual worlds. As anthropologist Tom Boellstorff writes in *Coming of Age in Second Life*: "Clearly a murder in Second Life was a representation of a murder; no actual-world person was harmed. But sex in Second Life, even forms of BDSM or edgeplay, were forms of sexual expression for many residents, leading to orgasm and even to long-term relationships."[13] Technologies are being developed that will make sex even more realistic. The Sinulator, a wireless female vibrator, can be controlled over the Internet. The Real Touch is a device that envelopes the penis, plugs into the USB port of a computer, and synchronizes with pornography being viewed—or, perhaps, with an encounter on Domina Island. (It even maintains an internal temperature of around 98.6 degrees Fahrenheit.) SL sex can have RL effects beyond orgasm as well, especially if an RL spouse interprets avatar sex as real infidelity and files for divorce.[14] Users sometimes refer to "sex in virtual worlds" rather than "virtual sex" to highlight these complexities. Some users also claim that "emotional bonds are as strong in Second Life as they are in the physical world," and that "cybersex can be as meaningful, intense, and erotic as physical sex."[15]

Reality is always bolstered by fantasies—how we perceive ourselves and others, how we interpret events, and how we manifest our goals and dreams all involve subjective elements as well as external objects, events, relationships, and meanings. But are the boundaries so blurred in SL that real lives are destroyed, as some commentators warned? And is there a domino effect, where people are swept away into sexual deviance by their online explorations?

When psychologists explored people's understandings of the relationship between their online and "real-life" sexuality, psychological and physical satisfaction between the two domains—RL and SL—seemed unrelated; *most* people hadn't "crossed over" from SL to RL with a partner or experienced a reduction in real-life sexual activity because of their online escapades. In fact, users reported that SL had positive effects on their RL sex lives.[16] SL is indeed used for sexual experimentation, though. In one study, for example, survey participants reported that they did not necessarily know where to go or how to seek partners offline for the practices they were interested in exploring. So while these users claimed to present themselves as the same gender, race, class, and age in SL as RL, they used SL to experiment with relationships and sexual practices. Group sex, bondage/BDSM, observing others, and costume play—practices included on the survey—are stigmatized in RL but "maintain a flamboyant virtual presence" in SL.[17] Most users expressing interest in these activities did not have RL experience, but nearly all of them had SL experience. Still, concerns about such experimentation initiating a slide into depravity are probably misguided. Another study of 217 people with SL avatars found the prevalence of "atypical" sexual practices to be fairly consistent with their prevalence in RL. Although many participants had experimented "at least once" with certain activities in SL—for example, 56 percent had been with a same-sex partner and 43 percent had tried group sex, which is higher than in RL—this did not necessarily mean they *regularly* engaged in these practices. While 48 percent of respondents reported engaging frequently in oral sex in SL, only 9 percent reported frequently having group sex. Participants in Second Life engaged in both common and experimental sexual practices at a "faster pace and with a larger number of partners than in real life," but their virtual sexuality was not exactly "filled with rampant illegal and transgressive sexual practices." Further, researchers found that a great deal of sexual involvement still unfolded in longer-term relationships and that most Second Life users do not "consider sex and sexual experience to be among their primary activities in the virtual world."[18] While popular print and online journalism have "often portrayed the Second Life BDSM, Gorean, hentai, furry, and ageplay subcommunities as sexual and even predatory in nature, Second Life residents' perceptions of these communities may differ substantially."[19]

Even in the most extreme places I visited, like "Fuck Hall," advertised as "forced rape orgy," most residents were chatting. Users wanted to socialize, share fantasies, and connect. It made sense, at least to me: Without the human element, it's just naked cartoons.

Outsiders tend to see sex and nothing but sex. But even communities based around sexual interests and practices are never *just* about sex.

LIVING THE LIFE (INTERVIEW, CLAYTON)

When we got our opportunity to be on a reality show, it came fast.

Some friends run a lifestyle website and had signed up to do a series on swinging with Playboy TV. They said the producers were already done casting but encouraged us to submit our information anyway. 'You'd be perfect,' they told me. So I wrote up a blurb about my wife and me and e-mailed it. Within an hour, someone from Playboy had e-mailed me back—they wanted a conference call that night.

Damn, I thought—I haven't even talked to Kristen yet!

So I went home and we talked. "What do you think?" I asked her. "Do you want to pursue it?" We've been together over twenty years. We communicate well and discussed our concerns. We grew up in Utah, in staunch LDS families. We haven't been active in the church for a while but knew there might be challenges and some fallout if we put ourselves on TV. But we decided that the worst thing that could happen was that the truth about us came out. That can be a good thing.

A few days later, we were on a plane to meet the casting agent. They wanted us to film for every episode, but with kids and work we were already busy. We ended up filming seven out of ten episodes of season 1. We interested the agent because we are an attractive couple, but we're also average, normal people. We work. We love being outdoors, playing sports. We're family oriented. That's part of what challenges people who don't know anything about the lifestyle—they think just freaks get involved, and that's not the case at all. Kristen and I wanted to portray swinging in a real light, not what you see in *Real Sex* or some of the other shows.

Swing was produced by people who worked on *Survivor*, but instead of a bug-infested island, we were sent to a mansion in California. Along with our friends, we were the "residents," the regular couples. They brought in a new couple every three days for a new episode. The show was unscripted, but they had games and activities planned to make things happen because that was the end goal. Or they would set up a dramatic situation to drive forward. They also asked us a lot of questions on film. You'd be talking for hours upon hours, sometimes two days, but then they'd condense it down into two or three speaking segments. They took care of us: our food was catered, and they had plenty of alcohol to keep things flowing. I'm torn on alcohol when it comes to the lifestyle in general. Sometimes it's okay for people to loosen up, but when it becomes a crutch to play, it's a problem for me. You shouldn't need to be drunk. For us, life is about experiencing as much as possible. Why numb your senses? One new couple had a big blowup on the show, and when the crew interviewed us, we said this happens when you get too drunk. You can't communicate what you want.

How they chose to edit it was frustrating. I complained to the crew that I thought the editing was misleading, and they said that every person on a reality show says that same thing. One day, Scott and Nicoletta were joking about a party in the past where I'd shown them how fast I could make a girl squirt. Well, the newbie couple started asking questions, and we were explaining how it worked. I wouldn't brag about something like that—this was in the context of a conversation. But, of course, they edited it so it sounded like my opening line to this couple was about how skilled I am at making someone squirt. That night, I made several of the girls from the house ejaculate; girls were saying, "See if you can do it to me." But not everything made it on tape for any episode. They definitely missed some chemistry. In fact, some of the sexual things that happened off camera would have made for the best footage.

We had already been in the lifestyle for seven years. Being on the show created a bit of pressure. They weren't forcing us to have sex with anyone, but we knew we're on their dime, we're here to do a job. We wanted to make things happen. Fortunately, we connected with some of the people and had some fun times. Was it tough having sex on camera? There were awkward moments, I'll admit. Once, I was getting a blow job, and when I opened my eyes, there was a big fuzzy boom mike in my face. That's weird. My wife had a similar experience. There was a play scene, and then suddenly we had twenty-five minutes to shower and get ready for the next activity. She showered with another woman to save time, but then the camera crew came in. So, Kristen and the woman thought they should do something sexier than wash their hair. They started lathering each other up and getting into it, and then they realize there's a microphone right there in the shower with them. They're trying to hurry but also trying to make it sexy, and there's a film crew crammed into the bathroom.

If you've been in group play, you know that funny things happen. Someone falls off the bed or someone laughs or makes a stupid face. But the crew wasn't used to any of this. They weren't from the porn industry. They constantly made jokes to keep things light and not get turned on. Once, we were all having sex and the cameraman tripped. We all just stopped and laughed, but he was distraught. Sometimes we found it distracting that they had to keep joking at the wrong times but then couldn't laugh naturally when something was funny in the moment. But we understood that they just had no experience.

Some scenes affected everyone. Once, Kristen and a few girls ended up on the bed, just the girls. It was hot. It was one of those moments where you're like, "Wow, this is what the lifestyle is about. . . . This heat, this passion." But this time there's a producer and his assistant there, watching, trying not to feel awkward. At one point, he asked his assistant, "This is hot, right?" And she said, "Oh my God, yes."

We brought our own camera and interviewed the crew members, which was interesting. They had started the project with their own prejudices about swingers, about what kind of people we would be. We overturned some of those stereotypes. They said, "We don't know how you've done it but most people would kill to have this life." It was validating for Kristen and me.

I work for myself, so I wasn't worried about my job when the show aired. Kristen and I also thought, if people see us in the show and want to say something to us, they have to admit that they watch it. They have some explaining to do also! Some of my brother's friends told him that I was on the show. They also confronted me. Some of them said, "Are you crazy?" But then they'd add, "You're a lucky man. I wish my wife was into that. That looks like so much fun." A few friends subscribed to Playboy TV just so they could watch us. They'd text me during each episode. My brother, though, still won't bring it up with me. We've never talked about it, even though I know he knows.

Our life has changed a bit. Sometimes, we can tell people recognize us, maybe at a gas station or restaurant, but they don't want to say anything. It's not the kind of thing you'd bring up to someone, especially in Utah! Maybe in Vegas, but not here. There's a local nightclub here where a lot of lifestyle couples go. When we go, we're recognized. That's weird for us, because we don't really think of ourselves as celebrities. Seeing our episodes is like watching home videos for me. But when people find out or recognize us, they want to take pictures with us. If we go to big lifestyle parties, we go to meet new people. But now instead of talking to us because they want to play, people talk to us because we're on television. Since being on the show, we've become more protective, often playing with our group of close-knit friends.

Kristen and I were religious when we were first married. I tend to ask a lot of questions about life, maybe even overthink things. As we've journeyed through the lifestyle I've changed dramatically from what I was fifteen years ago. My religion told me that if someone was gay, I should treat him differently from other people. But there are gay people in my life that I know and love and it isn't worth it to me to believe something like that. I don't believe what my religion told me about marriage, either.

When we left the church, we had to decide on our own rules, so we came up with honesty. That's the most important thing to us. For the lifestyle, though, Kristen and I don't have a lot of rules. We explored it together from the very beginning and are very invested in each other's happiness, whatever form that takes. Let's say we're at a party and she has no one paying attention to her and I've got tons of girls around me—well, it's not like that ever really happens [laughs]. But if she was miserable, then I'd do something else. If she's having fun watching me, or if we have friends around and she isn't feeling lonely, we just let each other pursue the moment. A perfect night is where we're both happy, even if we maybe just flirted with someone else and then went home together. We don't have expectations—we could go out for drinks with a couple and nothing could happen except for good conversation. Or we could have sex that lasts for six hours. Either way, it can be a great night. We want to wait for chemistry; we don't want anyone to force it. People who keep doing that will eventually be pushed away. It isn't fun anymore. So maybe people get into the lifestyle for the sex. That's what its about, right? We think, I'm married, and this gives me an opportunity to still have sexual variety. But the reasons we stay? The friendship. Meeting people from all different walks of life. The acceptance. The openness and honesty.

For me, this is also about a philosophy of life. Whatever you do, whatever you say, that should be where your heart is. Live the life you believe in. Don't make excuses when your behaviors don't match up to your beliefs.

We have two kids together; our oldest just turned thirteen, and our youngest is nine. We've tried to raise our kids with an overwhelming sense of honesty. That doesn't mean being blunt about our sex lives. We've had some friends we're so close to that they're an extension of the family. But when someone questions me on what I tell my kids, I ask, "Well, what do *you* tell your kids?" Some things, your kids don't want to know. At sixteen, they don't want to think about their parents having sex! But by the time they're twenty-five, or when they're dealing with relationship issues of their own, maybe they'll want to talk. Maybe they'll even say, "You were on a TV show? Are you crazy?" And then we'll explain why we did it, and why we made the choices we've made. We would never claim that our way of life is for everybody. But we will answer questions honestly. What if, when I try to teach my daughters to be smart with sexual choices, they say, "Well, you're a swinger, Dad. You can't teach me about morality." I'd point out that I might be a swinger, but I am still living an ethical life. When I have sex, I'm protecting myself, I'm making good choices, and I'm living authentically. When it comes to raising kids, you know, there are some absolutely horrible parents. They don't have sex with anyone but their spouse—I'll give them that. But they're abusive. They're neglectful. The truth is that how you have sex doesn't say anything about how you raise your kids. Parenting is parenting.

When people think about gay people or swingers, they think about the sex first. They don't think about what that person does for a living, or what kind of car they drive, or anything but what kind of sex they have. But what if you

approached every person that way, imagining the sex? What if your first thought on meeting someone was, "I wonder how this person has sex?" It would seem ridiculous. It *is* ridiculous. Yes, we are swingers. We have sex with other people sometimes, though not with everyone we meet.
But there's a lot more to us than that.

GROUP SEX AS PLAY

Some play golf or tennis, I swing, it's my hobby, outlet, job. It may not be for everyone but most can't say WHY. It isn't natural? It just isn't done? Well, it is a step out of the ordinary and that is another appeal for me. I'm no Thoreau but I don't fancy living a life of quiet desperation. This works for me, can't speak for others.[20]

You meet people who have had different sexual experiences who give you different tastes of different things. And you know, this friend of mine calls [it] porn education and it can be when you see other people experiencing different things. . . . And you know, do I want to try this, do I want to try that. And I am adventurous. I do like to try different things. . . . I do like different sexual adventures. And there'd be a lot more I'd like to go on.[21]

All orgies are *not* created equal.

In her research on straight-identified men who solicit sexualized encounters with other men on Craigslist, sociologist Jane Ward acknowledges the temptation to see them as "closeted" gay men. After all, if not for frequent references to beer, straight pornography, and aggressive sex with women, wouldn't these just be guys who like to have sex with guys? Well, maybe not. Beyond the same-sex activity, Ward argues, there are actually few similarities to "queer" culture in these men's hypermasculine and misogynist worlds. They describe themselves as "buzzed, horny, checking out porn," or suggest getting together to "fuck the hell out of my hot blow-up doll" or have "a bi/str8 dude circle jerk"—"a group of masculine dudes just sitting around stroking, watching a game, drinking some brews, jerking, showing off, swapping college stories, maybe playing a drinking game and see what comes up."[22] These guys aren't likely to be marching in a pride festival or responding to surveys aimed at "gay" men.

In other words: the beer, porn, and misogyny *matter*.

People who do the same thing can do it in vastly different ways.

Multiple sources of satisfaction must be considered when thinking about why participants are drawn to particular scenes or practices—and especially why they choose to stay and play, if they do. Group sex is organized spatially and socially to minimize risk, conflict, and stress, as explored in chapter 3. Although the specifics vary across communities, rules and expectations allow participants to experiment in situations where safety and danger are balanced. But there is more to consider, such as sexual styles, consumption preferences, aesthetics, ethics, beliefs about gender and sexuality, and understandings about why one participates in alternative sexual communities.

The lifestyle, for example, does not appeal to everyone. Some researchers argue that couples usually begin swinging in their late thirties after establishing careers and starting families; when these pressures are eased, people can focus on sexual fulfillment, and swinging presents a "nonthreatening" option for exploration.[23] Many twenty-something couples that I spoke with at lifestyle events, however, had a different perspective. They had already experimented sexually and were now contemplating their future relationships. Many desired to marry, for example, but imagined that they would experience difficulties being faithful over their life span; they wondered whether consensual nonmonogamy might provide an answer. But the reasons couples choose the lifestyle out of all the possible sexual outlets —and stick with it, if they do—are not reducible to sexual practices. In study after study, regardless of age, lifestylers highlight the importance of the friendships they develop as much as the sexual aspects of their experiences. Some of this may be an attempt to legitimize practices that are stigmatized and misunderstood—who can argue with friendship? But swinging is more appealing to some people than others. One group sex aficionado I spoke with disliked the lifestyle, for example, because of the extended socializing it involved; he preferred to use Craigslist, where one had fewer obligations to sex partners. Most lifestylers enjoy socializing as couples. Women claim to appreciate the atmosphere of female camaraderie rather than competitiveness, as well as the lack of male aggression. Women who are attracted to "femme" women may find the lifestyle appealing, as "girl-girl" play is commonplace (in fact, so prevalent that "straight" women can feel the need to explain themselves). In theory, lifestylers believe in female sexual equality and tolerance of sexual differences. Lifestylers also generally prize emotional monogamy and take steps to ensure that negative emotions like fear or jealousy are experienced in low doses, such as requiring same-room play, unanimous consent, or public demonstrations of commitment. As one woman said of swinging, "It's exciting but not emotionally dangerous."[24] (Individuals who are unable to "separate sex and love" may find themselves uncomfortable or unwelcome in some lifestyle communities.) Some participants enjoy being able to rebel in a safe environment. A woman quoted in Bergstrand and Sinski said, "If I feel like having sex with four men in a row I know I can because my boyfriend is sitting beside me and won't let anything happen."[25]

There are differences among lifestylers, of course. During the 1970s, the couples that escaped to Sandstone Retreat, hoping to change society through their beliefs and sexual practices, were different from the celebrity sex partiers at the Playboy Mansion. Researchers at the time distinguished between urban versus rural groups or "utopian" versus "recreational" attitudes.[26] Contemporary lifestylers differ in their sexual proclivities (such as "hard" versus "soft" swap or focus on girl-girl play), substance use (alcohol only or club drugs such as Ecstasy), musical taste (rock 'n' roll versus house/techno), social class or spending practices (partying at a Holiday Inn versus in a Vegas megahotel suite), play space preferences (on-premises sex clubs versus off-premises events, where participants host their own after-parties), or attitudes toward inclusiveness (open versus invitation-only events). Although the topic of differences between polyamorists and swingers can inflame an Internet forum for weeks—and in the end, a practice-based distinction can always be deconstructed—there *are* unique sexual styles, consumption practices, and aesthetics associated with the lifestyle.

If there weren't, the jokes wouldn't be so funny: "You might be a swinger if . . . you forget that some people still have pubic hair"; "you know which of your bikinis looks best in black light"; "you have over 100,000 frequent flyer miles on Air Jamaica"; "your friends know what kind of condom you prefer"; "you spent twice as long on your online profile as you did on your resume"; "all the men bring their wives to your bachelor party"; and so on.[27]

The same might be said of other alternative sexual enclaves—while sex is part of the appeal, it is rarely the only aspect considered. Group sex events can be segregated by sexual orientation or relationship status—gay, pansexual, bisexual, heterosexual, couples, singles. There are play parties catering to polyamorists or tantra practitioners. Sex parties can be based on the activities allowed, such as "sixty-nine" or "all anal." Some events, such as "Jack and Jill off," "safe sex," or "unsafe sex" parties, promote or reject discourses of sexual safety. Parties may be organized by theme, such as "dark party" or "slave auction." The Center for Sex Positive Culture in Seattle offers different options throughout the week: "Monday Madness" for weekday enthusiasts, "Asylum" for BDSM medical play, "Crowbar" for "the transmasculine community," and "(cat)FIGHT," featuring female wrestling. Some events are organized by what you wear, or don't: "Buff London," for example, is a weekly naked play party for gay men held at a nightclub; the same club also hosts "Hardplay" for men who are "into skinhead, army, leather, rubber or industrial." Xplore Sydney is a festival featuring "deep play" and ritual; the dress code is "Fetish—Hyper Sexy—Deviant." Myth Party, in New York City, sponsors "kinky," queer-friendly parties that are "a throwback to the anything-goes 70s"; the last event, according to the MythParty website, "boasted a human piñata (it's what you think it is), a pee-play section, unicorn activities, and a Dexter scene in which participants were drenched in fake blood." In New York City, one might also attend the "Nubian Party," for African American or Latino men only, the "Milk Chocolate

Party," for mixed-race guests, or the "Sticky Rice" party, for "young, hot, lean, in-shape Asian guys between 18–35."

Race, class, and age shape constellations of sexual practice, leisure, and consumption, as well as the social and political reception of alternative sexual practices. Exclusivity and upscaling are part of the appeal for some sex partiers who want to socialize within their own age group, social class, or ideal of attractiveness. A 2011 article on sex parties in New York City proclaimed: "The mega swinger clubs are dead. These artsy sex parties are where the young people are." Many of these participants balk at the term "swinger," not just because of the stereotypes discussed in chapter 3, but also due to an often erroneous belief that swingers do not exercise choice in their sexual partners. Given that the younger crowd is not necessarily married or even coupled up in committed relationships, heterosexual sex partying is a broader phenomenon than just "the lifestyle." Chemistry, in New York City, is a members-only event described as "a leader of the new crop of young, hip sex parties in the city." Attendees are still down for group sex, according to a journalist who attended:

> Upstairs the floor is covered with futons, and a thin, exotically dressed woman advertises tantric massages in the corner. The first person to get naked is a tall, strikingly handsome man in his early thirties who buys a rubdown. Watching him, two people undress and fall onto the futons, getting into rough and fast missionary sex. Waves of couples and threesomes follow, with some of the 15-odd people upstairs watching and gauging how they could get involved.[28]

Circuit parties are held around the globe, usually in metropolitan areas and sometimes coinciding with gay pride events. Attendees are primarily young and fit men with enough disposable income to travel. As with some of the more commercialized lifestyle events, there is a focus on a "party culture" involving travel, electronic music, costumes and themes, appearance, and an ideal of acceptance toward sexual diversity and recreational sex. (Although I've never seen a gay male couple at a lifestyle event, I have known lifestylers who traveled to circuit parties.)

There are play parties for senior citizens and play parties with age limits (such as "under thirty"). Carol Queen, a sexologist, writer, and activist who founded the Center of Sex and Culture in San Francisco, suggests that discomfort with older people having sex, especially at public play parties, is related to fears of aging and mortality. As BDSM is a highly skilled practice, older practitioners may find themselves most welcome at these events.

In BDSM play, inequalities are often explicitly eroticized. Anthropologist Richard Martin writes of visiting a German BDSM play space where rooms were themed for different types of fetishes: a clinic for medical play, a classroom, a torture chamber, a stable for pony play, a jail, and a confessional. Each of these spaces, he argues, draws "on everyday configurations of power and authority that underpin relations in a society that is officially egalitarian and experientially asymmetric."[29] But inequalities can be eroticized in less explicit ways as well. "Mandingo parties," or gang bangs featuring black men and white women, are influenced by a history of racial and gender inequalities, regardless of whether power is discussed by participants. In the United States, long-standing myths about black men's greater sexual prowess, larger penises, masculinity, and athleticism, along with a history of racial violence, fuel the erotics of a mandingo party. The hypersexuality of black men is not limited to the United States, of course; for example, one finds blackness/whiteness eroticized in Germany as well, although playing out in terms of local histories and politics.

SEX, DRUGS, AND RODENTS

"Deadheads," orgies, and acid. Quaaludes and 1970s swingers. "Poppers," fisting, and gay men. Youthful ravers, "puppy piles," and Ecstasy. (*Wati* and *otiv-bombari*?) Why do particular substances become associated with specific groups and forms of sexuality?

People oriented toward sex as "play" manipulate aspects of their environment to elaborate on and intensify their overall experience, taking a future orientation toward the kinds of sex and socializing they prefer. Occasionally, this includes altering consciousness through substances. Substances supposedly possessing aphrodisiac properties have long been the source of myth, from raw oysters to Spanish fly. Although the existence of true aphrodisiacs is debated, some substances do impact human sexuality more than others, either through prosexual effects, such as increasing arousal or intensifying stimulation, or inhibiting response. Substances can be natural or manufactured and work in a variety of ways on the human brain or body; the impact of any substance on human behavior and experience, however, is also shaped by individual and contextual factors.

"Party and play" (PNP) originally referred to sex while using crystal methamphetamine, although the phrase is now used more broadly to indicate sex under the influence of illegal substances. In the contemporary sex party scene, whether gay or straight, some participants use "club drugs"—MDMA/Ecstasy (E), ketamine (K), crystal meth, or GHB (G). These illicit substances may be combined with each other and with legal substances such as Viagra, Adderall, or alcohol. Group sex participants occasionally use other substances as well, depending on the context, such as hallucinogens or opiates. "Crack" cocaine is associated with hypersexual behavior and the disinhibition of users, but I do not consider it here because it is rare in "party and play" (or perhaps so stigmatized that I did not encounter references to it).

Recreational drug use triggers moralizing responses. But although drug use of any sort is accompanied by risks, whether a substance is legal or illegal depends on many factors, only some of which are related to its dangers. Legality varies by country, time period, and political, legal, and economic factors. Alcohol is currently legal in the United States, although it was illegal during Prohibition and remains illegal in some countries. GHB and Ecstasy were once legal in the United States and the United Kingdom but have become controlled substances. Legal drugs are used for "partying," often in combination with other substances. Viagra, Cialis, and Levitra have all seen incredible success in legal markets; all also have vigorous black markets. Teenagers have added Ambien to their list of party favors—sometimes it's easier to steal pills out of the home medicine cabinet than to find someone selling LSD when you're in the mood for hallucinations or out-of-body experiences.

Some substances and their users are stigmatized while others are normalized. Crystal meth is viewed as one of the worst street drugs in the United States, for example, while Adderall is regularly consumed on college campuses for both productivity and recreation. While there are differences—methamphetamine is more powerful than amphetamines like Adderall because it travels more quickly across the blood-brain barrier—both are nonetheless powerful stimulants. Patients taking prescription Adderall, or even legal methamphetamine in the form of Desoxyn, can be certain that other dangerous chemicals have not been added during the preparation process; prescribed dosage levels are designed to prevent dependency. Still, Adderall can be crushed and snorted, producing euphoria; misuse can lead to addiction, psychosis, and death. Crystal meth can be used at low dosage levels to enhance work or school performance.[30] Addiction, researchers point out, "is not an inevitable consequence of the mere self-administration of a potentially addictive drug," even a drug with a nasty reputation like crystal meth; even though "a large number of people experiment with potentially addictive drugs at some time, few develop an addiction."[31] Using too much of *any* substance can cause physical, emotional, and social problems; what constitutes "too much" varies across individuals, contexts, and substances.

Rather than labeling drugs "good" or "bad," then, let's focus on the fact that some humans throughout history have indulged in substances and practices (collective trance, rituals, carnivalesque inversion) to purposely alter everyday consciousness. Yes, people occasionally do things under the influence of drugs they wouldn't normally do—that's disinhibition. Just ask the flight attendant on your next overnight jaunt about the crazy things passengers do on Ambien—like eat *all* of the first-class dinners, urinate in the aisle, or have sex with the stranger in 4F. (Many airlines now suggest testing your sleep medications before flying.) As the literature on drunkenness shows, people also do things that they *think* they will do on that substance. But if substances were used only for their disinhibiting properties, any substance would do, and this is clearly not the case. In addition to tuning out that little voice saying "no," both legal and illegal drugs help people do things they *want* to do. People snort cocaine to stay up late, smoke pot to feel relaxed, or take MDMA to dance or have more intimate sex. Or they take Adderall to pass biology, Vicodin to get through holidays, and Viagra for "date night."

What we know, or think we know, about sex and drugs is shaped by dominant modes of thinking about sexuality. Unfortunately, the discourse of risk has permeated sex research such that it is difficult to fund studies of drug use that are not linked to HIV prevention, violence, or addiction. Urban gay men using crystal meth and barebacking at circuit parties have been studied for years as a "high-risk" group for HIV infection. We know far less, however, about gay men using crystal meth or amyl nitrates who do *not* have unprotected sex or about straight couples experimenting with GHB or ketamine at sex parties. Some groups are also easier to pinpoint for research. You're more likely to find studies on impoverished users of crack than on cocaine users who run Fortune 500 companies. And, as universities are disinclined to allow experiments where participants get high and have sex, researchers are limited to observing in naturalistic settings, surveying partygoers or others using public spaces where sex and drugs are linked, or interviewing people willing to talk openly about their drug use and sex lives.

Which brings us to sex, drugs, and—rodents again.

Rats are popular in laboratory research in this area because the physiology of erections and ejaculations in male rats is similar enough to that in humans to enable researchers to make predictions about the effects of certain drugs. Male rats have been given stimulants, such as cocaine and methamphetamine, and "downers," such as alcohol, MDMA, or other depressants, in experimental situations. Patterns of rat behavior under the influence of some substances parallel the patterns of human behavior. Some rats are more prone to substance abuse, just as some people are. When allowed to self-administer amphetamines, for example, rats who did so were high sensation or novelty seekers. (As rats couldn't be asked whether they enjoyed "wild and uninhibited parties," they were instead observed exploring a "novel environment." Rats doing so most thoroughly or with the highest levels of locomotor reactivity were considered "high responders" or sensation seekers.)[32] Rats given alcohol attempt to mount unreceptive females, even when "trained" not to,[33] and rats initially exhibit heightened sexual arousal on cocaine but develop a tolerance for it.[34] Similarly, infrequent human users of cocaine report spontaneous erections, increased sexual arousal, and intensified orgasms, while heavy users find their sexual functioning impaired.[35] Rats prefer sex while on crystal meth to sex without it, based on their tendency to revisit places where they received the drug. They also exhibit compulsive sexual behavior after taking meth, despite "learned negative consequences," which in this study was a form of "conditioned sex aversion" involving lithium chloride injections to cause "visceral illness,"[36] a procedure somewhat more cruel than asking teenagers to share masticated cheese snacks to discourage sex. Either way, rats that paired sex and meth, even only once, were less likely to be swayed from their goal—more sex—by stomach cramps. Human users report that crystal meth actually enhances sexual pleasure as well as influencing sexual compulsivity and inhibition, a finding that appears supported in rats. Like sexual novelty, methamphetamine triggers the release of dopamine in the brain, a "reward" that can be highly motivating.

MDMA inhibits copulation in male rats; it is sometimes called "the cuddle drug" because it produces similar effects in humans. In one study, however, rats given MDMA were then exposed to loud "techno" music, which stimulates the noradrenergic system and hypothalamic-pituitary-adrenal (HPA) axis more than slower music does. Researchers suggested that music activates regions of the brain implicated in reward and emotion, potentially producing intense pleasure responses; these chemical reactions could offset the dampening of desire associated with MDMA.[37] Ravers preferring the beats of Swedish House Mafia to the lyrical music of Taylor Swift will not be surprised that rats listening to "techno" while on MDMA were more likely to ejaculate than rats who had been given the drug without the dance music, nor will anyone who has attended a dance event and then been swept along to an "after-party" (or "after-after-party"). In fact, as MDMA is often combined with stimulants to intensify its effects, and stimulants tend to last longer than the "roll" of MDMA, one finds the likelihood of sexual activity to rise as dawn approaches (or noon, depending on the dose)—as long as the music plays on.

Since the 1990s, crystal methamphetamine has become increasingly popular in North American urban gay subcultures revolving around "sex based sociality," or "casual and group sexual interactions in bathhouses, public parks and sex parties." Crystal meth, researchers argue, enhances both sexual performance and sociality in situations requiring "high libido, sexual adventurism, self-confidence, focus, endurance, reduced discrimination in partner choice, and pain reduction."[38] Interviews with gay men in Manhattan exemplified this "elective affinity" between crystal meth and the social context: "I would meet a succession of people . . . and have sex with them, over and over again . . . without ejaculation"; "you can go on for days"; "I become very lustful"; "I feel indestructible." Several men described feeling "like a different person." An interviewee explained: "I can have sex with a group more easily—even if I am not attracted to some of the people in the group . . . so like if there is only two people in the room that I am really turned on to but there is two other people there, and you know, and they want me to take on all four of them, then I can and I am willing to."[39] Whether they sought such encounters weekly, monthly, or more rarely, respondents *targeted* crystal meth intake "in anticipation of intensive sexual interactions."[40] These men were not junkies or addicts; they planned, controlled, and perfected their usage. Some users experienced negative effects, such as sexual compulsivity, increased proclivity to participate in risky behaviors, and other psychological and behavioral changes that lasted even when the drug itself wore off. Nonetheless, because crystal meth helped them "participate more fully, and with more pleasure" in their sociosexual milieu, it gained a "therapeutic status similar to that of Viagra and other state sanctioned medicinal products."[41] Without a thorough understanding of the pleasurable or positive effects of a drug, researchers argue, interventions are unlikely to succeed.

Another study of 198 gay or bisexual male sex partners from New York City found that they purposely chose and mixed club drugs to enhance their sexual experiences. If they wanted to feel social, witty, and outgoing, for example, they took coke, G, meth, or E. Men who bottomed found ketamine to be numbing and relaxing, but less social. All of the club drugs, interviewees claimed, lowered their sexual standards, although for different reasons. Ecstasy increased sensual feelings and receptivity to touch, even from partners the men wouldn't find attractive otherwise; some men even reported feeling temporarily "in love" with their sexual partners. But if the men wanted "animalistic" sex, without any emotional ties? Meth, GHB, and cocaine made them "aggressively" and "voraciously" sexual: "I felt like I was devouring him, he was devouring me, almost violent"; "I just become an animal . . . go crazy"; "sexually, [cocaine] lets me step out of myself and do things I wouldn't do if I was level-headed . . . some of the kinky stuff."[42] Dosage mattered: just enough cocaine, for example, produced elation while too much caused anxiety and paranoia. Interestingly, the *sexual* peaks of cocaine, Ecstasy, and crystal meth occurred as users were "coming down"; for ketamine and GHB, the sexual peaks coincided with the drug's peak. The men were aware of these complexities, strategically timing their sexual encounters and combining drugs (such as meth and Viagra) for optimum performance.

The "Three or More Study" (TOMS) included over 1,200 Australian men who had group sex with other men in Sydney, Brisbane, and Melbourne in 2007 and 2008. Participants were generally well-educated, urban professionals, often identifying as gay, who used both personal networks and the Internet to find group sex partners. The men sought group sex out of desires for intensity and connection as well as to live out sexual fantasies.[43] Like the New Yorkers, they planned ahead for events and targeted their drug use; the anticipation itself generated pleasure. Amyl nitrates were reportedly used most frequently at the men's most recent group sexual experience, followed by Ecstasy, crystal meth, marijuana, and GHB (many of these were combined with performance-enhancing drugs such as Viagra). Again, like the New York sample, the TOMS partiers found drug use made them more interested in multiple, casual partners; drugs could "heighten the senses," allow them to "play longer," "stay hard," or "be fucked," or make them feel powerful and "less inhibited." One interviewee claimed that drugs made group sex "more animalistic": "It makes it dirtier; it makes it more thrilling, you know?"

Despite the widespread assumption that drugs primarily cause disinhibition, then, directly leading users to engage in risky sex, the picture is more complicated in both rats and humans. Whether a given rat experiences prosexual effects depends on physiological characteristics (such as its baseline sexual response and hormonal status), whether the drug is given "acutely" or "chronically," whether the rat has "learned" to be inhibited in particular situations,[44] and even what kind of music is piped into his cage. When thinking about sex and recreational drug use in humans, we need to consider the psychological and biological characteristics of users and the properties, dosage, and effects of the drug, along with a host of additional factors. The environment is important: is the setting safe and comfortable to administer the drug, ride out its effects, and engage in the types of sexual encounters sought? Amyl nitrates, for example, produce a euphoric rush lasting around two minutes and relax the sphincter muscles, useful for a quickie in a public park, especially if one fears being interrupted. Ketamine, however, is less ideal in a dangerous environment as it produces a dreamy, uncoordinated state; it is also easy to "k-hole" with an incorrect dose, briefly losing motor functioning. We must consider the available auditory or visual stimulation: What type of music is played? What kind of lighting is used? Don't expect to drop two tabs of Ecstasy in silence and under fluorescent lights and have a religious experience. The physical and relational needs of participants play a role: Do participants want "animalistic" or "sensual" sex? Do they intend to delay ejaculation or relax quickly into certain types of play? Do individuals need to overcome feelings of shame or fears of rejection? Do they want to bond with sex partners or remain emotionally detached? What types of social interactions are expected—extended flirtations or brief or nonverbal encounters, as one might expect in a bathhouse? Men and women may combine party drugs differently to maximize their experiences. Because most recreational group sex events rely on a cooperative, consensual atmosphere, overindulgence that results in miscommunication is discouraged. Finally, historical, political, economic, and cultural factors influence which substances are used, by whom, and toward what ends: cost, availability, the layers of meaning given to a particular drug at a point in time, people's expectations of its effects, and so on.

Whether any of these combinations of sex, drugs, and other practices generates identities or communities depends on even more factors. There is no essential connection between group sex and drug use. Drug use appears less in the literature on dogging, for example, perhaps because of the reliance on motor vehicles. Many BDSM events are substance-free, given an emphasis on safety and consent. Most people in every enclave probably do not use drugs, or they stick to alcohol. Not even everyone who enjoys circuit parties or raves uses drugs to enhance the experiences. These examples of sex partying, however, show how combinations of social, psychological, and physiological stimuli can coalesce. As sensation seekers in general prefer the company of others like themselves, and as both sexual activity and drug use provide intense stimulation, it makes sense that distinct enclaves develop. The types of substances preferred in such enclaves, rather than being random, are those that enhance participants' experiences. LSD, psilocybin, or benzodiazepines rarely appear in the literature on gay male sexual subcultures, for example; while these substances may enhance sexual activity for certain individuals, there is less affinity between their effects and the desired goals of *most* participants. People don't take drugs with the aim of shivering in a gutter or compulsively seeking anonymous sex in subways—although such negative consequences arise for some users. And while drugs can be taken to escape unpleasant memories, circumstances, or feelings, drugs can also be used to enhance emotional states or attain peak experiences, sexual and otherwise.

As one male circuit partier described his first experience: "It was like bliss."[45]

SMELLS LIKE TEEN CORRUPTION

Ecstasy tabs. Cheating. MDMA mixed into brownies. Girls kissing girls. Messed-up parents. Drug dealing. Revenge sex. Wrist slashing. Car crashes after driving while intoxicated. Fistfights. And, of course, parties.

There's a lot of drama, but it's the parties that make the British television series *Skins* so compelling—and infamous.

The boys in the series are skinny, often shirtless, and somewhat androgynous. The girls are also skinny. They all love getting high. Instead of having pillow fights at all-girl sleepovers, they do drugs and go to raves. They go to house parties, invited or not, leaving destruction in their wake. They fool around, forming drugged-up twosomes, threesomes, foursomes, and moresomes. When boys and girls collapse together, limbs entangled and exhausted at the end of another party, they perfectly illustrate the phrase "puppy pile."

The teenagers in the controversial series use partying to make connections, escape their troubles, fight boredom, and rebel against their parents and society. Nothing new there. Teens have been experimenting with sex and drugs for as long as "teenagers" have existed—that is, in societies where kids are no longer initiated into adulthood at puberty and given adult roles and responsibilities. This period of delayed production (in the workforce) and reproduction is often a time of experimentation with both sexuality and consumption. Teens might even form the largest group of sensation seekers. Although the nihilism associated with teen cultures may take different forms across countries or times periods, teenage angst and adventure has also long been a form of entertainment, from *90210* in the United States or *Amigas y Rivales* in Mexico to *Casi Angeles* in Argentina or *Heartbreak High* in Australia.

Skins supposedly inspired French teens to begin throwing parties themed after the series, called *Le Skins*. Some *Le Skins* parties are underground, with locations revealed only at the last minute like the early "rave" parties; others occur in private homes. In early 2010, Claudine Doury, a French photographer whose artistic work focuses on adolescence, was allowed a glimpse inside a *Le Skins* party held in a Parisian suburb. "This young guy's parents had gone away," Doury explained, "and he invited three or four hundred people on Facebook to a party in his house." The house had been carefully prepared to avoid damage, and a changing area was set up for guests. Attendees ranged in age from sixteen to twenty. A security guard had even been hired to manage the party, which cost twenty euros to enter (discounted to ten euros if partiers brought their own alcohol). The guard had the additional responsibility of directing amorous teens to the garden when they became sexual.

The teens call themselves "skinners" and trade the childlike aesthetic of the raver scene with its plush animal backpacks, furry leg warmers, and blinking pacifiers, for a more ragged "electro-trash" look, sort of like "Sid and Nancy do E instead of heroin." Doury's photographs focus on the bodies of the partygoers rather than their faces—girls in filmy dresses or nothing but bras and booty shorts, bare-chested young men in low-slung jeans. Some partiers have "Skins" or "Le Skins" painted on their bodies in graffiti-style lettering while others sport ripped hose, fishnet shirts, and boots or don masks in an assortment of styles, from Venetian to Mexican *lucha libre*. One young woman wears a gas mask; several young men appear in clown masks, paying homage to the show. Many of the teens in the photographs are in the early stages of embrace. "It was very practical," Doury said of the attire. "They know what to wear so they are not completely naked but so they can touch each other."

Themes of sexual exploration and social liberation emerge as justifications for the parties, recycled across time, nation, and neighborhoods. "It's completely free," Doury explains; the guideline was "no limits, no limits."[46] One of the young men she spoke with, Flavien, twenty, said: "We let ourselves go here, because there are too many restrictions for the youth." Sarah, also twenty, pondered: "It already existed in '68 with the hippies, maybe during repressive periods we turn to free sex."[47] The teens talk about sexual abandon, and some clearly indulge in intoxicants in the photos, although Doury makes it all sound rather orderly: "Delighted young men ask a girl if they can kiss her, and she usually says yes. If things progress, they head to the garden, where bodies sprawl across the grass." Some teens downplay *Le Skins* parties, claiming a few parties get wild but the rest are relatively tame, nothing out of the ordinary.

The parties are not limited to France, having spread to the United States and even back to the United Kingdom.[48] Commercial *Le Skins* parties are now held in nightclubs, rented event spaces, and even on a boat on the Seine; events may feature known DJs or bands and extravagant light shows. IDs are checked, sponsors and promoters scoop up entry fees, and there is less on-premises sex.

Supposedly, the party thrown by seventeen-year-old Rachael Bell from Durham, England, while her parents and siblings were on vacation, had a *Skins* theme—"trash the house." Rachael claims to have invited only sixty of her closest friends and that a hacker on her Myspace page was responsible for enticing uninvited teens to drive from as far away as London for the party. The number of skinners who turned out ended up being somewhere between two hundred and three hundred. Although Rachael and her friends tried to prevent party crashers from entering, "they just started climbing through the window." In hindsight, Rachael probably wishes she had picked a more benign theme—"toga," perhaps—because guests took this one literally. Elaine Bell, Rachael's distraught mother, described her house as "raped": "partygoers had stubbed cigarettes out on carpets, ransacked rooms, urinated on her wedding dress, scrawled on walls and broken light fittings by swinging on them."[49] In addition to this "orgy of destruction," a partygoer described "yobs having sex in every room in front of all to see."[50] Rachael was questioned after the party and reprimanded by police; she eventually reconciled with her horrified parents after fleeing to a friend's house for a few nights. The Bell family sought temporary housing while waiting for repairs to the estimated £20,000 of damage to the home. While the party got a lot of attention, the media focus was more on the wreckage than on youthful eroticism or revolution.

But there is another layer to the story that was circulated. Rachael was a middle-class girl living in a "respectable" neighborhood. She was supposed to be home studying for her "A-levels," the standardized tests taken to qualify for university entry. The party crashers, on the other hand, were described as "hoodlums" or "yobs," a British slang term for thuggish, sometimes violent, working-class boys (and occasionally girls). The degradation of Rachael's family home and the emotional scars it caused—"it was devastating, just devasting," her mother told the press—was newsworthy not only because teens experimented with sex and "drug-fueled mayhem," but because the social order was breached when they did so. Further, the breach occurred through the misuse of social networking sites, a concern about technological change corrupting youth that arises repetitively in stories of this sort around the world.

In 2007, the Pokémones of Chile became the focus of a media blitz. The Pokémones were described as an "urban tribe," although unlike hippies, punks, or Goths, they were considered one of the first such tribes of the Internet age. Supposedly inspired by the children's game Pokémon with its cute, colorful cartoon creatures, participants adopted an androgynous style. Both boys and girls sported anime T-shirts, piercings, dyed and spiked hair with bangs, and black eyeliner. "It's basically a fashion thing," a young man told reporters. "A Pokémone has a certain style and does *ponceo*." *Ponceo*, according to the pivotal report that appeared in *Newsweek*, was the term for the partying and sexual experimentation they engaged in, usually in public parks around Chile and primarily focused on oral sex with multiple consecutive partners or in groups. Heterosexual, same-sex—participants claim it is equal opportunity. "*Ponceo* is about having fun," a girl says.[51] Some of the parties are for those eighteen and under; the young age of participants is perhaps why their alcohol-free dance parties take place in the afternoons rather than late at night.[52]

Part of Pokémone style involves embracing technology, as the teens use social media websites and blogs to flirt, share information about events, and display evidence of their adventures. Though Pokémones use Facebook and MSN Messenger, like millions of other teenagers around the world, they really like Fotolog, a photo-sharing website. Chile had 4.8 million Fotolog accounts in 2008, more than 60 percent of which were held by twelve- to seventeen-year-olds. Teens who use Fotolog strategically, posting risqué party pictures that capture the attention of their peers and elicit the most comments, can become "the most popular users." This distinction then sometimes offers them an opportunity to attend *ponceo* parties as VIPs.[53]

Like the French teens attending *Le Skins* parties, Pokémones show off their bodies and trigger accusations of promiscuity and nihilism from journalists writing about them. Also like the *Le Skins* teens, they occasionally wax philosophical, though not necessarily political: "This is about being alive," a fourteen-year-old girl explained to a reporter. "It is about dancing, laughing, changing the words of the songs to something dirty." Well, she admitted, it's also "about making out with other boys." The youth do not support a common cause. "We're not for anything, but we're not against anything either—well, except our parents being mad at us for being Pokémones," a sixteen-year-old girl said. Not standing for anything might mean less disillusionment down the road, but it doesn't engender longevity; the Pokémones tribe was already pronounced dying by 2009.

Despite the apathy and disappearance of Pokémones, some commentators still insist that the movement had political connotations in a country where over half of the population is Catholic. The premarital erotic explorations of Pokémones—whether oral sex or just group gropes and kissing—are clearly in opposition to the conservative religious mores and traditional norms of their country and parents. Pokémones also represented emerging consumerist tendencies—sex partners are tallied ("This time I had seven partners") just like products purchased ("This week I bought two T-shirts and a webcam . . . and a new tongue ring").[54] The androgynous Pokémones generally came from the lower and middle classes and were seen as opposing *pelolais*, another youth group made up of girls who "dress fashionably," have long, often blonde hair with no bangs (quite important to both the kids and the journalists scrutinizing Facebook and Fotolog images), are from wealthy families, and attend private schools.[55] But in comparison with masculinized *flaites*—low-status, sometimes delinquent or criminal youth who adopt styles of music and fashion associated with hip-hop or rap—Pokémones claimed more respectability and spending power.

Media representations, of course, are motivated. This version of the Pokémones—sexually liberated, defiant, consumerist, technologically astute, and middle class—is certainly the one that spread across the Internet. As with many sensationalist pieces on group sex, one "news" story resurfaces on multiple websites and blogs, reworked with more blatant, attention-grabbing language each time: "rebellious teens," for example, become "Chile's Bisexual, Orgy-Having Pokémones." Some critics suggest that the *Newsweek* journalist who initially broke the story in the United States misunderstood the term *ponceo*—it translates as "kissing," they insist, not "oral sex." In a 2008 *New York Times* article on Pokémones, *poncea* is defined as "making out" and *ponceo* is "the one who pairs off the most." Other writers claim that *ponceo* is primarily "simulated sex" occurring at dance parties; this is certainly the case at the more organized events held in nightclubs rather than parks, where security guards monitor participants' behavior.

Some accounts of teen sex parties are urban legends. Sneaky Pete's interracial sex bashes of the 1950s may fall into that category. But surely, some kids "do *ponceo*"—and if they didn't before the news flash, they probably are now. Or maybe they're having "rainbow parties," playing "Two Minutes in the Closet," "Seven Minutes in Heaven," "Dark Shark," or other teen games organized around group erotic explorations. Maybe they are wearing "shag bands," color-coded jelly bracelets that supposedly signal a willingness to engage in certain sexual activities.

"Everything starts with the kiss," a fourteen-year-old Pokémone girl said.[56]

Are teens more sexually active nowadays than in the past? It is impossible, or at least irresponsible, to generalize—if only because of the complexity of the question. Only a few generations ago in the United States, and still today in some places around the world, "teens" were actually married, child-

rearing adults. And while we can't disregard the fact that social and technological changes do indeed contribute to an increasingly mediated, sexualized
culture, we should also realize that many times, media attention to a phenomenon can tell us more about our collective anxieties—as a society, as parents—than about objective dangers. Parents worry a lot about pedophilic
strangers lurking on the Internet, for instance, even though kids are much
more likely to be sexually abused by someone they know.

Even when media accounts are factually accurate, there are still reasons to
look at how stories are told, by whom, and to what ends. As with tales of
crazed Bacchus worshippers, Mau Mau rebels, or snacking Texas swingers, a
focus on transgressive sexuality elides the inequalities, fears, and politics
lying under the surface. Sexual leisure practices do indeed develop in combination with other styles of consumption and in relation to social categories
such as race, class, and gender, for reasons that are both practical (the use of
public parks, cars, or other people's homes when youth do not have private
space to retreat to) and political (such as the Pokémones' inclination for
sexual experimentation rather than outright delinquent behavior when rebelling against traditional authority). Tendencies to sensationalize the sexual
practices of certain groups of teens, especially those who can be identified
because they adopt a certain look, often stem from conflicting intergenerational anxieties. Parents, apprehensive about technological or social change,
wonder about the potentially new and insidious dangers their children face,
whether in the form of racial diversity, "rock 'n' roll," imported television
shows, or social networking (Facebook, Fotolog, Myspace). Is it easier for
today's youth to be lured away from their path, corrupted by the permeability
of social boundaries and the visibility and accessibility of other social
worlds? Stories about *Le Skins* parties and Pokémones are told and retold
because they cater to the audience's fears. Such stories can also be a way that
parents and other adults reassure themselves—"Whew, it's not my kid, she
doesn't wear bangs . . ."—or reaffirm social distinctions that are being questioned or challenged by social developments. Youth, worried about how to
forge meaningful, independent lives, find sexual exploration to be cheap,
accessible, and readily interpreted as rebellion—whether they become part of
an identified "phenonmenon" or not.

ANNABEL CHONG'S SHALLOW GRAVE

In 1991, four years before Annabel Chong starred in *The World's Biggest
Gang Bang*, a porn film in which she engaged in 251 sex acts in ten hours,[57]
she was a victim of gang rape in the basement of a London apartment building. At that time she was still Grace Quek, a young girl from the Philippines
on a scholarship at King's College in London, where she was studying law.

She was drunk and feeling adventurous, so she agreed to have sex with a man she met in an alleyway. She quickly realized that other men were present. The details of what happened next are "blurry," but she remembers "being forced to give them blow jobs" and being watched by a twelve-year-old boy who was encouraged by the others to join in. Suddenly, it "clicked" that she should try to escape; when she screamed, the boys ran. She was then rescued, half-naked, by a family who lived in the building.

After the rape, Quek dropped out of law school and began studying art and gender studies at University of Southern California. At age twenty-one, she took the name Annabel Chong and started appearing in porn films, where she became known for her intellect, sense of humor, and hard-core work such as anal sex and gang bangs—*I Can't Believe I Did the Whole Team* and *All I Want for Christmas Is a Gang Bang* were some of her earlier titles. In 1998, as *The World's Biggest Gang Bang* gained notoriety, I heard Chong speak at an *Adult Video News* event in Los Angeles. She was petite, almost fragile looking, but her vulnerability was worn like a challenge. Onstage, she quipped, "I like to have sex the way I like to shop for groceries. In bulk."

Chong recalls laughing when she first heard the idea for *The World's Biggest Gang Bang*. But after being reminded of the story of Messalina, the Roman empress who challenged a prostitute to a contest of having the greatest number of sexual partners in a day, she became inspired and accepted the job. "Female sexuality is as aggressive as male sexuality. I wanted to take on the role of the stud," she explained. "The more [partners], the better."[58] Though Chong received criticism from industry people at the time, her film sparked a trend in pornography that has lasted more than a decade. Her record was overturned within a year when Jasmine St. Clair took on three hundred men in twenty-four hours; St. Clair's accomplishment was also quickly surpassed. Chong was amused at the female competitiveness sparked by gang bangs. "It's usually the men who are bragging," she said, "and now women are doing it. . . . It's slightly subversive."[59]

Subversive was what she'd had in mind.

She reflected on the experience of filming *The World's Biggest Gang Bang* for an interview at Nerve.com:

> I guess the only word I could use to describe the event is that it was completely surreal. It was really bizarre watching so many naked men, nervous naked men in one place at the same time. In a very sick sort of way, it was kind of erotic, but I emphasize in a very sick sort of way. On the whole, I think I am glad I didn't sleep through the entire event. Because I went into it for the experience and if I slept through it, it would be kind of a waste, wouldn't it? I heard stories about girls who did it after me—how some of them were on Valium or just lying there looking bored. By falling asleep I mean just mentally switching off.

The gang bang was like "running a marathon":

You get the down time, you get the up time. It's very much the same physical process when you're on a roll and it's not painful, it's actually really enjoyable. Then it gets to the down time when it's not going at all and you just have to get yourself through that period and hit a good pace and then it's up time again. Yeah, there was pain. It was definitely a physical strain, I mean, not like vaginal pain but just general strain: my knees, my shoulders. And it's psychological too because I'm claustrophobic, so sometimes I would start to hyperventilate and we'd stop for me to take a breather, have some cold water.[60]

During the filming, security guards were stationed near Chong to remind the men to wear condoms and keep them from becoming aggressive. But most of the men were anxious, Chong realized, more concerned with being able to perform at all than with showing off or trying to dominate her.

In 1999, Chong became the subject of a documentary by Gough Lewis, *Sex: The Annabel Chong Story*. The conclusion of the documentary shows Chong revisiting the scene of her gang rape in London. For Lewis and many who saw the film, her participation in *The World's Biggest Gang Bang* was directly related to the assault, a way to work through the emotional aftermath and regain a sense of control over her body. Chong, however, resists embracing a straightforward link. At times, she claims that the gang bang, and her work in porn more generally, is an artistic, feminist statement about sexuality; other times, she attributes her decision to work in porn to a desire to be paid for sex because she was already promiscuous or to an "ego trip"—"All these guys . . . wanting to have sex with me."[61] In one of the more powerful scenes of the documentary, when questioned about whether she fears being infected with HIV, Chong declares sex "worth dying for." Then, as she comes into contact with movie producers, talk show hosts, and even her fans, she is treated like a throwaway, a joke. Sure, she might be willing to die for sex—but she seems destined to first be ground up for entertainment.

In her many interviews and appearances, including Lewis's film, Chong exposed layers of contradiction and revealed an intriguing complexity often denied those in the public eye. Some reviewers saw this as evidence that she was a psychological wreck: "sometimes like a defiant little girl seeking to shock with frank talk, sometimes an overwrought punk as she puffs on a cigarette, sometimes a lost soul, sometimes a would-be artist creating life as a work of outrage, feminism and politics, or openly self-destructive as she cuts her arm repeatedly with a knife."[62] Critics dismissed her feminist aims as misguided or failed: How could a feminist appear so confused and clueless about her own degradation? She might be waxing articulately about empowerment and freedom, but as the film reveals, she was never even paid in full for *The World's Biggest Gang Bang*. Even Chong seemed surprised by the disjunction between her beliefs and the way she appeared onscreen. "Was I really that depressed?" she asked after seeing Lewis's film. "Was I that vulnerable? But maybe I was."[63]

But was this complexity actually evidence of Chong's instability? Even though we don't all expose our inner pandemonium to the world or challenge ourselves to explore our personal life stories through transgression like Chong, aren't we all a mix of "messy" selves, sometimes feeling on top of the world and other times hiding under the covers? Couldn't any of us proclaim ourselves willing to die for a cause but still appear vulnerable as we charge into battle? Perhaps. Motivations and emotions are rarely simple. We can be empowered by the same things that wound us. What makes us feel strong one moment can later make us crumble. Our past is reinterpreted after new experiences. One of the biggest fallacies associated with feminism is that empowerment or freedom is inherent in any particular act, whether having casual sex, shaving one's legs, stripping, or becoming a CEO. It is, in fact, the feminist interpretations we make of these choices that matter. But we are constantly asked to impose singular meanings on our experiences, especially when it comes to sex—an ill-fated attempt to produce order out of inevitable chaos.

Many things are left out of such tidy stories. "I think on a subconscious level," Chong later said, "in retrospect, maybe there is an element of trying to take back control in the gang bang, but it's not something I was thinking about before the event." She also pointed out that her experiences after the rape in the legal system and National Health Service counseling systems were "incredibly dehumanizing"[64] —this part of the story, however, is often ignored in lieu of a neater cause-and-effect explanation focusing on the gang rape. Her journey in porn, she reflected, was also motivated by her desire to leave Singapore behind: "It's the idea of how far I can run away from home."[65] Further complexities arise due to outside circumstances—had she profited from the gang bang as much as promised or as much as the producers, would she appear more in control of her sexuality?

And is control what sex is necessarily about anyway?

Certainly, in the past few decades, sex has increasingly been framed in terms of control or power struggles—whether between men and women, nature and culture, desire and morality, health and pathology, or the perversity of the West and the repression of the rest. Power is indeed an important aspect of sexuality, and sexual exchanges always unfold within power relations. But sex is also a realm of play and experimentation. Creativity. People long to be transported. Overwhelmed. Entertained. Sometimes, people want to become someone different or try something different.

"If we ever have sex one more Friday night at 11 o'clock . . ."

Adventure, play, and exploration, like other facets of social life, cannot be removed from the social, cultural, political, and economic contexts that shape their meanings and position the individuals involved. Sexual adventure is gendered, for example: men are often expected to explore sexually more than women, although men and women have different opportunities available to them in actually doing so (this can vary by place and time, sexual identity, types of partners sought, etc.). Men and women also face distinct hazards and obstacles, personally and culturally. Still, with many other choices in life, we allow ourselves to experiment. We might try golf and find it boring or decide skydiving is too dangerous. But sex is often treated differently from other types of experimentation. In the contemporary United States, the sex you have is supposed to reflect your deepest, essential self. When a woman pursues transgressive sex, it is usually interpreted as even more problematic than when a man does, as either motivated by psychological weakness or damage or leading to it, or both.

Anthropologist Gayle Rubin argues that sex is "burdened with an excess of significance" in European and American history: for example, "although people can be intolerant, silly, or pushy about what constitutes proper diet, differences in menu rarely provoke the kinds of rage, anxiety, and sheer terror that routinely accompany differences in erotic taste."[66] Many theorists point to Christianity as a source of this sex negativity, although religion should not be used as a simple scapegoat. Throughout history and around the world, one can find non-Christian cultures with beliefs about sexuality that might be called sex negative. Further, in Christianity and other religions restricting sexual activity to particular partners or acts, sex is actually given deep meaning—its significance is not excessive or negative to believers. Secular individuals often retain such beliefs without the personal benefit of religious meaning behind them because the beliefs persist more widely in their social milieu. However, even if we lived in a society that ceased judging so many sexual desires as sinful or unhealthy and penalizing or stigmatizing individuals who deviate from a narrow range of accepted behaviors, we would likely not escape the fact that sexual excitement draws strength from power differentials, prohibitions, and contradictions. Our early relationships with (powerful) caregivers influence our ability to handle the tensions involved in attachment, such as that between dependence and independence. Although we continue to grow and change in the relationships that follow, desire can spark out of obstacles, conflicts, ambiguities, and even wounds. The crossing of boundaries—between inside and outside, self and other—gives rise to complicated emotions. Erotic life is messy and will remain so.

At the same time, though, while it may be true for all of us that unconscious tensions, needs, or wants surface in sexuality, the intensity of such intrusions varies. Some people are tormented for years by the same unwanted desires; others feel relatively undisturbed or find their desires and fantasies changing over time. Conflicts are resolved and wounds are healed. Or they aren't, but we move on anyway. Sometimes, change is dramatic or traumatic—a new psychic injury or preoccupation, perhaps, takes precedence in feeding our erotic life. Other times, change is unremarkable, just a shrug of the shoulders when something no longer turns you on.

In 2003, Annabel Chong retired from porn. She no longer gives interviews on her experiences in the industry. Her website now reads: "Where's Annabel? Annabel is dead, and is now replaced full time by her Evil Doppelganger, who is incredibly bored with the entire concept of Annabel, and would prefer to do something different for a change. From her shallow grave, Annabel would like to thank her fans for all their love and support all these years, and to let them know that she will never forget them."[67]

The young woman who once famously and tearfully declared sex worth dying for decided to do "something different." According to some reports, she's running real marathons these days and working as a web designer.

Chapter Seven

Fear and Bonding in Las Vegas (and Beyond)

Group Sex as Belonging, Status, Identity, and Affirmation

THE "MAN WHORE" (INTERVIEW, GREG)

For my friend Doug's bachelor party, he booked a huge suite in Vegas. There were five of us, including a guy named Jason whom I've privately called "Manwhore" since high school. Jason was a big, good-looking guy, about 6' 3" and very athletic. Well dressed, smart. He was kind of an asshole, but we all still hung out. He was fun to party with because he was always picking up girls. He could drink a lot and handled his liquor well.

Doug was on a mission to get laid before getting married. Friday night, we all got really drunk and no one hooked up. Even Jason decided not to, because the girls who were hanging on him weren't good-looking enough or something like that. By Saturday, the situation was dire. Doug was not going to be happy if he didn't have sex on this trip. Early in the evening, we met some girls in the casino. Doug started hitting on them hard but one of them really liked Jason—it was obvious. Jason looked good that night. He was even wearing a sports coat. So Doug decided he would take the other one. At that point, he didn't care. But she and her friend had already made a pact, and eventually, even though she liked the attention, Doug's girl told him the truth. She was not going anywhere with him unless her friend could have sex with Jason.

By this time, Jason was already off chasing other women.

Of course, now Doug was pissed—his friend had bailed on his bachelor party and he'd spent a lot of time on this girl—but he still wanted to get laid bad enough that we started hunting for Jason.

How do you find a manwhore in Vegas?

Everyone was drinking a lot of Red Bull and vodka. We looked all over the casino. Doug left several messages on Jason's phone. "Dude, come back. We have to fuck these girls." He also kept texting his girl, asking her to wait a little longer. We went to other clubs and casinos. Still no luck. Now the night was all about looking for Jason. We weren't focused on meeting new girls anymore or having fun.

When we found Jason, he was drinking at a bar in our hotel with two women. Doug said something lame to him, like, "Dude, you *have* to fuck that other girl. This is my last chance to get laid. This is it. It's your gift to me." Jason said he didn't want to fuck that one. He didn't like her. He had two girls at the bar and wasn't leaving.

Doug was angry. I don't remember much about the fight or what else they said to each other. Finally, the security guards told them to cool it. A few of the guys tried to talk Jason into "taking one for the team" but Jason turned his back.

The rest of us returned to the room to sleep. Doug was barely talking to anyone, but sometimes he'd go off on a tirade about how much of an asshole Jason was and how they weren't friends anymore. He muttered something about changing the key to the room, but we were all too drunk to seriously consider doing something that complicated. I think we were all both mad and envious of Jason.

A few hours later, the manwhore bursts in and turns on the light. He's with a petite, very young, very hot Asian girl. They're both wasted and loud. "Look what I won at the craps table," he yells. "She's got a great ass." He picked her up, carried her towards us, and lifted up her dress. The girl didn't say anything, just giggled a lot like a drunk college girl. We affirmed that she had a nice ass. One of the guys told him we were trying to sleep—we had the pull-out couches in the main room—so Jason carried the girl into Doug's room with her dress still hiked up and threw her on the bed. Doug and the other guy woke up. Doug yelled, "What the hell are you doing in here?" A few seconds later, we heard laughing.

Doug forgot that he was never speaking to Jason again.

I grabbed my camera and went in to check out what was happening. All three guys were on the bed. They were all muscled, big dudes, and the girl looked really waify by comparison. Doug and the other guy were touching her, while Jason kissed her and pulled off her clothes. He threw her dress on the floor and slid her underwear down her legs. She seemed very drunk but wasn't protesting. She kept laughing. I started snapping pictures. The guys noticed that her tampon string was hanging out, and they moved her around so I could get it in the photos. The bloody string grossed me out, but there I was, taking pictures of it to document Doug's success.

After taking pictures, I went back to the other room. That was when they started having sex with her. I suppose I could have joined in. Part of me wanted her and wanted to be on the bed with them. It was 5:00 a.m. She was naked and hot and we'd been talking all weekend about getting laid so I was horny.

But I just couldn't do it. I was feeling more sober at that point, and still hung over from the night before. I was also feeling sorry for the girl. It's not like she didn't want to be there but they weren't really being that nice to her. I've always been the voice of reason with that group, the one whose super-ego worked overtime.

There's not enough room, I told myself.

I went to sleep.

They all had sex with her and sent her home sometime in the night. I doubt they called a taxi for her. The next morning, there were bloody condoms all over the room and the sheets were bloody. The guys high-fived when they saw the mess in the daylight, celebrating, but the two of us who didn't have sex with her told them they were disgusting for leaving everything out like that.

I still think Jason brought her back to the room that night to share her with Doug because he felt bad about the fight. He was an asshole, especially to girls, and to all of us that night, but he was also a proponent of Doug having a "last hurrah." In the end, he was the one who delivered it.

"WILD BOAR DAY" AND THE *GUNABIBI*

In *Sex at Dawn: The Prehistoric Origins of Modern Sexuality*, Christopher Ryan and Cacilda Jethá argue that "socio-erotic exchanges" (or S.E.Ex) "strengthen the bonds among individuals in small-scale nomadic societies (and, apparently, other highly interdependent groups), forming a crucial, durable web of affection, affiliation, and mutual obligation."[1] The Canela, a Brazilian Indian tribe, is presented as an example of people who exhibit a "community-building, conflict-reducing human sexuality." The Canela practiced ritual group sex between multiple males and a female until at least the 1970s, minimizing jealousy and sexual possessiveness in relationships.[2] Quoting from anthropologists William and Jean Crocker, who first went to study the Canela in 1957, Ryan and Jethá propose that in a cultural context where sharing and cooperation is valued over individual accumulation and competition, "it is easy to understand why women chose to please men and why men chose to please women who expressed strong sexual needs. *No one was so self-important that satisfying a fellow tribesman was less gratifying than personal gain.*"[3]

Ryan and Jethá view the development of similar rituals of socio-erotic exchange across unrelated cultures—the Matis, the Mojave, the Tahitians, and so on—as evidence that such exchanges "probably serve important functions" for humans. In an ancestral environment, nomadic foragers lived in highly interdependent and "fiercely egalitarian" groups, sharing food and resources—and each other—to survive. Multiple intersecting sexual relationships, what Ryan and Jethá refer to as "promiscuity," although without today's negative connotations, created communities where children were cared for communally and men shared paternity.[4] In such an environment, women did not need to barter sex for male protection and access to resources; instead, female sexual availability increased "sharing, cooperation, and peaceful stability" in the group.[5] Asserting that "human sexuality probably evolved and functioned as a social bonding device and a pleasurable way to avoid and neutralize conflict" is not silly romanticism, they argue. Rather than being "noble," such a communal orientation was an effective way to survive given the conditions in which foragers lived.

Examples of "shamelessly libidinous behavior," Ryan and Jethá maintain, can be found "throughout the world, past and present," providing "voluminous scientific evidence" for "an alternative narrative of human sexual evolution" where women's libidos rivaled men's, paternity was not necessarily an issue, and nonmonogamy was the norm.[6] "Many explorers, missionaries, and anthropologists support this view," they write, "having penned accounts rich with tales of orgiastic rituals, unflinching mate sharing, and an open sexuality unencumbered by guilt or shame." (Although evidence for sperm competition in humans is presented to support their challenge to the traditional evolutionary narrative, the name is somewhat unfortunate, a Hobbesian interpretation of "each sperm for itself" that might have taken a different tone if named by a Canela scientist. So, even if reproductive access underlies these exchanges, a belief in shared paternity results in goodwill rather than competition—"the cells fight *in there* so males don't have to fight *out here*.")[7] Despite the fact that monogamous marriage, nuclear families, and the elevation of self-interest over cooperation are considered "natural," then, Ryan and Jethá suggest these are historical aberrations—a claim that has important social and political implications to those who wish to either liberalize or restrict sexual behavior. The development of agriculture, they surmise, initiated a significant departure from prehistorical human subsistence patterns of foraging and was responsible for these sea changes in human sexuality and social life, causing us to veer "into misery, scarcity and ruthless competition a hundred centuries ago."[8]

Ryan and Jethá's argument about human sexuality extends back into pre-history through debates about whether humans are more similar to chimpanzees or bonobos, primates that are both 98.5 percent genetically similar to humans. Chimps and bonobos also share 99.6 percent of their genomes with each other, although they have different reputations: Bonobos for being female dominated, peaceful, and oriented toward sharing; chimps as male dominated, violent, and hierarchical. Bonobos resolve disputes and bond through sex, sometimes in groups; chimps, on the other hand, rape and kill. For reasons beyond the scope of this book to evaluate, Ryan and Jethá embrace bonobos as more representative of ancestral human sexuality than chimpanzees. The traditional Canela way of life, with its bonobo-like lack of possessiveness and acceptance of—even insistence on—female sexual availability, thus serves as a fascinating foil to contemporary Western social organization and sexual mores, descended from the Victorian era. Their argument also probes tentatively into modern times, as they speculate that perhaps athletes who "share" women, musicians who sleep with their "most enthusiastic female fans," and even swingers are practicing similar types of S.E.Ex that "offer a measure of security in an uncertain world."

That there is an alternative narrative of human sexual evolution certainly seems reasonable, although I leave it to evolutionary psychologists, biologists, and historians to duke it out over the specific claims raised in *Sex at Dawn*. After all, whether humans are ultimately "supposed to be" monogamous is not at issue for me. My focus is on those humans who are decidedly not monogamous, and their ranks are full enough for me to have explored this topic for almost a decade already and probably for many more years in the future. Studying group sex means routinely encountering examples of women whose libidos rival men's and of nonmonogamous socio-erotic exchanges that create alliances. Ryan and Jethá's assertion that "our species has an innate capacity for love and generosity at least equal to our taste for destruction, for peaceful cooperation as much as coordinated attack, for an open, relaxed sexuality as much as for jealous, passion-smothering possessiveness" also makes sense. I am less certain, however, as to how these conclusions fit together—at least using the ethnographic data available to us. Does a community-building, conflict-reducing sexuality based on female sexual availability, nonmonogamy, and frequent socio-erotic exchanges necessarily lead to a particular kind of society (peaceful, cooperative) or experience of sexuality (pleasurable, less problematic, "unencumbered by guilt or shame")?

My reading of the Crockers' ethnographic work on the Canela, for example, was more ambiguous. Granted, the Crockers painted a compelling picture of tribal ideals based on sharing resources and minimizing conflict. Noncompetitiveness and cooperation were considered "manly" while fighting was associated with women, animals, and other Brazilian tribes. Multipartner sexual encounters were important in fostering such an environment, although sexual behavior was still subject to restrictions. Children were taught that sex was a "joyful" experience, and sexual joking was frequent. But virginity was economically valuable, and masturbation and homosexuality were thus forbidden. By age 6, female relatives sheltered young girls from gangs of boys who tried to experiment with them sexually. Girls began having sexual relations between the ages of ten and thirteen and boys between twelve and fourteen. If a young man had sex with a virgin, his kin paid a fine if he decided not to marry her; if the couple stayed together, the girl's family delivered a large "meat pie" to his house in celebration. Although marriage did not imply monogamy, young women lived apart from their husbands in the early phase of their marriages and faced restrictions on the age of their sexual partners and the frequency of intercourse, practices that presumably delayed conception. However, after her "belt-painting ceremony," which demonstrated her husband's family's acceptance of her, but before childbirth, a woman was expected to "please most men with her sexual favors." This period of a woman's life was also considered her opportunity for "great sexual freedom and fun"; after her first child, she curbed her sexual activity and took on more domestic responsibilities.[9]

Sharing one's body was a "cornerstone" of Canela cultural identity, behavior akin to offering meat, water, or other resources to tribe members. Some Canela women were recruited for *kuytswe'*, or ceremonial multipartner sex. The film *Mending Ways: The Canela Indians of Brazil* (1999) uses video shot over several decades to chronicle the changes occurring since the Crockers' initial visits, spinning a story about the demise of traditional sexual practices under the force of Western materialism. In one segment of the film, a narrator describes Wild Boar Day, a festival where men who have reached puberty participate in sequential multipartner sex with selected women in the fields—like a "pack of wild boar"—while the women's husbands remain in the village. A Canela man recounts his experiences:

> The great thing about Wild Boar Day is that it means that a man has a chance to have sex with a woman who has refused him in the past. And the women have to yield so the men will have good memories of the festival. Still, it's just this one time, not every day. So a woman can even be generous to an ugly man. Yes, the women enjoy it because it's a joyful game, an ancient and honorable custom.

Another man boasts, "During the Fish Festival, we had six women for our group. That's a lot of women. Many, many men had sex with them. All the men were satisfied and none of the women were worn out. It gave me great joy." While few women speak in the film, one woman discusses watching the men's preparations for Wild Boar Day: "I loved all the men," she says.

"They were so handsome in their wristlets and other decorations. They were so beautiful and there were so many of them."

"I like this way very much," a man declares.

Under the weight of additional detail, however, the "web" formed by this system of socio-erotic exchange appears fairly coercive at times. Sexual generosity was more easily practiced by some individuals than others, for example. Canela husbands often encouraged their wives to participate in ritual group sex, which Ryan and Jethá interpret as evidence of a lack of jealousy. "Anyone who can pretend not to be jealous as his wife has sex with twenty or more men is someone you do not want to meet across a poker table," they joke. But the Crockers' ethnographic work suggests more emotional ambivalence. When a woman was recruited for *kuytswe'*, Crocker explains, "her husband must not be jealous although he increasingly objects these days, and maybe always did even in aboriginal times." Women chosen to participate in ritual group sex—serving up to twenty or more men in the Crockers' ethnography but reported as "maybe fifty" in the film—describe being "taken away" from the village. Sometimes, these women earned payments of meat from the men. But why was the woman featured in *Mending Ways* chosen twice for *kuytswe'* and others not chosen at all? Why were payments (or gifts) necessary in a society where people were expected to freely share resources, from bodies to meat pies? Were women who traded sex for meat different from the women who were "taken away" or the women who "loved all the men"?

Some festive occasions allowed for more female choice than others, but few women wanted to earn a reputation for being "stingy" by declining to participate. Women could gain popularity, lovers, and resources through participation in sequential sex. A woman who refused to share her body was considered stingy and antisocial; not only would she be seen as undesirable, but she risked violence if she did not change her attitude: "a group of men will waylay her to teach her to be generous." "Young girls rarely resisted carrying out their sequential sex obligations to an assigned ceremonial men's society," the Crockers write, "but when they did, they were taken forcefully into it anyway."[10]

The system of nonmonogamous socio-erotic exchange did not mean an absence of power struggles or hierarchy. Despite a noncompetitive ideal, men jostled for status, even during sex: "There were stories of fierce men pulling weaker ones away from women in the very act of sexual intercourse and simply taking over." Canela men and women gossiped about one another's sexual abilities and, given the small size of the community, knew many intimate details about one another. Pressure to conform is heightened in small groups where dissent is handled with violence; gossip can be a subtle means of either resistance or intimidation. Most disputes in Canela society supposedly occurred between spouses, although Crocker claims that women are "so secure" in their social positions that "they can afford to be irritable, changeable, and demanding, while their husbands must put up with such treatment." But isn't putting up with someone who is "irritable" different from being ambushed by a group of men as a lesson in sexual "generosity"? In fact, the Crockers refer to the Canela extramarital sex system as their "most immediate and therefore their most effective institution of social control," although they also point out that we are all coerced, to some extent, as we are socialized into the expectations of our cultures. Whether one faces the repercussions of being labeled "stingy" or "slutty," the underlying social mechanism is one of disciplining individuals into the expectations, norms, and power structures of a community.

Ryan and Jethá would agree that conflicts can arise between individuals' desires and the interests of the group. What is most essential to their argument is that the sexual practices of the Canela promoted a "fiercely egalitarian" and cohesive community that ensured the survival of its members. This might involve suppressing self-interest in some socio-erotic exchanges, even though people likely still displayed preferences for certain partners in other interactions. Certainly, Canela beliefs and practices prioritized the group over the individual in ways quite different from those of contemporary Western culture. Maybe I can't imagine being *kuytswe'* on Wild Boar Day, but perhaps a traditional Canela woman would laugh at the possessiveness of a "same room, soft swap" lifestyle couple, let alone monogamous American spouses. Maybe, as *Mending Ways* suggests, internal conflict increased after contact with the outside world, when belief systems clashed, power dynamics changed, and the economic basis of Canela life shifted. "Waylaying" persisted among some villages but disappeared in others. Possessiveness became more pervasive. From a traditional perspective valuing sexual generosity, the jealous husband who beat his wife for taking part in Wild Boar Day acted aberrantly, inappropriately, and even irrationally. Yet despite the assumption that tribal societies were internally harmonious until explorers, missionaries, or capitalists intruded, the reality is that we don't actually know how people felt in the past about Wild Boar Day or anything else. Canela men talking about Wild Boar Day in the 1950s, 1970s, or 2000s are still Canela men talking to Westerners after contact and in a modern world, regardless of whether they are wearing loincloths or traditional face paint. The Crockers note that while forced participation in multipartner sex was reportedly rare during the 1930s and 1940s, force was increasingly necessary during the decades leading up to the 1980s, when the practice was finally abandoned. Perspective, then, can sometimes be the difference between peaceful cooperation and highly effective social control.

Let's consider another ceremony based on socio-erotic exchange. In the late 1920s, anthropologist William Lloyd Warner spent three years studying an aboriginal tribe he called the "Murngin." The Murngin, now properly referred to as the Yolngu, reside in Arnhem Land, in the northeast part of the Northern Territory of Australia. Conflict and violence in the region was frequent, usually erupting over disputes about women or during "blood feuds." Ceremonies were symbolically opposed to warfare for the Murngin and thus used to maintain peace over a large region and across the many different tribes. According to Warner, the Murngin practiced group sex and partner exchange during an elaborate ritual known as the Gunabibi, which lasted several days. The Gunabibi included songs and dances, prayers and chants, and symbolic costuming (fertility, totemic, etc.). The ceremony, believed to keep participants from becoming ill or injured, was rooted in beliefs about kinship and connection; a ceremonial exchange of wives was the "grand finale."[11]

The socio-erotic exchanges occurring in the Gunabibi reduced conflict and increased social cohesion. The Murngin were an age-graded, clan-based society where marriages fortified alliances between clans. Marriage was permitted between one set of cross cousins, the mother's brother's daughter, but prohibited with the other set, the father's sister's daughter. The terms "brother," "father," and many other kin terms were used widely to include distant relatives, however. The resulting kinship system was complicated enough to stir up decades of debate among anthropologists, causing distinguished scholars to hurl insults at each other over competing genealogical charts (the academic equivalent of a blood feud).

Gunabibi ceremonies drew men from distant clans, and sorting out the complex kinship ties required a bit of discussion even for these cultural insiders. "When a local man discovers that a certain visitor from a far clan is his tribal brother," Warner explained, he sends his younger brother, bearing gifts, to inform the visitor "that he may have the local man's wife for ceremonial copulation at the end of the Gunabibi ceremony." The recipient, through his own younger brother or a messenger, then "offers his own wife in exchange, and also sends presents."[12] Men could set up the swap in less formal ways, but ceremonial wife exchange supposedly occurred only between distant kin. Given that brothers shared property and respected certain prohibitions against fighting, recognizing men from distant clans as such was strategic. Some of Warner's informants also suggested that the ceremony functioned as a safety valve, a form of sanctioned deviance that made for more stable social relations: "It is better that everybody comes with their women and all meet together at a Gunabibi and play with each other, and then nobody will start having sweethearts the rest of the time."[13]

Each night of the ceremony, after the evening meal, women danced and were given presents by the men they were assigned to for Gunabibi. Ideally, there was no sexual contact between the ceremonial couples until the final night, although Warner admitted that for some, copulation "starts early in the ceremony, and in the minds of the natives it is purely a pleasurable act." Such early meetings were supposed to be secret, but "it is generally known which people are having these assignations in the surrounding bush or jungle, and many broadly humorous remarks are passed by both sexes about their various lovers."[14] Unofficial trysts took place in relative privacy, like everyday sexual relations. Ceremonial sex, on the other hand, took place in front of witnesses who played supporting roles. For example, after a man "has had sexual intercourse with another man's wife, the latter male comes to him and puts his sweat on the legs and arms of his wife's partner so that the one who has been with his wife won't be 'sick' from it." Men painted their bodies with blood in preparation for the final night, as in other important rituals. The sexual position used in the Gunabibi ceremony also differed from the customary one: "The woman sits on the ground on the back of her buttocks. The trunk of the body leans back and at an angle from the legs, with the hands on the ground in back of the body to support it. The man puts his legs under hers and his hands around her so that the pudenda meet in closer contact than if he lay on her."[15]

Participation was supposedly obligatory; anyone who objected was told that he or she would become ill. Men reported threatening women who balked at their assigned partners. "We don't take this blood out of ourselves for nothing and paint ourselves with it," a man explained. "We don't sleep that night, and if a woman says, 'I won't go to that corroboree [ceremonial meeting] place with you,' the man says, 'If you don't go with me you are going to be dead.' Sometimes we kill that woman by magic, and throw spears at them if they won't do it."[16] Some women had sex with several men at the ceremony, Warner notes, because "as always a larger proportion of men than women attend."

Warner claims that Murngin women exercised independence and power in their role as wives: "She is not the badly treated woman of the older Australian ethnologists' theories. She usually asserts her rights. Women are more vocal than men in Murngin society. Frequently they discipline their husbands by refusing to give them food when the men have been away too long and the wife fears they have a secret affair." But he also reports on women being beaten or murdered for suspicion of infidelity, "stolen" for wives, and traded to other men during political and economic negotiations— fates hardly equivalent to being sent to bed without dinner. And while the men told Warner that there were "no cold women"—that is, all Murngin women were willing to have sex—he also notes that male pride was such that "no man would admit that women were not interested in him."[17]

Or, apparently, a man might rely on spear pressure.

One cannot fully understand the meaning of the Gunabibi ceremony without studying the kinship system of the Murngin in depth and developing a more nuanced understanding of gender relations at the time. This part of the ceremony is not practiced among contemporary clans, however, and the existing data is sparse, as is also the case with the Canela Wild Boar Day and many other instances of non-Western group sex. But Warner's analysis of the Gunabibi differs from many accounts of ritual group sex because he focuses on the complexities of social interactions. Participants negotiate with and occasionally resist each other from different perspectives—local, visitor, husband, wife. The point of the ritual group sex associated with Gunabibi was to build, express, and maintain relationships—a function that group sex fulfills in both myth and actual practice—even if there is no ultimate agreement as to whether this is accomplished or for whom. Among other Australian aboriginal tribes, group sex was also reportedly used for the purposes of social cohesion, as when tribes were signing peace treaties, when men were leaving for battle, or to avoid a raid—"a woman would be sent over for the sexual use of the whole group of men." Again, participants reported varying interpretations and experiences: women did not necessarily mind sexual relations under everyday conditions, for example, but expressed "dislike and disgust" at being with hostile men. [18]

Ryan and Jethá do not discuss the Gunabibi ceremony because the Murngin are not "immediate return foragers" and thus not "representative of our hunter-gatherer ancestors" (as they believe the Canela to be). The Murngin, they assert, "are not typical even of Australian native cultures, representing a bloody exception to the typical Australian Aboriginal pattern of little to no intergroup conflict." [19] The Marind-anim of southern New Guinea, on the other hand, have a single paragraph cameo; their wedding ceremony is offered as an example of paternity uncertainty and nonmonogamy that challenges the traditional narrative of human sexual evolution. This argument is reasonable given Marind-anim sexual practices, beliefs about reproduction, and acceptance of foreign children as their own. Additional details, however, again complicate any general claims about their society or sexuality. Their internal affairs, for example, were described as relatively peaceful and egalitarian, and they allied with many of their neighbors, albeit in a somewhat fickle manner. [20] It was best to stay on their good side—the more distant tribes whose villages became frequent headhunting destinations would debate whether Marind-anim were "peaceful." Violence aside, despite frequent nonmonogamous socio-erotic exchanges, available evidence also suggests that their attitudes toward sexuality were neither completely open and relaxed nor fully encumbered by shame and guilt.

Granted, it is impossible for any researcher to survey every society and more could be written about each of these groups. Complexity is often lost, to some extent, in representation. But arguing either for or against a functionally "promiscuous" human past isn't just about compiling data but telling a story—and as we have seen repeatedly in this book, stories can be political. Stories about sexuality become central to debates about human nature: Are we naturally promiscuous or monogamous? Are we sharing, loving, and cooperative or selfish, violent, and individualistic? Are we more like bonobos or chimps? Are we more like the Canela, the Murngin, the Marind-anim, or the "real housewives" of Beverly Hills?

Here, the devil really is in the details. Polyamory activists have championed bonobos as our closest ancestors, for example. But what happens when researchers found that bonobos sometimes hunt, kill, and eat other primates? Journalists report that these "hippie cousins" of the chimps have a "carnivorous dark side."[21] And when females were observed exhibiting a keen sense of social order, acting differently around alpha females and using sex to make hierarchical alliances? These once egalitarian and "peace-loving" bonobos were exposed in the media as "sleeping their way to the top." Did bonobos change? Or did the story told about them become more complex? As Ryan and Jethá point out, representations are motivated: "Nothing sells newspapers like headlines of 'WAR!,' and no doubt 'CANNIBALISTIC HIPPIE ORGY WAR!' sells even more, but one species hunting and eating another species is hardly 'war'; it's lunch."[22] Of course, they are correct. Stories are told with a purpose and the details presented—or left out—matter. Ryan and Jethá also dismiss overly general questions about human nature; it depends on the context, they insist. Yet oversimplication and homogenization is, in fact, what happens with the Canela and the Marind-anim in *Sex at Dawn*. The traditional sexual practices of both groups support Ryan and Jethá's arguments that monogamy was not the only norm in human populations and that socio-erotic exchanges can contribute to community building and conflict reduction. But to further imply that these exchanges were homogeneously experienced—whether as pleasurable, gratifying, shameless, unflinching, relaxed, etc.—or result in peaceful, cooperative, or egalitarian societies requires overlooking numerous details and perspectives.

Maybe the real story is always complicated.

Group sex is as much about the group as the sex, but group bonding through sex, when it happens, is not necessarily conflict-free or associated with any particular outcome.[23] Group sex can promote connections and strengthen bonds among all participants, among only some participants, or among some participants at the expense of others. Some men and women are enthusiastic participants in such exchanges while others respond to social pressure, bribery, or coercion. The wish to be accepted by a group has a counterpart in the fear of rejection and the very real dangers that can accompany exile—being "put on the prairie" when there are no other options for survival is quite a different threat from losing favor with a peer group in a more individualistic society. Nonetheless, some individuals in any society are more susceptible than others to threats of exclusion.

S.E.Ex is a reality, but it isn't equally rosy for everyone.

GROUP PROCESSES AND SEXUAL VIOLENCE

On December 16, 2006, twenty-two-year-old Megan Wright killed herself in her bedroom. Her mother, thinking Megan was napping, found her daughter's body covered with blankets on the bed like a pile of laundry. Megan had suffocated herself using a plastic bag.[24]

Six months earlier, in the spring of her freshman year at Dominican College in New York, Megan was raped in a campus dormitory. When she woke up wearing different clothes than she'd worn the night before and discovered that she was bleeding vaginally, she went to White Plains hospital, where a rape examination established that her "substantial injuries, including bruising and lacerations, indicated forcible rape." The nurse on duty that day said that "in fifteen years of practice, [she] has rarely seen a victim evincing more physical trauma than Megan Wright."[25] Megan believed she had been drugged at a party she attended with friends earlier, as she could only vaguely recall sensations from the assault, like a "nightmare."

A campus surveillance camera provided some evidence of the evening's events, as it showed Megan "stumbling down the hallway" before being led into a room in Hertel Hall, first by one man, and then joined by two others. After a long period of time, one of the men came back into the hallway. He waved a poster at the camera that read, "I want to have sex." It was signed, "Megan Wright."

After viewing the surveillance tapes, a detective on the case decided not to prosecute, believing the signature could indeed have been Megan's. An examination of the handwriting, however, suggests that she was likely intoxicated even if she did sign her name, knew that she was signing a statement consenting to sex, or understood that there would be multiple men involved. Authorities did not interview the young men involved, and the case was not pursued. Wright's parents later sued Dominican College for mishandling the case, including failing to inform Megan that her assailants left the college. She hadn't returned for her sophomore year because she was worried about running into the men on campus.[26]

Megan's experience is unique because she took her own life, not because she became a victim of gang rape. The statistic that one in four women will be raped during her college years is widely cited; there is debate over this number due to a lack of consistent reporting and varying definitions of sexual assault in surveys, although competing statistics—one in five or one in six women—do not range too widely. Many of those rapes involve multiple assailants or witnesses. While each case of gang rape on campus is unique, patterns emerge. First, the perpetrators are often men who are unlikely to commit violent crimes in other settings. Why do relatively privileged young men—well educated and from socially upstanding families, athletes or fraternity members with professional futures—gang-rape when they would likely balk at robbing a gas station? Second, there has historically been a reluctance to view campus gang rapes as crimes. Like fraternity members, athletes are involved in a disproportionate number of rapes and sexual assaults. Dr. Claire Walsh, director of the sexual assault recovery program at the University of Florida, stated that when athletes are involved, "the entire group will fall behind the accused and deny any offense has been committed." In every case, she said, "they will deny there was gang rape" and insist that it was just "group sex."[27] Why do these men repeatedly believe they did nothing wrong? And why do authorities often agree with them, sometimes even suggesting it was the victim's fault for putting herself in a situation where things were likely to get out of hand?

Some researchers suggest that such rapes are manifestations of patriarchy, arguing that many men "have the attitudes and beliefs necessary to commit a sexually aggressive act" and rape "can be viewed as the end point in a continuum of sexually aggressive behaviors that reward men and victimize women."[28] But if this is the case, why do some men gang-rape while others do not? Even in cultures or settings where rape is frequent, some men publicly oppose sexual coercion. And why are gang rapes more likely in particular settings?

When anthropologist Peggy Sanday learned that one of her students had been gang-raped at a fraternity house, she drew on her previous research on rape patterns around the world to analyze "pulling train" on American campuses. Structural factors such as the way reported sexual assaults are handled, she argued, make some campuses "rape prone." Fraternity initiations, rituals, and parties may draw on sexist ideas and images or even downplay violence against women. In 2010, for example, a video posted on YouTube depicted Delta Kappa Epsilon pledges at Yale University marching through campus chanting, "No means yes! Yes means anal!" After the Women's Center accused the fraternity of "hate speech," the DKE president apologized, calling it "a serious lapse in judgment by the fraternity and in very poor taste."[29] Whether college authorities, campus personnel, or other students challenge such messages affects the sexual environment; some colleges make awareness of sexual violence a priority while others pretend it does not exist.

Other aspects of campus social life can make rapes more likely as well; for example, "party cultures" based on the denigration of sexually active women or the acceptance of high levels of coercion to get women to say "yes" to sex, such as plying them with alcohol or drugs at campus parties. GHB, ketamine, or other "date rape drugs" make women easier to coerce and can affect a victim's ability to recall the incident. By the time a rape is reported, it is often too late to test for substances. But the issue is thorny, as some young women purposely use substances to overcome sexual inhibitions. Drinks do not have to be forcibly poured down women's throats at parties. Many college students dose themselves with GHB for fun. Allegations that women cry rape to deal with morning-after regret—even though false rape accusations rarely occur—complicate the issue. Further, while a woman may consent to part of the experience, such as having sex with one of the assailants, withdrawing consent is not always possible when she is outnumbered or things get "out of control."

The men who had sex with Megan Wright knew consent was an issue: why else go to the trouble of preparing a statement and showing it to the surveillance camera? Other assailants, however, seem not to realize that consent is required when participants are "partying" (even though most legal definitions of consent require an individual to at least be conscious) or assume that consent has already been obtained. Shaming individuals who "pass out" is common practice among college students; part of the ritual involves making the intoxicated party eventually bear witness to his or her lack of control. Remember shaving off your roommate's eyebrows, stuffing a cold hot dog in his mouth, and photographing him with his pants around his knees? "Markering"—writing on an unconscious person's face or body with a permanent marker—has been popular for decades. Supposedly, you can also make a passed-out-partier "pee his pants" by submerging his hand in a cup of warm water. In my college days, we had to anxiously await double prints from the one local drugstore willing to develop nude pictures; Facebook now provides instant gratification. For some young men, having sex with a woman while she "sleeps it off" may feel like an extension of this tendency to see an inebriated person's body as fair game for such violations, treated as jokes rather than assaults.

But group rape is also about *belonging*. Focusing on the group processes involved helps us understand why individuals who do not exhibit psychopathology can be influenced by their environment or a group leader to participate in activities they would ordinarily avoid. Individual fraternity members who were interviewed after gang rapes, for example, were found to know "the difference between right and wrong, but fraternity norms that emphasize loyalty, group protection, and secrecy often overrode standards of ethical correctness."[30] Sanday argues that gang rapes are a way that "insecure" young men bond with each other and become part of a group. Young men may enter college already accepting cultural beliefs supporting male dominance, such as that heterosexual male desires are naturally aggressive and uncontrollable ("boys will be boys") or that women should act as gatekeepers ("she was asking for it"). When a young man then joins a fraternity, the initiation experience and house activities further affect his identity and beliefs. His insecurity and desire for belonging makes him vulnerable to peer pressure to prove his loyalty.

Fear of being rejected by the group—or a desire to gain acceptance, status, and recognition within it—can be as much of a motivation for gang rape as the desire for sex or dominance over women. Dumisani Rebombo, now a South African gender equality activist, took part in a gang rape at fifteen years old. At the time, he faced ridicule because he was poor and did not own goats or cattle, and because he had not been circumcised in the traditional rite of passage. "There was constant jeering that I wasn't a real boy," he says. A group of local boys suggested he help "discipline" a girl in the community, and Rebombo saw an opportunity to improve his situation. Despite "trembling" with fear, he recalls, "I made the decision to agree to it. I was given beer and I smoked. I remember that, after the act, it was reported to the whole soccer team and my friend and I were given a standing ovation."[31] Rebombo was allowed to associate with the other boys afterward and "did not think much of the incident" for decades, until he began working for an NGO and listening to women's stories about sexual violence. He decided to return to his hometown and asked the woman for her forgiveness. Although it had taken him twenty years to realize he had committed a rape, the young woman told him that she had "never been the same."[32] Rebombo's willingness to discuss his motivations and publicly recount his experience is rare and valuable, illuminating the variability in how an event can be interpreted.

As "scoring" with women is often a sign of heterosexual prowess, men participating in group sex scenarios maintain a superior status to both women and to men who don't "prove" their heterosexuality. Men may fear having their sexuality called into question if they do not participate. During group rapes, participants often "ritualistically take turns, converse about taking turns, watch each other, and engage in simultaneous sex with victims." The use of a "symbolic penis"—a bottle, broomstick, or baseball bat—is common as a way to emasculate and degrade victims of either sex. *Not me.* Witnessing is central: the rape may "be experienced by participants as a dramatic contest in which one's peers evaluate one's sexual, or masculine, prowess" and thereby prove themselves worthy of belonging.[33] But acts of sexual violence can also become "celebratory dramas," where the group creates an atmosphere of "recreation and fun."[34] Convicted gang rapists describe feelings of "male camaraderie" during and after sexual assaults, for example; the assaults also provide a sense of adventure. One man said participating in gang rape was "the ultimate thing I ever did."[35]

Purposely engaging in an irrevocable and forbidden "bridge-burning" act, or participating in intense physical or emotional trials, can be part of the process of taking on a new identity as the member of a particular group.[36] Sometimes, initiations involve violence directed toward an outsider; other times, the initiates themselves undergo the tests to prove commitment to the group and establish hierarchy. Mara Salvatrucha 13, or MS-13, is one of the most violent, fastest-growing, and well-organized gangs in the United States, with an estimated thirty thousand members operating in thirty-three states. For males, initiation into MS-13 may require being "jumped in," or beaten for thirteen seconds by gang members, or committing a physical assault, rape, or murder to prove competence. Female recruits may be given the additional choice of being "sexed in," or gang-raped by existing members. MS-13 members have been associated with numerous high-profile gang rapes, including a 2002 assault on two young deaf girls in Massachusetts. Many other gangs have been linked to group rapes as part of their initiation process. There are political aspects regarding how such attacks are reported and to which groups they are attributed, but group sexual violence as a means of fortifying hierarchy and connection is widespread.

"Hazing" is practiced worldwide in militaries, fraternities, sororities, and other institutional settings. Sex has a number of features that make it ideal for ritual incorporation, as it involves the boundaries of the body and the self (even if both are variable) and may already be shrouded in mystery, secrecy, taboo, or fear. Many—although certainly not all—hazing rituals are sexualized, and can involve manipulation or torture of the genitals, penetration with objects (dildos, candles, wooden poles, etc.), forced nudity, the ingestion of body fluids or their application to the body, and humiliation. Some practices are widely reported: for example, in the United States, the "elephant walk," might require initiates to walk in a line while holding the erect penises of the men in front or back of them, or require each man to insert a thumb into the anus of the man in front of him. Other practices may be unique to a particular group, embellishing on general themes of pain, deprivation, disgust, or humiliation. Same sex contact carried out in a special space and time (such as "Hell Week") is not necessarily interpreted the same way as it is in other contexts. Hazing can be dangerous; deaths due to hazing or "ragging" have occurred in the United States, Japan, Russia, the Philippines, India, and elsewhere. Individuals may choose to undergo initiation rites in order to belong to the group, but get more than they bargained for because of the secretiveness involved; some individuals have committed suicide to escape ongoing hazing. Yet despite deaths and injuries, negative public opinion, and potential legal penalties, people continue to undergo, replicate, or produce hazing rituals. Most of the time, hazing does not cross the border into abuse or violence, and if hazing were only interpreted as abuse, it wouldn't keep reappearing. The point here is that witnessing and being witnessed in sexually transgressive situations can be emotionally powerful, impacting both individual and group identities.

Whether we draw on psychoanalysis, attachment theory, or another way of explaining how humans create and maintain emotional connections, some relational strategies are more successful, culturally or personally, in a given time and place. Bonds might be created through affection—love, respect, friendship, and so on—and obligation. Bonds can be created imaginatively through practice, such as ritual, or suffering. What some researchers have called "trauma bonds"—"strong emotional ties that develop between two persons where one person intermittently harasses, beats, threatens, abuses, or intimidates the other"[37] —can be remarkably stable. On the other hand, bonds created through shame, anger, humiliation, or fear can be weakened if one of the parties becomes stronger and more independent. Cycles of abuse can be found in the life histories of many, though not all, perpetrators of violent crimes. Conscious and unconscious desires to overcome past experiences of shame and humiliation, take revenge for previous hurts, or feel a sense of power or control over one's life can underlie both the processes of bonding with others and the selection of others with whom to bond. The impact of a charismatic leader—especially one who demonstrates aggression against noncompliant group members—can be exponential if the group is composed of individuals who are processing emotional wounds. But, as is evident in instances where men without such abuse histories gang-rape, sometimes the quest for acceptance is all one needs.

Many elements of the group process—the desire to belong, the influence of a sadistic and charismatic leader, the thrill of adventure, and a link between sexual activity and group identity—came together in South Africa during the reign of the "Jackrollers." The Jackrollers were a gang led by Jeff Brown, a notorious South African criminal. (Despite his notoriety, however, there seems to be relatively little information available about him; his mythological status is itself revealing of how some stories are retold.) In 1987 and 1988, Brown supposedly became known as the "most feared man in the township" of Diepkloof, a relatively affluent area of Soweto.[38] In addition to abduction, car theft, and bank robbery, the Jackrollers were known for *ba dla abantwana* ("they eat the girls or children") and for raping girls and women in public places.[39]

During the 1990s, "jackrolling" became popular among other youth gangs in South Africa. According to researchers, jackroll was different from ordinary rape because it was recreational. Rapists did not try to conceal their identity and jackroll was committed in public places such as "shebeens (informal township bars), picnic spots, schools, nightclubs and in the streets"[40] as a way to develop reputation. Racial and class conflicts, as well as political unrest and a lack of cohesion in black communities, set the stage for street gangs to become a means of surviving and claiming identity for disenfranchised youth. The political, economic, and educational systems were stacked against them. One young black man, forced to leave school and earn his living stealing car parts, was quoted as saying, "If you were nowhere in the past, so will you be nowhere in the future."[41] Left without legitimate job opportunities or outlets for creating a meaningful life, young men turned to gang membership and jackrolling to increase self-esteem and gain status among peers.

Though jackroll is purportedly less of a problem today, South Africa's history of colonialism and apartheid continues to shape patterns of sexual violence. Authorities are often reluctant to intervene in "corrective rapes," meant to "cure" lesbians of their sexual orientation, or in sexually violent relationships.[42] Rapes are underreported and inconsistently prosecuted; when cases make it to court, perpetrators tend to receive light sentences. In some surveys, South Africa ranks first for number of rapes per capita; in 1995, South Africa was named "rape capital of the world." There are also high incidences of child and baby rapes, some of which are motivated by beliefs that having sex with a virgin can cure AIDS. (Up to one in eight South Africans may have been infected with HIV, giving South Africa a dubious status as the nation with the highest number of HIV-positive citizens.) Anti-rape organizations estimate that a woman is raped every twenty-six to eighty-five seconds in South Africa, depending on the source; gang rapes are said to account for 75 percent of all cases.[43] In 2002, Rachel Jewkes and Naeema Abrahams, researchers at the South African Medical Research Council, detailed the problems with arriving at accurate rape statistics: differences in popular and legal conceptualizations of "rape," inconsistencies in reporting, and diverse methods of data collection across regions. As statistics are repeated in the press, on blogs, and by human rights organizations, they can become decontextualized. The finding that a 1999 survey of 1,500 schoolchildren in Soweto found a quarter of the boys interviewed calling jackrolling "fun" is widely reported, for example, although the original study is elusive. Yet Jewkes and Abrahams believe that existing statistics on rape and attitudes toward sexual violence, however variable, are more likely the tip of an "iceberg" than overinflated.[44] In 2010–2011, 56,272 rapes were reported in South Africa, an average of 154 per day. In 2013, Jewkes, now acting president of the South African Medical Research Council, was interviewed following a violent gang rape and murder in Bredasdorp. Between a quarter and a third of South African men still admit to rape, Jewkes stated, suggesting little progress even though the issue has been politicized for twenty years.

Because attacks now usually involve groups of friends rather than organized gangs, they may be referred to as "group rapes" instead of "gang rapes"; the term "streamlining" sometimes replaces "jackrolling."[45] In a country fighting high levels of poverty, unemployment, disease, and violence, youth face daunting political, economic, and social problems. Sexual aggression is still one of the few recreational outlets for marginalized young men.

We could call this society "rape prone."

Is it surprising that the Rape-aXe—an antirape female condom—originated in Cape Town? The device, unveiled in 2005, is inserted like a tampon. When an attacker attempts penetration, sharp barbs grasp his penis, causing severe pain and preventing him from urinating until the device is surgically removed. The assailant will thus be identified when he seeks medical attention. How a woman is supposed to relay this information to a potential attacker is unclear, and in situations with multiple assailants, she might face continued violence as retaliation. Still, Rape-aXe inventor, Sonette Ehlers, stated, "The device should become part of every woman's daily routine, just like brushing her teeth."[46] While critics call the invention "vengeful, horrible, and disgusting," it is at least somewhat kinder than a device created in 2000 by Japp Haumann, a South African man, which deployed a spring blade to cut off the tip of the penis.

And it beats slowly evolving a counterclockwise, corkscrew vagina like a duck's.

Gang rape can establish the identities of the perpetrators in relation to each other, symbolizing belongingness to a group and status within it. Violent group sex can also dramatize the relationship between perpetrators and victims.

In 2005, South African immigrants were blamed for spreading jackroll to the English town of Northampton. After five gang rapes in ten days, police warned women to be careful on the streets. Suspects were said to be black and young, with heavy South African accents. The media reported on the random selection of victims, who were supposedly abducted by car, and the growing panic of residents.[47] Townspeople were "terrorized" at the possibility of being victimized as sport, especially on the sole basis of ethnic difference. But when three men were eventually arrested in connection with the case, they turned out not to be South African and not to identify themselves as "jackrollers."

In the United States, a similar panic emerged after the rape of Trisha Meili, the "Central Park jogger." On April 19, 1989, twenty-eight-year-old Meili was found in a gully, near death after being beaten with a metal pipe and a rock and having lost around 80 percent of her blood. Later that evening, police picked up a group of teenagers who supposedly confessed to Meili's assault, among other crimes, as amusement, a diversion they called "wilding": "It was fun"; "It was something to do."[48] Meili was *not* an easy victim to blame. Sure, she'd been out jogging alone, but she wasn't swilling beers at a neighborhood pub or doing a drunken striptease at a frat party. There was no logical motive in the wilding story—no stolen car or money, no disrespect by the victim, no infringement on the attackers' territories or property—and no clear reason why Meili had been victimized, something that was reportedly "chilling" to residents of New York City and people around the country. She was simply an outsider.

Meili survived but spent six weeks in a coma and emerged with severe brain damage. She remembers nothing about the attack. After a high-profile, emotional trial, five of the young men went to prison.

In 2002, the men were cleared when Matias Reyes, a convicted rapist, confessed to Meili's rape.

The details of Meili's case were certainly disturbing. Yet in 1989, 3,254 rapes were reported in New York City—almost nine a day. A week after Meili's attack, a black woman was raped, beaten, and thrown from a rooftop by a group of black men. She "miraculously grabbed hold of a television cable, where she dangled, naked and seriously injured, until she was rescued by neighbors."[49] Her story was not widely reported until commentators began to question the incessant coverage of the "Central Park jogger" story. Some critics argue that stories with white victims and black assailants automatically garner more attention; others suggest that racial slant can be affected by the local politics and fears of the day. In 2007, for example, Channon Christian and Christopher Newsom, a young white couple, were gang-raped, tortured, and murdered after a carjacking in Knoxville, Tennessee. Their assailants, one of whom was a woman, were all black. Once again, the gruesome story received little national attention until protestors—joined by white supremacist groups and conservative bloggers—questioned why the media was ignoring the murders. But, as one public defender mused in response, "Why is this worthy of national news coverage? Unfortunately, this probably happens in major metropolitan areas every month."[50] His point is clear, if disquieting: until the Christian/Newsom murder became entangled in debates over racism, hate crimes, and the objectivity of the media, the story simply didn't have an angle that differentiated it from all of the other rapes, tortures, and murders happening every day around the world.

So what was the angle that made the Meili story an object of rabid consumption by the American public for months on end? Race certainly played a part, although it was not the full story. Headlines such as "Teen Wolfpack Beats and Rapes Wall Street Exec" or "Wolf Pack's Prey: Female Jogger Near Death after Savage Attack by Roving Gang" went beyond race, contrasting the identities of Meili and her supposed attackers in terms of age (teen versus adult), social class ("wolf pack" versus "Wall Street"), employment status (gang versus executive), and leisure choices (roving versus jogging). These differences between the victim and her alleged attackers reflected highly politicized and emotional social divisions. Meili's story also evoked the powerful fear of gang rape as cold-blooded recreation, with a victim so dehumanized by perpetrators that collective sexual violence becomes "just something to do" when you can't afford a movie.

Being overwhelmed by an out-of-control horde with no respect for human pain, dignity, or life is perhaps a primal fear. Responses to these crimes hark back to discourses discussed in chapter 2 of group sex as a force destructive of civilization, symbolizing social and moral corruption. This fear, in fact, propelled the "Central Park jogger" case forward even in the face of shoddy evidence. Although the real rapist acted alone, many people still remember Meili as the victim of a horrific gang rape, and the term "wilding" has entered the English lexicon.

Even more chilling than the frenzied, aimless horde, perhaps, is the organized, purposeful one. When gang rape becomes a tactic of war, it is precisely this fear that is mobilized.

"WE WILL DESTROY YOU, ALL OF YOU": MASS RAPE AS TERRORISM AND GENOCIDE

Doctors without Borders is an international medical humanitarian organization that sends volunteers to more than sixty countries where warfare or
disasters threaten the population. DWB maintained a presence in Sudan from
2003 to 2011, where thousands of people were affected by the conflict between the Sudanese government, aided unofficially by Arab militias known
as the Janjaweed and Darfur's non-Arab, or "black," tribes, especially the
Fur, Massalit, and Zaghawa ethnic groups. Roaming Janjaweed militias systematically targeted non-Arab blacks by burning their homes and villages,
destroying crops and livestock, stealing food or other resources, killing civil-
ian men, and kidnapping and raping young women and girls. The two main
ethnic groups of the south, the Nuer and the Dinka, also warred with each
other. By 2005, experts estimated that approximately 1.9 million people had
died due to violence, disease, and starvation stemming from the conflict.[51]
Some refugees escaped to camps in Chad, a country that has also seen violent
conflict. Others set up mud huts and tents made of plastic scraps in isolated
desert areas.

     During the Darfur conflict, DWB estimates that 82 percent of rapes in the
area—of which most were gang rapes—occurred when women ventured
away from their refugee camps or villages to graze their cattle or seek food,
water, or firewood. Riding camels or horses, the Janjaweed surrounded the
women, who were unarmed, on foot, and often accompanied by babies or
children. Women who tried to escape could have their arms or legs broken.
Sometimes the women were raped and killed; sometimes they were raped
and left for dead or helped back to camp by their companions. Other rapes
occurred when the Janjaweed stormed camps and villages, as women attempted to flee with their children. Designating daily chores thus became a
ghastly calculation of life and death. Gathering food was essential. Protecting
the camps around the clock was also critical. So who was sent out? As one
report suggests, "Families face the decision of who should bear the brunt of
assault—if they send their sons, they will be killed. If they send their daughters, they will only be raped."[52]

     The actual prevalence of rape during the conflict in Darfur is difficult to
determine. Some victims did not survive. For those who did, reporting a rape
made them vulnerable to police harassment, fines, and rejection by their
community. Given the extreme stigma, rape victims are considered "tainted"

or "unmarriageable" and may be abandoned by husbands or families. A woman from Silaya describes being abducted from her village with eight other women in July 2003: "After six days some of the girls were released. But the others, as young as eight years old, were kept there. Five to six men would rape us in rounds, one after the other for hours during six days, every night. My husband could not forgive me after this, he disowned me."[53] Rape, another Sudanese victim explained, "is a shame, and women will hide this in their hearts so that the men do not hear about it."[54] This "social death" and loss of respect in the community was frequently considered more traumatizing than sexual violence, resulting in widespread silence among women who were able to keep their experiences private. A refugee explained that she would not dare go to a gynecologist even when she arrived in the Netherlands, out of fear that the doctor would write down what had happened to her and her community would somehow discover her secret.[55]

The numbers that *were* reported are sobering. In March 2005, DWB reported that more than 28 percent of the women they interviewed reported being gang-raped and that they had treated almost five hundred rapes in four and a half months.[56] Halima Bashir, a doctor attempting to draw attention to rapes committed at a school near where she worked, was abducted and gang-raped by Janjaweed in retaliation—three men a night until she was rescued.[57] Over 89 percent of women in Darfur have undergone infibulations for cultural and religious reasons—a form of female circumcision where the labia majora, or outer lips of the vulva, are sewn shut, leaving just a small opening for urine and menstrual blood. The procedure, which is designed to ensure chastity and prove virginity, may also involve removing the clitoris and the inner lips of the vulva. Injuries caused by forced intercourse are thus often quite severe.[58]

Pregnancy resulting from rape brings more suffering: women who do not know the name of the father of their baby can be arrested for "illegal pregnancies" and charged with "fornication";[59] married women can also be charged with adultery. Some pregnant victims were given the choice of either paying 15,000 dinars to the police (approximately fifty US dollars, or around two months' salary) or being raped forty more times.[60] Some women committed suicide on finding themselves pregnant through rape. Others killed the infant after birth. Still others raised the children, a new generation with a new family drama. Babies born as a result of rape were believed to be Arab, not black, which accounts for warnings given to victims: "We want to wipe you out" or "We want to finish you people off."[61] Messages were written on— and *in*—women's bodies: "You blacks, you have spoilt the country! We are here to burn you. . . . We will kill your husbands and sons and we will sleep with you! You will be our wives!"

"We will make a light-skinned baby."

Violence in Darfur peaked in 2010. The southern area of Sudan seceded on July 9, 2011, prevailing in a long battle for independence and becoming the Republic of South Sudan. By early 2012, the United Nations reported a "cautious improvement" in Darfur as around one hundred thousand refugees reportedly returned to the region, setting up squatters' camps when their homes and villages no longer existed.[62] Conflicts in the region have persisted, however, and DWB continues to aid refugees fleeing from the border zones of Sudan into South Sudan and Ethiopia.[63] Although the target of Sudanese military forces has shifted to the Nubans, an ethnic group living in the mountains that was aligned with southern rebels before the split, humanitarian reports from the area suggest that gang rape continues to be a problem, reinforcing boundaries of belongingness and exclusion.

Martial rape has been viewed as an unavoidable by-product of violent conflict, resulting from the misuse of power by psychologically conflicted or unstable individuals or "undisciplined troops." The gang rape and massacre of civilians is sometimes committed by rogue individuals, as in the 2006 Mahmudiyah killing and gang rape of a fourteen-year-old girl by US Army soldiers in Iraq, or by isolated military units, perhaps even following orders, as with the Charlie Company at My Lai during the Vietnam War. Wartime rape can bond together young men who are expected to be brave but who may feel fearful, lonely, and vulnerable. Some perpetrators are willing participants; others obey orders or go along with the group out of fear of exclusion or retaliation. The combination of risk, secrecy, and emotional ambivalence is powerful. Soldiers may feel hatred for the "enemy'" but have mixed emotions toward their own country, leaders, or peers for endangering their lives or requiring the loss of comrades. Conquered women (and men) become "easy and fulfilling targets" on which soldiers can release aggression.[64]

But when organized by a military and systematically deployed against specific ethnic groups, mass rape becomes a tactic that should be distinguished from the sexual violence unleashed for centuries against prisoners of war and political prisoners. Mass rape of civilians occurred during the Nanjing Massacre in China, in the former Yugoslavia, in Rwanda, in the Democratic Republic of Congo, and elsewhere. For both perpetrators and victims, mass rape is more symbolically and emotionally loaded than isolated outbreaks of sexual violence, as it is meant to send specific and repeated messages to the populations in conflict. In mass rape, according to philosopher Claudia Card, there is a dual target: the victim and the community. The victim is raped for who she is and then used to warn others in the community about the risk of noncompliance with soldiers' demands. For the victim and the men and women connected to her, the experience "breaks the spirit, humiliates, tames," and produces a "docile, deferential, obedient soul."[65] In the context of already violent conflict, the exclusion of the victim is proof of the perpetrators' ability to permanently undermine the population. She is living evidence of inferiority.

Mass rape thus works as a form of terrorism. Social media and networking sites such as YouTube and Facebook have been demonized for retraumatizing victims as their stories spread across the Internet. But victims can be retraumatized regardless of the state of technology. Often, that is the very point of nonlethal violence. For a gang rape to send a message, there must be an audience, and in mass rape, the audience for those messages increases in size. News certainly travels more quickly when soldiers upload video directly from cell phones to YouTube than when assailants wield handmade machetes in lands without electricity. But even then, messages of mass rape are effectively disseminated to the populace. Survivors share their stories or are identifiable through their injuries, a resulting pregnancy, or abandonment by their families. People may be forced to witness rapes. Those who do not experience or witness the violence directly are meant to hear tales, reinforced by preexisting fears about the enemy. When the Serbs moved in on Kosovo, their sexual cruelty toward Bosniak women was already known. As one woman said, "I wasn't afraid of the killing. I was afraid of the raping."[66] If five supposedly ethnically motivated sexual assaults could "terrorize" an English town, and if *one* woman raped and left for dead—no matter how gruesome—could change New York City "forever," it is difficult to imagine the impact of thousands of targeted, bloody attacks.

Mass rape in warfare can also be a means of genocide. Genocide can be accomplished through mass murder, "killing individual members of a national, political, or cultural group," or "decimating cultural and social bonds" such that a group's identity is destroyed.[67] In his 658-page tome, *Worse Than War*, Daniel Goldhagen surveys outbreaks of genocide around the world. Mass rape, coupled with "excessive cruelty," is one of the tactics included in his research. During the Bosnian war, Serbs reportedly raped twenty thousand to fifty thousand women. The Serbian leadership used a combination of "rape camps" and roaming rape gangs to terrorize Bosniak[68] Muslims and as a strategy of ethnic elimination. Raped women were polluted, shamed in their home communities and in the eyes of their assailants. The repeated raping of women in the camps was designed to ensure that at least some of them became pregnant; those who did were sometimes incarcerated and forced to carry the fetuses to term. Victims reported rapists who sang or celebrated during the attacks. A Bosniak woman recalls her attackers saying, "Fuck your Turkish mother," and "Death to all Turkish sperm." Another woman was told: "You will have a baby. You will bring new life. It will be Serbian. . . . Just Serbian people. We will destroy you, all of you."[69]

As such measures were believed to be producing future generations of Serbs, this example might seem to return to the simplicity of arguments about rape as a primal reproductive strategy. Yet if we dig deeper, we find ourselves in territory far afield from Thornhill's ducks and scorpion flies, in a world of meaning.

Forced pregnancies can shatter ethnic and community ties. Had the Serbs been operating under a "one-drop rule," or a belief that children of mixed ethnicity should be assigned to the group with lower status, forced pregnancies would have increased the Bosniak population rather than shrinking it. But for these rapists, who were also occasionally the fathers of children, the goal was ostensibly to produce a future with more Serbs and fewer Bosniaks, a commitment to their ethnic group exceeding personal evolutionary legacies. Although some Bosniak women raised the children they bore from such violence, others abandoned them in orphanages. These orphans, who are now entering their teen years, face emotional and legal difficulties in contemporary Bosnia and Herzegovina. Schools and social life may be segregated by Serbs, Bosniaks, or Croats. The long-term effects of being without a fixed ethnic identity in such a social milieu are still unknown. In Darfur, pregnancy was often similarly a goal of mass rape, as ethnicity is traced through the father. Janjaweed attackers reportedly told rape victims they wanted to produce "Arab" children who could repopulate the land. But Dinka leaders also stressed women's reproductive role in war, and their soldiers demanded access to women's bodies as "national property." The saying, "I should have as many children as I can in case I die in war," was widespread.[70] Babies born from wartime rape face unpredictable futures, regardless of which ethnic group—if any—claims them. "Janjaweed babies" may be killed or abandoned. Those who survive face challenges in their communities and families. "I will love the child," one woman said, "but I will always hate the father." Some women tried to hide the fact that their children are born of rape—"If the color is like the mother, fine. . . . If it is like the father, then we will have problems. People will think the child is an Arab."[71]

Pregnancy is not always a goal of mass rape, however. In the Nanjing Massacre, Japanese soldiers were ordered to kill women after raping them. Soldiers systematically sought out young women, who were gang-raped, mutilated, and murdered. These soldiers cut off breasts and stuck bayonets or sticks of bamboo into women's vaginas. Pregnant women were bayoneted in the stomach. Survivors understand the message of the sexual violence similarly—through such violent interventions in reproduction, the "future" has been stolen from them. Yet precisely *how* this future is stolen, and through which types of violence, is linked to beliefs about ethnicity and heredity, gender and sexuality, as well as existing systems of social control.

In the neighboring countries of Burundi and Rwanda, Hutu and Tutsi have murdered each other for decades. In Burundi, Tutsi killed thousands of Hutu in 1965, over one hundred thousand in 1972, around twenty thousand in 1988, and three thousand in 1991; Hutu and Tutsi each lost around twenty-five thousand in 1993. In Rwanda, Hutu killed around ten thousand Tutsi in

1963 and around eight hundred thousand Tutsi in 1994. In this latter conflict, mass rape was deployed as a means of genocide, with estimates of between 250,000 and 500,000 women raped. Tutsi were supposedly taller, thinner, more beautiful, and more intellectual than Hutu, who were portrayed as short, stout, and suited for physical labor. Because Tutsi women were thought to manipulate both Hutu and foreign men with their beauty, propaganda was used to incite sexual violence against them. Hutu Power cartoons featured Tutsi women engaged in orgies with Belgian troops. The Rwandan minister of justice, Tharcisse Karugarama, noted that perpetrators justified violence against Tutsi women in part by claiming that Tutsi women despised Hutu men and believed themselves to be superior to Hutu women. Hutu women even encouraged their husbands to rape, "humiliate the victims," and enact vengeance for perceived acts of dishonor.[72]

In these outbreaks of ethnic violence, mass rape was regularly coupled with the murder of the victim; babies and children were killed along with their parents. Women (and sometimes men) were raped with spears, knives, or other objects instead of, or in addition to, penises. Goldhagen references a Human Rights Watch study of Hutu raping based on interviews with victims which found that rape was often accompanied by ritualistic mutilation of the sexual organs: disfiguring the vagina with boiling water or knives, penetrating the vagina or anus with weapons, cutting out unborn children, slicing off breasts, and slashing the pelvic area. One woman described her experience after being raped by Hutu men:

> When he finished he took me inside and put me on a bed. He held one leg of mine open and another one held the other leg. He called everyone who was outside and said, "you come and see how Tutsikazi are on the inside." Then he said, "You Tutsikazi, you think you are the only beautiful women in the world." Then he cut out the inside of my vagina. He took the flesh outside, took a small stick and put what he had cut at the top. He stuck the stick in the ground outside the door and was shouting, "Everyone who comes past her will see how Tutsikazi look.[73]

Goldhagen found her story so disturbing that he almost left it out of the book; however, he included it to illustrate his point that perpetrators of mass violence are not dispassionate or clinical. In such acts of "excess cruelty"—gratuitous physical, verbal, and symbolic violence—Goldhagen believes that we can read the specific messages sent to the victims by the perpetrators as well as see evidence of the preexisting beliefs, prejudices, and fears held by each side.

Group sex is mythically associated with breakdowns in social structure. Because participation requires abandoning inhibitions, individuals involved are feared to risk a loss of individuality and self-control, insanity, and even death. When group sex *begins* with violence, as in gang rape, it can stir fears that the disintegration of human culture has already begun and is about to rage out of control. Yet, as we have seen here, even violent group sex is highly organized and shaped by social processes. More information is necessary to fully analyze these examples of gang rape, and some of these narratives are contested in addition to being incomplete. Alternate cases from around the world might have been chosen. But although limited, this discussion sheds light on the symbolic potency of group sex more generally. Whether we are talking about aborigines at a Gunabibi ceremony, college athletes, Jackrollers, or soldiers, group sex can reflect existing relationships and forge new ones. In violent gang rape, the conflicting perspectives of perpetrators and victims, and even among perpetrators, are often relatively clear. Other group sex scenarios, however, still involve participants with diverse aims, social positions, and experiences and can thus similarly be used to realize human desires for respect, status, and identity.

"GROUP SEX IS TRIBAL" (INTERVIEW, JAY)

Group sex, to me, is tribal. There's this connection between people, this bonding that happens. There's a lot of affectionate touching, not just sex. It's really special. One thing I've noticed as I've gotten older is that being open sexually is less about sex and more about family. I have people to share the aging process with. We are all experiencing changes in our sexuality, and it's nice to have people to talk with about it. And, you know, your family changes as people die. When you're in your seventies, the people around you are *dying*. I've already lost two partners in their sixties. Desire is still important, but now I really crave the intimacy. Sometimes you don't need pounding sex, but someone to just be with you while you take care of yourself. My past sexual experiences have taught me that. Sometimes, I just look around the room at all these naked old people and think about how lucky I am to have people to share this phase of my life with. I know now that getting old doesn't mean the end of sex or of intimacy with others. It's different but still satisfying.

I don't worry about loss. Even though I'm almost eighty, I know that I'll find women to connect with, even if I somehow end up single again. I'm a sexual man and I like myself. Deep down, I enjoy who I am. I know there are women out there who will be attracted to me at any age. I went to check out an old folks' home, because I'm moving into one soon, and the woman who runs it told me, "Jay, you're lucky you're bringing your girlfriend because if you came here alone, you'd be inundated with casseroles!"

My partner is almost sixty, and I've opened her up to new experiences also. I took her to Hedonism and she had oral sex with a woman right by the hot tub while I watched. We've been together a few years and are still exploring. I'm visual. I love watching my partner fuck, though she is less comfortable with it. We had sex with another man a few times. At one point, I was watching from the couch and I could tell she was getting turned on. I enjoyed them being together. But she felt horrible guilt about it later. "I'm supposed to be in love with you," she said. Some things get easier as you age, but other things stay the same—like the need to check in with each other. I think she was worried about my feelings. But I enjoy watching so much that I don't need to always be in the middle of things. I'm thankful to have a committed partner who understands my need for occasionally being sexual with others and accepts it.

I go to fewer sex parties nowadays, though they are still fun and exciting when I do. I threw a party for about twenty people a few weeks ago. The youngest person was a sixty-five-year-old woman. I introduced her to BDSM. She'd been with other men before with her husband in the room. He's eighty-four and likes to watch her have sex with other men while he masturbates. They've done that for a while. But she'd never had someone take the time to really expose her to all the sensory aspects of BDSM, like bondage or feathers.

Sometimes things happen more slowly when it's a bunch of old folks, but people still play. Our parties are loving, accepting. It's not just about getting off, because some of the guys don't even get off! But the women are still hot and have lots of orgasms. Most importantly, everyone laughs together.

BONDING AND ITS DISCONTENTS

In a group sex environment, there's a different thing that happens. When you are having sex 1-on-1, there's an immediate, close sort of thing. Just "you and me," sort of personal intimate contact. But in a group sex situation, you magnify that. It's not about "you and me," it's about us [waves his hands to indicate others]. There's a community, a tribe, a bunch of people who share something. [74]

Bachelor parties ostensibly originated as a way for sexually inexperienced young men to learn about sex before their wedding night. Few men need such instruction nowadays, although the ritual persists among some groups of men. In the United States, bachelor parties can take place at strip clubs or feature strip shows at private homes; occasionally, the bachelor participates in sexual activity with performers, privately or in front of the group. Bachelor events might also involve seeking attention or sex from women in everyday settings. Although some brides are accepting of the bachelor's possible transgressions, others are resistant beforehand or notably hurt afterward. The bachelor's willingness to participate in the ritual anyway, however, is an important declaration of solidarity with certain male friends. How far he is willing to go in terms of sexual activity and whether he is willing to keep secrets from his future spouse can be similar statements. Yet even taking part in the ritual does not guarantee that bonds among the men will be preserved; in fact, the bachelor may change status in the group afterward.

Humiliation of the bachelor is sometimes a goal during parties. He may be stripped, taunted, or tempted onstage at a strip club in the name of "fun," but these sanctioned forms of aggression can also be seen as symbolic punishment for his betrayal of group loyalty through his upcoming marriage. While working as a stripper, I observed firsthand the challenging emotional position into which many bachelors were thrust during these celebrations (not to mention the difficult position of the father of the bride, closeted gay friends, etc.). The stress did not necessarily mean the experience was unpleasant; ambivalence can contribute to excitement if the balance is right. Although it is impossible to generalize extensively about bachelor parties and the social dynamics involved, the point is that while participating in either erotic or sexual activity can be an important means of demonstrating or experiencing belongingness to a group, developing and maintaining status among group members, and claiming identity, these interactions can be fraught with ambivalence and even hostility. Bonds can also be created between some individuals at the expense of others without overt physical violence.

When group sex occurs among an apparently heterosexual group of men and a woman, the scenarios are often termed "homoerotic." Sharing the body of the woman (or women) is believed to be arousing because it draws erotic power from feelings the men have for each other but cannot express directly. But while unacknowledged same-sex desires might exist, it would be a mistake to overlook the other processes and attachments involved. Medical anthropologist Carol Jenkins found that even though institutionalized men's cults have vanished in Papua New Guinea, masculinity is still seen as vulnerable (and valuable) and intense male bonding occurs, sometimes to the detriment of marital bonds. Boys learn about sex from older boys, search for girls together, and eventually may move into group sex scenarios (called *lainap*, "lineup," or *singel fail*, "single file") that are biased toward multiple males and a single female. Jenkins's research team included both male and female interviewers. Men talked about *lainap*, which often took place after meeting women at discos or video parlors, in detail with the male interviewers —"All the young fellows who go around together have turns on one woman. . . . She wouldn't know that we are having turns on her until we have gone to a place where there's no house or no people around and then we start having sex one after the other." The female interviewers found it difficult to elicit stories of group sex from women, however. Because the women considered the sex rape, it was shameful; women bear the responsibility of avoiding male advances and *lainap*. Occasionally, women took part willingly or were paid to participate; if more men joined in than they expected, however, women believed that they had no choice but to submit. In these scenarios, the woman became a form of "booty," shared between men in particular ways—successful, dominant men allowed older men and younger male relatives to "have a chance" (*sans*) at sex with her, for example. The men formed a line, watching each other perform while they took turns having sex with her, occasionally engaging in anal sex with each other as well. "Instead of fighting over a woman," Jenkins writes, in *lainap* "the men show their capacity to cooperate, enjoy each other's sexuality, and totally ignore the woman."[75]

Like many other anthropological examples, Jenkins's research troubles the applicability of a heterosexual/homosexual division across cultures. Condoms were not always used in *lainap*, and participants could be exposed to STDs or HIV directly or through the mixing of body fluids. But while women who contract HIV during *lainap* do so through heterosexual contact, Jenkins points out that when men are infected through the mixing of semen during such events, neither homosexual nor heterosexual transmission makes sense of the circumstances.[76] Same-sex activity, which the men explained as a result of overstimulation, or "going crazy," is not overtly connected to claims of sexual identity (gay, straight, or bisexual) and emerges in a context where male same-sex relations have historical, cosmological meaning.

Even when men do not have physical contact with each other, there is more to consider than repressed sexual desire. Researchers working with Mexican migrant laborers in Northern California found that almost half visited prostitutes while in the United States and 13 percent reported participating in a bonding ritual where several men had sex with the same prostitute in succession. Afterward, the men referred to themselves as *hermanos de leche*, or "milk brothers."[77] Sharing a prostitute could be a financial decision, but it could also be related to feelings of loneliness experienced by migrant laborers, many of whom have left wives and families in Mexico.

Sociologist Clifton Evers suggests that men on sports teams "are familiar with bonding through their bodies"—they "go through physical pain together . . . train together . . . get inked-up together."[78] Group sex, consensual or not, can become another way of forging connection through *doing* rather than talking or sharing emotions. Athletes who share women often display a surprising lack of jealousy toward teammates during these encounters—at least when it comes to women who fall into the "share" category. Desmond Morris, known for applying a zoological perspective to human behavior, suggests that sharing sexual conquests serves a leveling function, even temporarily, when ability or compensation varies across players; Ryan and Jethá refer to this as "prehistoric egalitarianism."[79] English "football groupie" Amanda

Hughes (a pseudonym) began having sex with famous soccer players when she was eighteen. "Once you were in a player's hotel room," she explained, "he would encourage you to allow his mates to join in. I never understood why—the argument seemed to be that it was 'only fair' that they have the same as he was having." Sometimes a player's friends would "suddenly 'appear' in the bedroom doorway," she explained, "and it would be assumed you didn't mind." Hughes was never gang-raped, but she also did not protest when teammates arrived.[80] Yet as we saw in violent scenarios, bonding does not preclude conflicting interests or competition. As in campus rapes or *lainap*, some women report acquiescing to unwanted group sex with athletes out of fear or helplessness—cooperation can result from the expectation of coercion.

In Thailand, visiting prostitutes serves as a "rite of passage" for some groups of young men. As a way to demonstrate heterosexuality to their peers, the young men visit brothels alone or in groups; condom use in such situations is inconsistent. The men vie for status through both drinking heavily and boasting about sexual conquests, leading one researcher to analyze the excursions as "an avenue for one-upmanship, competition, and demonstration of merit." Another researcher, though, maintains the outings are "an opportunity for irresponsible fun," to escape from a restrictive social environment, and a way that friends demonstrate support for one another. These explanations, however, are not mutually exclusive. Both researchers note the influence of peers on patterns of condom use and sexual activity—men were sometimes ridiculed for insisting on condom use, for example, and men admitted that they would rarely turn down a friend's request to visit a brothel. Given local beliefs about male sexuality as impulsive, nonmonogamous, and risk oriented, along with cultural norms valuing "community and social harmony," it is unsurprising that men claim to make independent decisions while at that same time exerting powerful influences on one anothers' behavior.[81]

While the sexual practices of working class men, migrant laborers, and street prostitutes have been studied around the world, often in the name of public health, far less is written on more privileged individuals. This pattern is related to scholarship norms, but also to the fact that privilege affords invisibility. If I were able to share the details of the many stories I've been told about relatively privileged American men arranging sex for friends, colleagues, clients, or club members, this section would be far longer: raffles and contests at retreats where the winner is treated to sex acts while the others watch, prostitutes competing for the chance to accompany a wealthy man into private quarters by displaying sexual skills, golf "tournaments" where politicians were served beds of well-paid Barbie look-alikes along with their sushi and Cristal—in exchange for other gestures of good will, of course. Given the transgressions required by participants when illegal behavior is involved, *all* are implicated—the man who wins the favors of a hooker, reaping momentary sexual rewards or status, is simultaneously the group member who is most at risk of exposure and thus the most dependent on the others for protection.

Sex workers and groupies probably know some of the most intriguing private details about the wealthy and powerful men of this world. But even though a few women make headlines by divulging these secrets, why do so many others keep their mouths shut? Bonds are not created just between the men in consensual group sex scenarios, but also between the men and women. Women's participation in group sex, especially encounters involving many men, is often skeptically or simplistically attributed to coercion or psychological dysfunction. Yet professional athletes—and even high-school competitors—can attest to the fact that some women seek these central roles and even compete for them. Professional Australian surfer Nat Young wrote about the sexualized and masculinized beach culture in his 1998 autobiography. During his teen years in the early 1960s, he spent his time surfing on Collaroy Beach north of Sydney and thinking about sex. While a few girls surfed, they did not necessarily have sex; by default, "sexual intercourse became a group activity, involving several surfers and one of the more promiscuous girls who hung around the scene." The sex was consensual, as Young tells the story, and although the girls "weren't well-respected in the normal sense of the word," "strong ties" developed between them and the young male surfers.

> The Grunter was really into group sex and we all greeted her with open flies every time we saw her getting off the school bus. This began happening a few times a week on a regular basis, then every weekend when all the crew at Collaroy would join the queue. . . . Other girls from our beach started to get a bit jealous of all the attention the Grunter was getting and some decided it was better to join her if they couldn't beat her. The competition was terrific. "Brenda the Bender," "Sally Apple Bowels," the list got longer and longer and we had plenty of activity down at the beach in between riding waves. [82]

In some cultures, sexually active women can make no claims to deserving respect (and safety), or very weak claims to it, whether in the eyes of their peers, relatives, or the law. In other locales, respect becomes an axis of distinction. But the belief that women *should* want men's respect "in the normal sense of the word"—and should align their sexuality with mainstream norms in order to get it—can cause us to overlook the complexity of motivations involved and the benefits some women perceive in stepping outside of gendered expectations. Pamela des Barres, a classic 1970s groupie turned author, reminisced that although groupies were thought of as "sluts" by outsiders, the women sought more than sex. They wanted to be part of something "important" and close to the "incredible musical brilliance" of the performers.[83] Some women still relish the glamour and rewards that come with having powerful associations or enjoy the pursuit and conquest of men they find highly desirable. "Jersey chasers" follow most professional sports teams. NFL groupies fill entire hotels in cities that are hosting important football games. Sex with multiple players is just another menu option. CEOs may find themselves similarly pursued by women, although given that the business of running companies is rewarded independently rather than as a team sport, group sex scenarios may vary. Women also willingly engage in group sex with men who are not famous or wealthy for reasons ranging from the desire for protection to their own sexual pleasure or adventure. Just as all men's participation in group sex should not be reduced to homoerotics, all women's participation cannot simplistically be attributed to low self-esteem, masochism, or other psychological disturbances—even if homophobia or misogyny emerge during some of the encounters.

Although not all women want to bargain for "respect" in the traditional sense, respect becomes a recurring topic in discussions about groupies in the United States and Europe. Groupies should "respect themselves." Players should "show some respect." Hughes suggests that players be taught basic courtesy to avoid scandal: "show a girl some respect, be nice and don't ignore her the morning after."[84] But the "morning after" is light years away nowadays, especially given the ease of replacing a woman who is too demanding. Another groupie is already on her knees. ("Gutter groupies," one writer suggests, are women willing to do almost anything to service an NBA player, including providing oral sex in the parking lot of the arena.)[85] In some ways, talk about respect reflects the lack of bonds created during exchanges, especially in an atmosphere of seemingly endless supply and constant turnover. On the flip side, the days of waiting, like des Barres did, until one's conquest retires from the public eye to report on his anatomy, sexual preferences, or skills are over. Websites and message boards allow contemporary groupies to share personal and practical information about athletes, rock stars, and other celebrities. Digging through GroupieDirt.com, for example, you can find some interesting nuggets and an occasional gem: Eminem supposedly once hired a "groupie wrangler" to cull the herd of hopefuls and asks to videotape the sex on his cell phone. The members of Whitesnake like "to line their women up and take turns." Kid Rock loves orgies and fisting. The band members in Orgy like to have orgies. David Bowie likes orgies (but not airheads). Sting likes orgies (and hookers). And so on.

But the game is still played with a set of unwritten rules. Groupie Kat Stacks, for example, became a "divisive" figure in the hip-hop community by talking too much and too scandalously while using more expletives than a gangster flick. Stacks, a former Florida stripper, started propositioning celebrities on Twitter and then reporting about the sex on her blog, calling out men for having a "little ass motherfucking dick" and even publicizing rappers' phone numbers if it did not go well ("harrass that fat motherfucker"). With a quarter of a million Twitter followers and over twenty million hits on her blog, Stacks found an audience—and trouble. In 2010, she was assaulted by two men on video. The men demanded that she "apologize" and "watch her mouth," possibly in retaliation for insulting the rappers Fabolous and Lil' Bow Wow. Considered one of the "most hated" contemporary groupies, Stacks is frequently called a "ho" who "exploits" rappers for fame. Her position on the matter, however, is that she is standing up for women by publicizing her exploits and didn't do anything more than what "most rappers rap about, hoes . . . and spending money." If one is going to seek fame through controversy, though, even if only for fifteen minutes, it is probably best to have a green card—Stacks was deported to Venezuela after spending two years in jail for residing illegally in the United States. [86]

A TALE OF TWO PARTIES

The Minnesota Vikings found themselves in hot water in 2005 after some of the players rented yachts and hookers for an evening excursion on Lake Minnetonka. (*"If it floats, flies, or fucks . . ."*) In hindsight, the athletes should have hired their own crew as well, because while their antics didn't shock the working girls flown in from Atlanta and Florida for the occasion, the small-town crew members were appalled at the party that began shortly after pulling away from the dock. Alarms were initially raised when the women used the downstairs rooms to change into G-strings. Then the lap dances started. Dancing became "grinding," grinding became "groping," and groping became full-scale "debauchery," escalating until the captain ordered the boat back to shore several hours ahead of schedule. The crew members were responsible for identifying seventeen Vikings players and providing juicy details about the party to police investigators: naked women, a man performing oral sex on a woman on top of the bar, men receiving oral sex in deck chairs, and a sex toy demonstration in the lounge. [87] Fred Smoot, a defensive back signed to the team earlier that year, was exposed as the player "manipulating" the double-headed dildo into the vaginas of two women while teammates shouted instructions. Smoot was also declared the "ringleader" of the event. Although he denied the masterminding allegations, Smoot had indeed signed the contract with the boat rental company. His teammate, Lance Johnstone, used a credit card to cover the security deposit.

Each year, rookie players planned a party for the veterans of the team. This wasn't the first time that strippers or hookers had been recruited for the traditional festivities, nor was it the first time that Vikings players stripped down and partied with girls on Lake Minnetonka. Publicly chartering the two 64-foot boats from Al & Alma's Supper Club was a mistake, however. As a former Minnesota Viking explained to *Sports Illustrated*, in the past, they used a boat that one of the players owned. These commercial yachts, on the other hand, were usually rented for romantic moonlight cruises, not sex parties; the employees, portrayed as "innocent" in court documents by the lawyer for Al & Alma's, hadn't ever seen a lap dance before, much less a live dildo show. "To have a wild party out there," the former player said, "it doesn't take a genius to figure out that's a horrible idea."[88]

The "Love Boat scandal"—named because sports talk-show hosts played the "Love Boat" theme when discussing it—was an instant media favorite. Smoot and a teammate eventually pled guilty to "disorderly conduct" and "being a public nuisance on a watercraft" and paid thousand-dollar fines. The NFL imposed a one-game check fine on the players—a harsher punishment in financial terms, given that Smoot's penalty was $82,352.

Smoot was supposedly disliked by his Eden Prairie neighbors for failing to pay his homeowner's association fees, neglecting to water his grass, and throwing loud, late-night parties with lots of "naked ladies in the hot tub" (according to a teenage boy living nearby).[89] But had he not bungled the logistics of the rookie party, he might have still been quite popular with his teammates. After all, from another perspective, the "Love Boat" incident could be an example of community-building, conflict-reducing sexuality. Smoot was a newcomer, trying to win favor with the more established males on the team. He was being paid a large salary and hadn't proved himself yet. The rookies were presumably footing the bill for the evening's entertainment, an act of generosity. Morale was low among the Vikings, as recent weeks had seen team bickering, an angry owner, a proposal for a new $790 million stadium defeated, and a depressing 28–3 loss to the Chicago Bears. Instead of claiming a hoped-for status as a Super Bowl contender, the team was facing the harsh reality of being considered "the biggest flop of 2005."[90] If there was ever a time when group cohesion was at stake, this was it. The message Smoot sent to his teammates when he asked the hookers to lie on the floor and share the purple double-dildo wasn't quite the same as what Annie Sprinkle hopes to convey to her audiences during her "Public Cervix Announcement." But it was a message of solidarity, nonetheless, with ardent audience participation. If the Vikings players hadn't disastrously clashed with the "outside world"—from the "innocent" servers and boat captains of Al & Alma's, to the local police, to the higher-ups at the NFL, to the general public, each of whom had different grievances—the sexual practices engaged in during this annual tradition probably would have brought great joy to the team.

As for the Vikings players' female consorts, much less is known. The working girls most likely knew the culturally acceptable ways to be "generous" with their bodies—which are supposed to be exchanged only for love, indirectly for material goods such as shoes, diamonds, cars, or houses, or occasionally for pleasure (though not too frequently or enthusiastically). They simply chose to accept money instead, possibly the reason they didn't talk to the press.

The United States is a large, highly stratified society that can only be compared tongue in cheek with a small-scale tribal group such as the Canela. Smoot had signed a six-year deal with the Vikings for $34 million, including an $11 million signing bonus, an amount of money that most upscale escorts couldn't dream of earning (without marrying a football player). The party, though based on an ideal of female sexual availability, would have unfolded differently in a context where such sharing was a community-wide norm rather than an aberration. My point, however, is that even when socio-erotic exchanges among group members contribute to community building and conflict reduction, this doesn't necessarily tell us anything about sexuality or society more generally. What sex means, or does, depends on the context and perspective. It matters whether you're the rookie teammate, the veteran player, the blonde escort squashed into 14B, the brunette hooker sipping cocktails in first class (rewarded for last year's generosity), the young waitress horrified at being asked to give a lap dance, or the captain wading through used condoms on the deck of the boat. It matters how many of these parties you've been to already—while sports commentators couldn't get enough of the salacious details, Smoot later told an interviewer that the party was "overrated." (I'm with Smoot—on that detail, anyway. The proceedings sound tame for the amount of press it received.) It matters whether you are analyzing the evening from the perspective of a journalist, evolutionary biologist, social psychologist, feminist theorist, or all of the above. And it matters what story you want to tell about sexuality.

Consider "key parties."

Journalist Terry Gould suggests that modern swinging originated among World War II air force pilots as a way to cement bonds between families in case one of the men was killed in battle, a claim that seems to have originated in the work of sexologists Dwight and Joan Dixon in the 1980s.[91] The frequency with which this account is put forth in popular discussions of swinging shows that it strikes a nerve, possibly because tracing swinging back to these highly skilled and "often extraordinarily attractive" risk takers ("with every pilot carrying a set of genes that was probably in the top 1 percent of the nation," Gould asserts) is appealing to current-day lifestylers. Another reason this chronicle is retold is probably because it ascribes a social purpose to behavior often viewed as deviant. Swinging as a form of socio-erotic exchange that strengthens communal bonds sounds almost virtuous, no longer just a kinky or selfish way to spend a Saturday night. And finally, the account resonates because it is at least partially true—for some participants, important bonds *are* created through these sexual exchanges—regardless of whether air force pilots figured that out first. Gould traces the term "key club" to the same military legacy, although he points out that "it remains unconfirmed whether airmen actually threw keys in a hat, their wives then randomly choosing one and making love with the owner."[92]

Ryan includes the story of the fighter pilots in *Sex at Dawn* and blogged about it for *Psychology Today*. Ryan quotes from Gould's interview with the Dixons, proffering swinging as an example of how "these warriors and their wives shared each other as a kind of tribal bonding ritual." Yet although he doesn't claim outright that the pilots transacted these swaps using a key-based lottery, he doesn't mention the ambiguity either; he also invokes the film *The Ice Storm* (1997), which includes a memorable key party scene with disastrous effects.[93] This gloss is inconsequential in terms of his argument about socio-erotic exchanges as a means by which humans build community and reduce conflict. Similarly, whether some Inuit women thought that "wife exchange" in the name of hospitality was a bad idea or whether some Canela women resisted tradition and had to be taught generosity does not detract from a claim that monogamy is not the human evolutionary pinnacle. But when the story being told shifts from being about what sex does for a community to assuming how it *feels* for participants—when mate sharing is "unflinching," sexuality is "relaxed" or "unencumbered by guilt," or behavior is "shamelessly libidinal"—these details begin to matter quite a bit.

In middle school, we played a game called "Two Minutes in the Closet"—a group of boys and girls sat in a circle around an empty Coke bottle, which was spun to determine with whom we would retire to the small, dark space (in our case, not a closet but a basement laundry room). Given that my partner and I sat in silence, surrounded by dirty socks, for what felt like eternity the only time I participated, we were lucky we weren't playing "Seven Minutes in Heaven." But despite this preteen experience in (relatively) random partner selection, and even though I have attended hundreds of erotic events, I have never been to an actual key party, been invited to a key party, or interviewed someone who has *personally* attended a key party, whether in the 1960s or in the decades that followed. I haven't found reliable scholarly accounts of key parties, though they are sporadically mentioned. Such a lack of evidence screams "urban legend," although as with other scandalous but unverified sexual practices from "rainbow parties" to the "soggy biscuit game," once the idea is out, someone, somewhere has tried it—even if only a writer at Nerve.com, "doing it for science."[94] Call it the power of suggestion. (Now that I've written these words, maybe I'll find out that key parties happen all the time and I'm just not making the cut.) I've heard of lifestyle events with themes of "key party" or "lock and key," where participants draw a key that fits the lock assigned to another guest—but the new pairs do not even necessarily hook up, much less leave the premises together. I've heard of dozens of other creative party themes, some of which are specifically designed to get guests unclothed or interacting quickly. Overall, though, the logistics of a true key party just don't fit the desires of most contemporary American lifestyle couples for ongoing negotiation between spouses, consent to each encounter, and bifurcating domestic space from space used for sexual recreation.

This doesn't mean that there aren't people who eroticize random, even anonymous, sex or who do not want the responsibility or hassle of choosing their partners—there are plenty. They just don't need to throw a key party to get it. Craigslist and Grinder work just fine. Sex clubs with dark rooms. Bars and nightclubs.

Stories are told for a purpose and circulated because they strike a chord with the community consuming them. Tales about key parties, I believe, often betray both outsiders' and participants' ambivalence toward randomness or absence of choice in contemporary swinging. In fact, one of the myths that lifestylers routinely confront is that they are open to any and all sexual partners; certainly, both this assumption and lifestylers' defensive responses to it is affected by negative connotations of promiscuity. Lifestylers also repeatedly confront myths that women must be coerced to participate, even though they place an overt value on female agency—"wife swapping" went out of style long before "free love," and the contemporary lifestyle isn't *either*. (In fact, women's freedom to choose their partners is often so emphatically stated that it is difficult to even broach the topic of power differentials that impact men's and women's experiences in the lifestyle, even if the spears have been laid aside.) If one wants to argue that female sexual availability and frequent socio-erotic exchanges produce a social milieu where sexuality is relaxed, shamelessly libidinous, and nonpossessive, though, key parties certainly make for a better example than the couple locked in the bathroom at a swingers' party, negotiating heatedly about which couple they should invite back to their hotel room and whether doing so would be "taking one for the team."

Key parties, bachelor parties, Wild Boar Day, Gunabibi ceremonies, and Smoot's "Love Boat" excursion are all examples of how community members forge and sustain relationships through group sexuality. The process, however, is complex—and I believe that it always was, whether or not it appears that way from a modern vantage point. (For some individuals, the possibility of opting out of traditional practices they find unfair or unappealing is one of the benefits of industrialized, capitalist, mobile and fragmented societies.) The sexual exchanges engaged in by the Canela contributed to community building and conflict reduction—but so did those of the Murgin and the Marind-anim. Bonding is not inconsistent with the existence of hierarchy, power, or competition, as bonds can be created out of fear as well as affection. Sometimes sexual bonding rituals reaffirm existing hierarchies or spawn new ones; other times, "sharing" momentarily levels an unequal playing field. Socio-erotic exchanges might be ritualized or casual, violent, affec tionate, or indifferent; some individuals may benefit more than others even when everyone consents. Bonding can bring some individuals closer while others are literally or symbolically excluded. The social impact of such inclusions and exclusions varies depending on one's position—whether the unsuspecting woman at the center of a *lainap*, the young man pressured into visiting a brothel, the executive who turns down his opportunity to lick a whipped-cream bikini off an escort at a retreat, or the wife-to-be sitting home while her fiancé rages in Vegas. Individuals participate for varying reasons, from a belief in sexual generosity to the desire for pleasure, to gain resources or because of a lack of options. One can encounter danger, even violence, in sexual activity even as one also, at times, experiences "great sexual freedom and fun." As sexual experiences are interpreted and reinterpreted, what sex does or means for a group and for individuals depends on a broader social, political, historical, and economic context. Both Rebombo and the woman he raped told stories of shame and fear, although he did not interpret his act as criminal until years later. Among some tribes, sexual practices labeled "deviant" and suppressed by colonial forces actually increased in importance and frequency for a time, even if driven underground.

Is it only because I live in an individualistic, capitalistic, competitive society that my thoughts immediately turn to my own selfish preferences when hypothetically contemplating a key party: *Do I really have to have sex with that irritating guy whose keys I just picked? Is he going to crash the car or ask me to cook him breakfast? Does my husband remember that he's not allowed to have sex with anyone else in our home? No other woman can see the dozens of animal print outfits I left slung around the bathroom like the aftermath of a big game safari—how embarrassing—maybe they can have sex in the SUV instead? Why couldn't I have drawn the other set of BMW keys, the ones belonging to the hot new neighbor?*

Might I be overlooking the significance of such an exchange because, unlike ancestral foragers, the tribal Canela, or air force pilots, my survival is not directly interdependent with the "group" whose shiny keys are beckoning from the bottom of the bowl?

Now, maybe if I were being offered a meat pie . . .

Case Study: A Life Fantastic

Some theorists suggest that public and group sex was central to the processes of identity formation that eventually burst into the US gay liberation movement of the 1970s. Activist Patrick Moore asserts that "in the 1970s gay men used sex as the raw material for a social experiment so extreme that I liken it to art." Sex, he argues, became like theater or performance art, a means of "creative exploration and expression."[1] But why sex? And why group sex in particular? Certainly, the development of gay male identity in the United States has a multilayered history that might be traced differently through rural and urban populations or across social classes and races. Men have been having sex with other men in parks or bathhouses as long as there have been parks or bathhouses, and not all gay men of the time participated in sexual culture or saw it as a path to social change. This section is not meant to generalize about all gay men, then or now, but to illustrate how forces combined at that historical juncture to make group sex meaningful as a mode of personal and political rebellion for a specific population.

For many same-sex-desiring men in the United States living midcentury, life was about invisibility. This had not always been the case. In *Gay New York*, historian George Chauncey argues that the late nineteenth and early twentieth centuries saw an "extensive gay world" taking shape in New York City, where "fairies" interacted with sailors in the Bowery and lesbians gathered with bohemians in Greenwich Village. In the 1920s and 1930s, antigay laws were instituted as a response to the challenges this growing visibility posed to the social order. Gay life was forced underground. As gay men adopted styles of masculinity enabling them to "pass" instead of performing openly as "sissies" or "fairies," they were demonized: "The fact that homosexuals no longer seemed easy to identify made them seem even more dangerous, since it meant that even the next-door neighbor could be one."[2] In the

1950s, as well as being a crime, homosexuality was considered a psychological disorder. Many establishments did not allow openly homosexual patrons; police harassment, entrapment, and arrest were common. If discovered, men with same-sex desires risked violence from gay-bashers and ostracization from families and friends. "The dangers gay men faced increased rapidly in the postwar decades," Chauncey writes, yet at the same time, new bonds were being forged among them. The growing gay enclaves in cities since the turn of the century provided safety, connection, and some degree of escape from the closet.

In the 1960s and 1970s, gay men continued migrating to urban centers seeking relief from social and familial pressures. Organized resistance to antigay legislation and public violence was already underway in New York; so, too, was the creation of what historian Jeffrey Escoffier has dubbed a "new gay sexual culture," which "gave gay men a chance to learn about sex and about other gay men in a public setting rather than in more furtive personal encounters." Watching others was educational and exciting. The sheer availability of sexual encounters—especially for men who had grown up with a sense of lack and shame—was also thrilling. A man could "cruise someone on the way to work, pass a phone number to him, and meet him for sex in the office during lunch time"; men could "dart off into doorways for quick blow jobs and orgasms." New York's raunchy sexual landscape, from Christopher Street to Fire Island, Escoffier writes, "generated a rich body of personal stories and in later years achieved a mythological status—marked iconic references such as 'the trucks,' 'the piers,' and 'the tubs.'"[3] Individual experiences, along with stories of those experiences, were shared, generating a sense of belonging.

Participating in public sexual culture was about pleasure but also about developing new understandings of bodies and desires. Although illegal until 1976, when the Consenting Adult Sex Bill was passed, bathhouses had operated in the United States since the turn of the century. Police periodically raided bathhouses, but they were still safer than outdoor locations. Ira Tattleman argues that while some saw the baths as an extension of the closet—gay men pursued orgasms but remained relatively invisible unless raided—others saw the baths as places where men could finally express themselves "outside the language of a homophobic society" and "experience commonality." Patrons gained confidence by watching other men and learned about sex "as performance, technique, and mutual satisfaction." Patrons shed outside identities and followed a uniform dress code, wearing a single white towel; the dim lighting required them to "favor other senses over sight." Bathhouses also displaced a focus on speech, as "behavior was coded by location, posture, eye contact, and hand gestures." Water, which engaged on a tactile level, and continuous music enveloped patrons in a "timeless" and "secluded" world that helped "loosen long-imposed restraints" on their sexuality.[4]

Group sexuality engaged in at the sex clubs, bathhouses, parties, and other public sex locations on each coast became "at heart, a form of political resistance to a so-called 'normal' world that attempted to control queerness through shame."[5] Through witnessing and being witnessed, gay men participated in rites of passage and initiation rituals. Sociologist Michael Pollack argues that "homosexual rites," such as fisting, "combine individualistic elements with others which reveal a collective belonging."[6] "In spite of their communal, affirmative nature," he writes, "specifically homosexual orgies are first of all actions of apprenticeship and promotion of individual sexual freedom."[7] For some participants, gay male leather communities permitted them "to be something not allowed in more ordinary life," providing empowerment and companionship on the "long struggle toward selfhood."[8] This newfound affirmation of the self was coupled with a sense of belonging. S/M could "initiate" a gay man into a community of men with particular ideas about what it means to be masculine and gay at a given point in time and into a new physical relationship with his body beyond the "disdain, shame, and hatred" patriarchy had heaped upon it. Although the body is tested and marked in BDSM, it is also "resurrected."[9] Participants could achieve new awareness and personal transformation. The desire to be witnessed in such rituals is not simple exhibitionism, Tim Dean notes, but a wish "for cultural rather than individual sanction that is particularly important in the case of nonnormative or stigmatized erotic activities."[10]

The Catacombs was an underground gay BDSM club that operated out of a private residence in San Francisco during the 1970s. Events were invitation-only. Anthropologist Gayle Rubin describes the Catacombs as a place that engendered "camaraderie and loyalty" and allowed for "intense bodily experiences, intimate connection, male fellowship, and having a good time." Patrons engaged in "wild excess," serious physical trials, and playful Crisco fights or poppers-sniffing contests in an environment that offered acceptance, protection, and comfort. Part of the legacy of the Catacombs, Rubin believes, was "a very deep love for the physical body" and "its capacities for sensory experience."[11] The Catacombs also "offered men the opportunity to further diversify and specify their sexuality whether or not they perceived any political implications to doing so. Instead of generic homosexuality, it delineated a community of men who were drawn to masculinity, fisting, and S/M." Even then, differences arose. "Some old-fashioned leathermen," Patrick Califia writes, "thought fisting was dreadful and had nothing to do with S/M. They were not about to get Crisco on their leather. Some fisters thought S/M was violent and extreme. Old-guard leather was a beer and bourbon scene; fisting was MDA and poppers." Mainstream gays and lesbians were often hostile toward both BDSM and fisting, worried such practices would thwart their attempts at assimilating with heteronormative culture. [12] Despite the divisions and disagreements, however, sexuality provided a realm for identity construction among men that would become important in the decades to come.

Although there were overlaps with the sexual ideals of 1960s "hippie" youth movements, the notion of sex as a means of political rebellion took on a particular shape and importance in these gay male worlds of the time. In a context of violence, illegality, stigma, pathologization, and isolation, group sex became a route to intense feelings of liberation—not for all men and not the only route, but an important one nonetheless. In some writing of the time, witnessing each other, or being witnessed, during group sex or in bathhouses became an explicitly political act. The magazine *Fag Rag* debuted in 1971. Charles Shively contributed articles such as "Indiscriminate Promiscuity as an Act of Revolution" or "Cock-Sucking as an Act of Revolution." He positioned "gay male sexuality and sensibility as the central tools for revolutionary change in America" because they posed challenges to "the morals (monogamy) and institutions (marriage and the church) that were at the center of American capitalism." "The greatest empire in the world fell apart because of self-indulgence and lack of personal discipline," Shively reasoned. "Now if cock-sucking could bring down Rome, think what we might do to Capitalism and the American system of imperial terror . . . SHOW HARD. MAKE DATE." [13]

The utopian ideals of sexual revolutionaries were not always realized, of course. Even before the AIDS epidemic, some gay men criticized the objectification and competitive masculinity expressed in public sexual cultures. The figure of the "clone" [14] —a tough, macho, muscular man—displaced stereotypes of gay men as effeminate but was accompanied by pressure to live up to a narrow physical ideal. Clones followed masculinized sexual scripts emphasizing anonymous, experimental, occasionally rough sex, often in groups. Sexual performance became a competitive way to claim status. Some critics claimed the focus on sex made for shallow relationships; socializing revolved around sex partying rather than intimacy or sustainable connections. Transgression provided only ephemeral thrills, and after their orgasms subsided, the men remained isolated, sometimes experiencing even more self-loathing. Drug use progressed throughout the 1970s, occasionally enhancing men's experiences but sometimes becoming excessive to overcome inhibitions, escape emotional pain, or engage in ever more extreme sexual practices. For some men, then, the culture "delivered acceptance, even spiritual transcendence, while for others it was filled with cliques and cruelty." [15]

In 1976, one of the more infamous New York City clubs, the Mineshaft, opened alongside the slaughterhouses of the meatpacking district. Patrons entered through an unmarked door, where a guard controlled entry. The activities became progressively more extreme as one moved farther inside—

first past the "glory hole" wall and fisting area, then down another stairway into a basement featuring bathtubs for "piss pigs" and dark back rooms, where men who were less attractive or more interested in edgier activities congregated.[16] Escoffier analyzes the Mineshaft as an entertainment complex where paid performers created grand sexual spectacles for patrons but also acted as "coaches" and guides. The "real" and the "fantastic" were separate realms; the Mineshaft was "a portal into an erotic fantasy world" where patrons could enhance their sexual pleasure and stimulate their imaginations.[17] Other theorists, however, took a less celebratory view of the extreme S/M found at the Mineshaft, arguing that it wasn't liberating or creative but instead a manifestation of deep psychological wounds. Journalists of the time described scenes that, when decontextualized, supported interpretations of degeneracy rather than playfulness: "a circle of men stand around a bath tub, urinating upon a semi-nude man who fondles his penis and moans, 'Piss on me, Yeah, piss on me.'"[18] "The cluster of bathtubs was an otherworldly sight," Moore writes, "and the piss pigs lying in them, ready for use, seemed to have reached an altered state not just from whatever drugs they might have been using but from the act in which they were absorbed. Their pleading eyes looked elsewhere."[19]

In 1978, outspoken activist Larry Kramer published *Faggots*, a satirical look at gay male culture that became one of the best-selling gay novels of all time. His characters seek sex incessantly at places named the Toilet Bowl, the Meat Rack, and Fuckteria, believing that plunging into the "pit of sexuality" is a necessary part of "the faggot lifestyle—to find abandonment and freedom through ecstasy."[20] One of the characters eventually finds himself voyeuristically watching a man

> fucking himself by sitting on a stationary twelve-inch rubber dildo while being bound hand and foot, the dildo impaled to a cross, the cross mounted on a stage, and the fellow also sucking the cock of a gentleman clad entirely in chain mail, except of course for his genitals, which were exposed, and enormous, and holding in his hand while mouth-fucking the impaled acolyte, not one but two hissing rattlesnakes, reputed to have been defanged but dripping something from their mouths nevertheless, all of this witnessed by forty-nine other members, each donged with grease, each jerking off either himself or a fellow clubber.

He then has an epiphany: Was he going to be left endlessly playing "'Can You Top This?' every time he wanted to get his rocks off?"[21]

How far did they need to go to bring down an empire?

Some critics declared the revolution a failure. Author John Rechy, who based some of his novels on his own sexual exploits, wrote, "What kind of revolution is it that ends when one *looks* old, at least for most? What kind of revolution is it in which some of the revolutionaries must look beautiful?

What kind of revolution is it in which the revolutionaries slaughter each other, in the sexual arenas and in the ritual of S&M?"[22] Sex alone, even transgressive orgy sex, proved unable to overthrow heteronormative society just as, for the hippies, it wasn't enough to vanquish capitalism. As Rechy acknowledged, unrelenting "outside pressures" from the straight world, such as hatred or "imposed guilt," meant that radical gay male sexual cultures could never live up to their promise as a "noble revolt."[23] With the dawning of the AIDS epidemic in the early 1980s, bathhouses and other public sex spaces became demonized as "killing fields" rather than sites of liberation, revolution, or salvation. Even men who had experienced a "baptism" in the public sex culture of the previous decade, such as Marco Vassi, grew disillusioned. In 1985, the Mineshaft was closed by the New York City Department of Health. Sexual encounters become "weighed down with a roster of questions about safety and the nagging aura of self-destruction and shame."[24] In his retrospective commentary, Moore acknowledges that while repression may lead people to respond creatively, it also creates emotional damage, "meaning that the sexual explorations of the 1970s, while creative, would also be marked by extremity."[25] The "triumphant act of coming out and living an open life does not erase the damage done by living in fear during one's development," he cautions, and the more destructive side of the 1970s sex scene must be analyzed in "the context of men who faced enormous emotional challenges."[26]

Still, the process of claiming space, participation in group sexual rites and rituals, and the experience of witnessing and being witnessed in transgressive sex, led at least some gay men—albeit relatively privileged ones—to construct powerful cultural critiques. As they finally began to "explore their sexual fantasies in public," they started to envision a world "where homosexuality was not demonized but celebrated." They began to "learn from and support other men, exchange ideas, build community structures, and raise a political ruckus."[27]

Further, the relationship of emotional wounds to sexual pleasure is complex. Pain and pleasure transform into each other. One's man degradation becomes another man's ecstasy. Barry Charles, known as "Troughman," describes being a "piss pig" in the Mineshaft as "sexual heaven." His first night in the tub was intensely exciting: "I knew I was never going to get over this moment of identification with my innermost sexual desire and I never have."[28] Charles resists explanations for his love of watersports: "One part of me would like to go into the psychology of it, and another part of me says, no, just enjoy it." The point, for him, of the public "piss orgies" he participated in—which he did not abandon after the Mineshaft closed—was to indulge his "central sexual turn on"; the point of his activism was to push boundaries and increase tolerance of sexual practices and desires. "What's the point of gay politics if it's not about sex? What's the point if you can't do it?"[29]

Some writers and participants embraced sacred sexuality as the next step, a cultural progression toward a more authentic existence. In 1984, Canadian biochemist Geoff Mains published *Urban Aboriginals*, a book using tribal themes to critique Western culture's disavowal of the body. After exploring the West Coast gay communities in Vancouver and San Francisco, Mains had come to believe that alternative sexuality could have a significant impact on society. Gay leathermen, he argued, had created a new tribal culture based on both universal, primitive human capacities and experiences that evoked extreme sensation or emotion. As leathermen shared erotic and sexual scenes with each other, they also enabled magical connections, healing, and transformation.[30] *Leatherfolk*, a volume released almost a decade later, also highlighted the potential for erotic practices to serve as initiation rituals or tools for spiritual growth, valorizing some as "magical," "tribal," "primal," or "primitive." One of Purusha's followers, Ganymede, writes: "Intense erotic experience often leads to alteration of consciousness and transcendence of limitations. Through it comes the divine release of ego, pride, and attachments, and the healing of deep psychological wounds."[31] The focus on cultural transformation was still present: "Raising one's personal Kundalini power through direct sexual stimulation," Ganymede argued, is "the most potent tool for transformation we have available." Contributors also stressed the need for reflexivity and continually increasing one's self-knowledge to avoid becoming abusive in sexual relationships.[32]

Despite assertions that gay sex is about politics, spirituality, or cultural evolution, *most* sex between men occurs outside of the spotlight of such discussions and does not necessarily carry those meanings. Men meeting on Casual Encounters for group sex, for example, don't necessarily feel baptized into commonality or consider themselves to be routing the "American system of imperial terror" as they do so. One man in the room may indeed feel liberated; another man may consider himself straight and live in fear that his wife will discover his secret life. The sexual behavior and beliefs of a mere slice of the gay population easily become sensationalized through the discourse of both inspired activists and their opposition. For right-wing opponents of gay rights, a focus on sex can be used to delegitimize political claims. Stereotypes of gay men as "sexually deviant" or insatiable can also become self-fulfilling prophecies: as "gayness" becomes associated with certain types of transgressive behaviors, those behaviors provide a means of defying heteronormative expectations and claiming identity.

Transgression, always lashed to the taboo.

Some writers are nostalgic for the utopian ideals of pre-AIDS gay sexual life, despite the limitations. What might have happened, Moore wonders, if AIDS hadn't cut the experiment short? What was begun then was in the service of revolution, he points out, not self-destruction: "Is it too late for us to pick up those threads of revolution and become artists again?"[33] To do so would not mean recreating the 1970s but once again imagining new possibilities. "Creating and maintaining a public culture of queer sexuality in a heterosexist society," Wayne Hoffman argues, "is a political act in any decade." Young gay men today, he argues, cannot even imagine the experiences of freedom and communion felt in the back rooms of 1976.

Then again, could a young man of the 1970s imagine gathering with five thousand other openly gay men for a weekend circuit party, wearing silver booty shorts, and strolling through the barricaded streets of New Orleans arm in arm with his lover while local businesses compete for his "pink dollars"? Could he imagine 65,000 gays and lesbians from around the world congregating at the Circuit Festival in Barcelona for twelve days of parties, dancing, and sex in dozens of languages?

Hoffman believes a renewal in public sexual culture occurred in the 1990s that represents not "a step backward in gay men's sexual development—either *to* the days of liberation or *from* the horrors of the epidemic—but rather a step ahead in time *toward* a new kind of sexual and political expression."[34]

But what exactly does this new kind of sexual and political expression look like?

Chapter Eight

From Revolutionaries to Rock Stars (and Back Again)

Group Sex as Rebellion, Liberation, and Entertainment

Here, when we go to parties, of course our bones are shaking, but we go with shaking bones. And I'm telling you, we are scared . . . every time the doorbell rings, *delet mirize* (your heart sinks). . . . *Could it be [the morality police]*? It's scary. But you know, we have to do something . . . to remind ourselves, Hey, we are alive!
—Iranian woman [1]

There are two levels where we can lead our lives. The real and the fantastic. We have to disco and do drugs and fuck if we want to live fantastic!
—The Devine Bella, *Faggots*

It's liberating to watch other couples fuck. There's something primal about it. We watch them and either have sex in a private room or, less often, have sex in full view of the others. It's terribly exciting to have sex while others watch. It's the closest thing to being a rock star that most people will ever experience.
—American swinger, male [2]

WELCOME TO THE JUNGLE

When Iranian American anthropologist Pardis Mahdavi first visited Tehran in the summer of 2000, she expected to encounter the Iran she grew up imagining. Her family remembered violence and extremism, and these were the images that stuck: "women clad in black chadors, wailing and whipping themselves," "black bearded men with heavy hearts and souls," arranged marriages, and the fierceness of the "morality police." But while she encountered this repressed side of Iran, she also heard stories of and witnessed signs of what some friends and informants called *enghelab-e-jensi* or *enghelab-e-farangi*, a sexual or sociocultural revolution. Her interest in how an "insatiable hunger for change, progress, cosmopolitanism, and modernity" was being linked to sex by young Tehranians sparked the beginning of seven years of anthropological study.[3]

During repeated visits, Mahdavi found that despite the strict moral policies of the Islamic Republic, young Iranians were listening to music, dancing, drinking alcohol, and socializing in new ways. Western dress and makeup were ubiquitous. She attended parties where famous DJs played techno music, Absolut vodka and Tanqueray gin were served, and female guests mingled with "western guys." Although house parties were common among the middle and upper-middle classes, lower-class youth threw parties in abandoned warehouses or at secluded outdoor locations, serving homemade liquor and playing music on "boom boxes" or car stereos.[4] Young Iranians also indulged in premarital and extramarital sexual escapades. As a twenty-three-year-old man explained: "In Iran, all things related to sex had a door, a closed one. Now we, this generation, are opening them one by one. Masturbation? Open it. Teenage sexual feelings? Open that door. Pregnancy outside of marriage? Open it. Now the youth are trying to figure out what to do with all these opening doors."[5] Understandably, young people experience confusion in the face of competing ideals and desires—traditional expectations versus contemporary temptations—and the stakes of personal decisions remain high. In 2004, despite nationwide attention to the public execution of a seventeen-year-old girl suspected of having premarital sex, Mahdavi nonetheless found many young women willing to lose their virginity in order to participate in the changing sexual culture.[6]

Like youth in other countries who lack private spaces to retreat to, some Iranian youth reported having sex at parties and in cars (which sometimes allowed them to escape the morality police) out of necessity. But some also purposely sought group sex. Shomal, in northern Iran, had a reputation as a popular destination for these sexual explorations. One informant told Mahdavi that young men and women "go there, deep in the jungle, and have lots of sex, with lots of people; it's really something to see. I love it." Another young man said: "Have I ever had group sex? Well, yes, with a few women at a time, but who hasn't done that? But I've watched really elaborate orgies too." He had observed "a big group orgy in Shomal," after being convinced to attend by a girl he knew.[7]

Although Mahdavi did not visit Shomal, she attended other sex parties in Iran. One evening, she accompanied her friend Babak to a party held in a huge garden with beautiful hanging trees. "Welcome to the jungle," a young man said as he greeted her. After stripping off her Islamic dress, including her head scarf and manto, she followed the men further into what felt like "the hanging gardens of Babylon." Babak squeezed her arm and whispered into her ear, "Take a deep breath, Pardis." As they walked closer to the swimming pool, she noticed it had been drained of water. Voices drifted up from the bottom of the pool. With surprise, she realized that "a full-blown orgy was taking place." As Babak took off his shirt and "started to wade into the group of young people," Mahdavi perched herself on the diving board, which seemed like a safe place to observe: "I continued to watch as bodies moved from one trio to another. A group of five men and women huddled together below me. I couldn't tell who was kissing whom, and I couldn't see how much oral or penetrative sex was taking place, but it seemed that most of the people were completely naked, and from the movements I could see, it looked as though half were having some kind of sex."[8]

Another sex party Mahdavi attended was held at a garden estate outside of Tehran, hosted by a young woman whose parents had gone on religious pilgrimage to Mecca. Upon arrival at the property, she heard techno music coming from a bathhouse. She followed her friends inside. When her eyes adjusted to the dim lighting, she saw "forty or so young people present, all naked or in undergarments, kissing, touching, dancing, and some having oral, anal, and vaginal sex." She watched groups of men and women "engaging in sexual acts with both genders," until she felt faint from the heat. She began searching for the friends she had arrived with, who had disappeared into the steam. The young woman was "kissing and being kissed by three men." Mahdavi was unable to find the man who'd driven them; later, she learned that he had been in a back room procuring Ecstasy.

When talking about their weekend adventures, some of Mahdavi's informants focused on the recreational aspect of the parties: "[There is] alcohol, there is sex, there is dancing, there is—it's just fun! It's what we do for fun!" Others viewed the parties as a representation of "all things Western," a way of gaining status and claiming a cosmopolitan identity; some also expressed ideas about sex as freedom that harked back to ideas underlying the sexual revolution in the United States. Still others claimed parties offered escape and "eased the pain" of living in Iran. As one man said, "Sex is the main thing here; it's our drug, it's what makes our lives bearable, that's what makes parties so necessary."[9] "If we don't live like this, we cannot exist in the Islamic Republic," a woman declared. "We hate our government, despise our families, and our husbands make us sick. If we don't look fabulous, smile, laugh, and dance, well then we might as well just go and die."[10]

But the new sexual culture in Iran, Mahdavi believes, is not simply an embrace of Western consumerism and morality nor merely an escapist hedonism, a "last resort." Urban young adults, the focus of Mahdavi's inquiry, made up about two-thirds of Iran's population; they were mobile, highly educated, underemployed, and dissatisfied with the political regime at the time. Some were directly involved in politics. Many used the Internet to make connections, blog about their frustrations, and peer into youth cultures elsewhere around the world. Willingly taking risks with their social and sexual behavior, as these Iranian young people were doing, was viewed as a step toward social and political reform—not *just* a means of escape and excitement. After all, the consequences of partying in Tehran were different from in Los Angeles, despite similarities in flashy dress, electronic music, and group sex. Iranian youth had "restricted access to social freedoms, education, and resources (such as contraceptives or other harm-reduction materials)" that might minimize the risk of some of their behaviors.[11] If caught, the punishments many young people would receive from their parents would likely be harsh. The punishments meted out by the morality police could be harsher. If caught drinking, for example, youth could be detained and sentenced to up to seventy lashes. Premarital sex could be punished by imprisonment and lashings; unmarried men and women caught in a car together could receive up to eighty-four lashings each. Although physical punishment has decreased in recent years, Mahdavi notes, young people are still detained and harassed by the morality police.[12]

Yet stories of being apprehended and arrested by the morality police were sometimes told with pride; occasionally, even parents were pleased that their children stood up for their beliefs. Some young adults courted run-ins with the morality police in the name of activism, boredom, or both. One couple caught having sex at a party were arrested and forced to marry. When Mahdavi talked with the twenty-two-year old woman involved, the woman explained that she and her new husband were trying to annul the marriage. Despite her ruined reputation, however, the young woman mused that her experience was "almost worth it": "The sex was great, and the excitement and adventure of doing what we know we aren't supposed to be doing, then being caught! Well, and it makes a great story."[13] Mahdavi's informants claimed that they were *living* the social and sexual changes they desired, reminding her that their "revolution was not about momentary acts" but was "a way of life." This way of life included social gatherings and behavior that "could be viewed as hedonistic" but were also "a necessary part of constructing a world over which they had control, a world they could live in rather than in the world of the Islamists, who would have them stay home and obey."[14] As another young woman said before attending a sex party:

> It's all about *laj bazi* (playful rebellion). Here, when we go to parties, of course our bones are shaking, but we go with shaking bones. And I'm telling you, we are scared. Everyone is. No matter what they tell you, they are scared, from the moment they leave their homes; and every time the doorbell rings, *delet mirize* (your heart sinks). *Could it be?* You ask yourself. *Could it be them?* It's scary. But you know, we have to do something. Something to get back at them,

something to remind ourselves, Hey, we are alive! Hey, we have a say in our lives![15]

But although the social and sexual revolution in Iran has brought change, especially in how young people express themselves, Mahdavi asks, if some of the repression dissolved, "would young people still resist this way?"[16]

Contemporary sex partying is often thought to be linked to the spread of Western values and practices even while taking on local forms and meanings. At times, even the idea that group sex is a Western phenomenon becomes important to participants, adding layers of meaning to the encounters as modern, fashionable, or evil. After the Queen Boat scandal in Egypt in 2001, thirty-five members of the US Congress wrote to Hosni Mubarak to protest the treatment of the men, who were tortured and subjected to examinations to determine whether they had had anal sex. In response, the Egyptian newspaper *Al-Ahram al-Arabi* ran a headline that translated as, "Be a pervert and Uncle Sam will approve."[17]

Some sex partying is certainly related to processes of globalization, as citizens from wealthy nations have the privilege of traveling to other locales to escape restrictive laws or take advantage of cheap labor. Tourism is regularly promoted as the answer to poor nations' economic woes; beliefs about natives' unrestrained sexuality in certain locales reinforce patterns of labor and leisure. It is not surprising that Jamaica became home to the notorious Hedonism resorts: "Unleash your wildest desires with open minds, open bars, and open relationships." Other well-known lifestyle resorts exist in Mexico and Spain; lesser known, perhaps, are the resort in Pattaya, Thailand, or the swingers' cruises offered off the coast of Turkey. Gay circuit parties have spread around the globe; as these events can last for several days, many host cities find them economically advantageous. The porn industry, similarly driven by the desire for cheap labor and the erotics of otherness, has extended into Asia and Eastern Europe (Warsaw, Poland, was the site of the Third Annual World Gangbang Championship and Eroticon in 2004).

Sometimes, sex partying draws on Western symbols, themes, or discourses regardless of where it takes place. As I was finishing this manuscript, I had the opportunity to talk with a Pakistani businessman at a rooftop bar in Los Angeles. We drank mojitos while he told me about underground "key parties" in Pakistan. From what he had heard secondhand, they sounded similar to the key parties of 1970s American folklore—where couples supposedly deposited their car keys into a bowl and each woman drew any set of keys except her own, leaving the party with the man whose keys she selected. But in Pakistan, he told me, couples use hotel keys; in the name of discretion, no one would actually go back to their own homes or drive their own cars. Unfortunately, even though he provided a few leads, I was unable to find participants willing to talk with me. Still, the reappearance of the key party in such a context—whether rumor or practice—is a fascinating example of cultural appropriation. The French sociologist Michel Fize suggests that the interest in *Skins* shown by French youth proves that they are casualties of pornography: "We're living in a pornocratic world where sex is everywhere, in thoughts, words, images, and deeds. This is leading more and more young people into unconventional sexual practices." For some adolescents, though, the parties are described as a way of expressing themselves and resisting authority, paying homage to the 1970s United States in ethos as well as practice. As a *Le Skins* partygoer declared: "We live in a society full of rules, control and conventions. Some people burn cars to revolt but we don't hurt anyone. We stand for eccentricity and free love."[18]

But sex parties aren't *just* Western creations. Group sex has been depicted in art and literature for centuries, and some of those portrayals are celebratory. Some symbols and meanings loop back on each other—even portrayals of orgies as "tribal" or "Roman" can't easily be traced to a singular origin at this point in history. Over the years I researched this book, I also heard tales about secret group sex parties for men in the South Pacific and rental houses in Dubrovnik serving as temporary, mobile sex clubs. Films about swinging in Israel and India appeared. The electronic dance music scene, with its focus on multiple sources of sensory intensity, has spread around the world. Three-day events, club drugs, and sensation-seeking youth seem to beget after-parties and group sex wherever they coalesce. Unfortunately, it remains difficult to find participants from non-Western countries willing to talk about their recreational experiences with group sex. Mahdavi's scholarly account is a rare find.

Baudrillard claims we live in a post-orgy world. What he means is not that orgies no longer occur but that the deep referential meanings they once had have been vacated, beginning with the political events of the 1960s and accelerating as the global spread of capitalist consumerism ensured that homogeneity and surface desires would win over authentic difference and pleasure. "The myth of sexual liberation is still alive and well," he claims, but the state of ecstatic transcendence once possible through transgression has become mere simulation, just another form of pornography.[19] We haven't been liberated by our revolutions, sexual or otherwise, but rather, the linear progression of history has concluded. There is no longer any end game to believe in—no salvation, rapture, utopia, or apocalypse. Postmodern culture has become based on an endless play of surface signs, and meaning has sold out to capitalism: "Closing down, closing down! It's the end-of-the-century sale. Everything must go! Modernity is over (without ever having happened), the orgy is over, the party is over—the sales are starting. . . . But the sales don't come after the festive seasons any longer; nowadays the sales start first, they last the whole year long, even the festivals themselves are on sale everywhere"[20]

Baudrillard's reference to the orgy, then, recalls a lost world of possibility, mystery, and even deep passion. His reliance on ideas of staunch male/female difference is irritating to many theorists; he also makes problematic statements about transsexuality and troublesome distinctions between "primitive cultures" and "our post-modern world." But if we grit our teeth through those sections, his writing can still be provocative. After all, he isn't the only one who mourns the supposed intensity of past political movements or human relationships; he isn't the only one who laments a lack of depth, truth, values, goals, or ultimate significance in contemporary life. And he isn't the only one who views sex as a realm where these losses are palpable. In fact, there will probably be critics who view the activities discussed on every page in this book as evidence of such a demise of the rightful meaning of sex.

"We're not for anything, but we're not against anything either."

Free love, of course, means something different in the Parisian suburbs of 2012 than in San Francisco's Haight-Ashbury of 1968, the gay baths of New York City in the 1970s, and the millennial jungles of Shomal.

But *what*, exactly?

WELCOME TO KANDYLAND

Visiting the Playboy Mansion was a teenage dream.

But while I ticked off visits to other famous residences before turning twenty-five—the White House, Buckingham Palace, the Vatican—the Playboy Mansion remained elusive.

When people talk about the Playboy Mansion today, they are referring to Hugh Hefner's property in Los Angeles, a 22,000-square-foot house located near UCLA and the Bel-Air Country Club. The property was purchased in 1971 for just over a million dollars, though its current worth is estimated at around $50 million.

For a while, I hoped that maybe having worked as a stripper and writing a book on male desire would secure my invitation to a Playboy party. I imagined myself sipping cocktails and talking politics with Hef and whichever clique of famous authors and musicians currently gathered around him, perhaps slipping off to call Gay Talese and compare notes if the action began heating up in the grotto.

But the invitation never came.

One day I discovered that my friend Amy[21], a fitness model and professional pole dancer from California, had been to the mansion numerous times. I begged her to take me. "Sign up online," she told me, directing me to the website of the Karma Foundation. "You can go with me and my girls when you get the sponsored ticket."

She assured me that I wouldn't see sex of any sort at the mansion but that it would be a worthwhile experience anyway.

After some research, I learned that Hefner is now often a contracted guest at private parties hosted by other groups. The Karma Foundation, for example, founded in 2005 by entrepreneur Eric Stotz, is a networking organization hosting charity events for groups such as the Humane Society of the United States, the Marconi Foundation for Kids, and Journey Forward. But these aren't your average charity socials. Karma selects luxurious or "unique" settings, such as the Playboy Mansion or the *Celebration*, a 125-foot mega-yacht, and hires performers like Snoop Dogg, DJ Paul Oakenfold, or P Diddy. As part of their aim is to "throw the sexiest, classiest and most outrageous high-profile parties," they also unabashedly recruit eye candy; Kandy Masquerade, for example, advertised that "over 1000 of the sexiest girls in the world" would also be in attendance. Most of these girls, who do not work for either Playboy or the Karma Foundation, attend the party on "sponsored tickets." To obtain a free ticket, thousands of girls compete in several invitation rounds; if selected, a girl is expected to pay her own transportation and lodging costs, along with a twenty-five-dollar donation to the featured charity.

The Karma Foundation has been criticized for primarily benefiting already wealthy individuals. Much of the ticket cost, detractors say, goes toward the event rather than the featured charity. The foundation's stated aim—"to provide our member base with remarkable upscale lifestyles that enrich their lives, expand their networks, and benefit noble charitable causes"—seems frivolous to some, an opportunity for rich executives to mingle with underwear-clad, twenty-something girls in the name of goodwill. And the "four pillars" of the foundation—networking, revelry, philanthropy, and ultimate access—have been called elitist, given a membership that is invitation-only. This is, however, the *point*: "our Members prefer to socialize and party with other like minded individuals." Stotz acknowledges his critics: "There are certainly people out there who question Karma's philanthropic side, or who'd rather we soften our sexy image." But there is something to Stotz's philosophy that rings true to American pop culture and certainly to the legacy of Hefner's empire. As Stotz told *Business Today* in 2009: "One thing that doesn't change, even during a recession, is that everybody wants to hang with the cool kids, to do cool things. People still want a taste of the lifestyle that Karma offers, to be part of an amazing experience—people are 100% experience driven. With Karma, I get to be the cool kid throwing the parties. It's pretty awesome."[22] With general admission tickets to the parties at the Playboy Mansion running $1,000 or more and private tables or cabanas priced at around $10,000, Stotz is banking on just how much people want to "hang with the cool kids."

I wanted to hang with the cool kids, too.

So I applied for a sponsored ticket. Creating the online profile was fairly straightforward. Height, weight, hair color, eye color, measurements. I uploaded two photos. Then I spent several hours writing and revising my answers to the essay questions on the profile, trying to second guess what types of responses would make me stand out.

> *Question: If you were a Kandy, what kind of Kandy would you be and why?*
> *Answer: If I were a Kandy, I'd probably be a Nerd, because in my everyday life, you'll always find me surrounded by books! I love learning and writing*
> *. . .*
> *Question: Tell us about yourself and be creative. Your background, lifestyle, goals, three wishes in life, experiences would all be appropriate subject matter.*
> *Answer: I'm a cultural anthropologist who writes on sexuality in the United States . . .*

I poured it all out, discussing my research on stripping and monogamy, my goals (which I linked to furthering the project of sexual freedom pioneered by Hefner himself), and how much it meant to me to set foot on the grounds of the historic Playboy Mansion. If I was going to mingle with intelligent, successful guests, I surmised, I might as well highlight the fact that I was also well educated, well read, and able to converse on more than which celebrities would be in attendance that evening. *Right?*

The invitation still never came.

I missed Kandy Masquerade, the annual February party celebrating Mardi Gras.

When I called Amy to lament my luck, she asked, "Did you put up a picture?"

"Yes, of course. And I filled out everything. I wrote some damn good essays."

"You wrote *essays*? What are you talking about? What picture did you use?"

When we hung up, I sheepishly returned to the site, logged in, and deleted my essays. I also deleted the photos I'd put up—publicity headshots taken after the publication of my first book—and replaced them with some snapshots of myself in a bikini.

My invitation came—a sponsored ticket for Kandyland 2009, an annual Karma party held each June, described as "a cross between Willie Wonka and Alice in Wonderland."[23] I was thrilled.

Within a week, I was on a cross-country flight to Los Angeles.

Amy designed our outfits. The five of us attending together dressed as Hershey's Kisses in silver metallic bikini tops and "microminis," basically a four-inch ruffle of fabric that sits on your hips. (While wearing one, you never sit down and try not to think about your rear view). Our handmade chokers were designed to look like the candy packaging, with a white label and blue lettering: HERSHEY'S KISSES.

The night began with a shuttle ride from a parking garage, where the staff first checked IDs and issued wristbands, making sure none of the girls had scored a free ticket fraudulently. There were hundreds of girls in line—candy canes, lollipops, and snow cones—but no other Kisses. I was relieved. That would be worse than showing up in the same dress as your ex's new girlfriend on prom night.

Upon arriving at the mansion, we swarmed out of the shuttle bus like candy falling out of a trick-or-treat bag. In the confusion, I bumped into a larger-than-life black man. "Are you the welcoming committee?" he asked. His friends laughed.

We took our place in a line of people, almost all girls, twisting around the side of the mansion.

"Wow, that guy looked like Snoop Dogg," I whispered to one of the Kisses.

She looked at me with pity. "That *was* Snoop Dogg," she said.

The line began moving forward. We were greeted by Oompa Loompas. We took photos with them. Beautiful girls passed out smoky drinks. We took photos with them, too. We posed again for photos along the walkway leading to the tents on the lawn, underneath a glowing Cheshire cat.

The first thing I learned about the mansion was that it was pure folly to wear stilettos on the grounds, which were primarily cobblestone. As a stripper I had acquired the ability to keep my footing almost anywhere in heels, including rickety tables with a diameter of less than twelve inches; negotiating the steps behind the mansion with a drink in my hand and reporters aiming news cameras at my friends and me, however, was a bit more disconcerting.

The second thing I learned was that when men expect bunnies, they see bunnies—even if you're really a soccer mom on a free ticket. The male guests seemed confused as to which of us were working and which were tourists like themselves, so we posed for dozens of photos with random men (some of which can still be found on the Internet). I enjoyed feeling like a star, although part of me was nervous: was I destined to spend my entire fifteen minutes of fame in a micromini?

We ducked inside the steamy, low-ceilinged grotto. Two girls were topless in the water, but there was no real debauchery in sight. The rocks were slippery, so we sat down to have our picture taken by a blonde girl dressed like a cupcake (her bikini top appeared made of whipped cream and sprinkles). As I stood up again to retrieve my camera, I bumped my head on one of the rocks, nearly falling into the pool. *Treacherous.* Taking a last, nostalgic look around before ducking to follow the Kisses outside, I imagined the cesspools of celebrity DNA that had formed in the nooks and crannies over the years. Despite my claustrophobia, I felt a certain reverence for the cave walls that had once sheltered Warren Beatty.

The third thing I learned was that the bathroom situation was dire. After waiting an hour in a line inching forward as if the bathroom housed the only mirror at a party where "over 1000 of the sexiest girls in the world" wanted to look their best—which it *did*—I finally realized that there was a row of portable toilets outside. Portable toilets had never figured in my Playboy Mansion fantasies, but by my third trip to the bathroom that evening, I was grateful for them. The bathroom and porta-potty lines provided an opportunity to meet other girls who were there on free tickets. Many were from Los Angeles, although Karma events really do draw women from around the globe. A beautiful young girl from Turkey had flown in just for Kandyland at her own expense. Her family threw her a party when she received the invitation, she told me. Now, she was overwhelmed at being in the United States for the first time and starstruck over the mansion. She didn't even realize *she* was part of the draw for many of the paying guests.

Hef's cabana was under the main tent. We meandered over, and I caught a glimpse of him through a tangle of lace and limbs as young girls eagerly tried to catch his attention. He sat on a couch, wearing his trademark pajamas and flocked by beautiful blondes, just as you'd expect.

I was *really* at the Playboy Mansion.

The Kisses wanted to dance. They'd been to parties here before.

The fourth thing I learned—after taking photos on the dance floor, on a Victorian couch, with the Turkish girl, and underneath a life-sized lollipop—was that Amy was right. The real action doesn't happen at the mansion, at least not on Karma nights and not for us. Maybe the VIPs and the real centerfolds were invited into the main house to frolic in the bedrooms. But for the masses, confined to the backyard and pool area, a visit to the mansion is about taking pictures and socializing. If you're looking for sex, you'd probably have more luck at the after-parties, which spread across Los Angeles like fireworks almost every weekend. Early in the evening, I received a few business cards with suite numbers on them. As the clock struck midnight, the invitations came more swiftly. The Roosevelt Hotel. The SLS. The Mondrian. A Hollywood Hills mansion. Amy herded us toward the front of the house, as regulars at the parties knew that one should catch the shuttle long before the party ended at 2:00 a.m. or risk standing in line for hours with hundreds of other half-naked women, freezing and with no free champagne in sight. Once back on the shuttle bus, we'd make our after-party plans.

Unfortunately, when I dug the invitations out of my purse, I realized I'd lost my camera.

Stotz wasn't lying. Kandyland was an experience. I've gone back to the Playboy Mansion five times—twice to Kandyland, twice to Kandy Masquerade, and once for Kandy Halloween—and I've lost my camera twice more. I still have no photos in the grotto. At the last party I attended, Kandy Masquerade in 2012, I finally saw the game room and the famous monkeys.

But still, no sex.

Karma's events are *sexy*. For some people, that's enough. For others, it's already too much. As a newscaster from Fox 11 described the parties: "If I had to narrow it down to one thing . . . it would be the sex. No, I'm kidding! When I say sex, I mean that it's sexy. You guys do that sexy thing really well." But sexy has a point. Sexy, as long as its promise isn't fulfilled, keeps us coming back. For some people, "sexy" is even more appealing than sex. I certainly didn't hear any complaints from the male guests that the lingerie-clad girls weren't getting down and dirty in the cabanas.

This wouldn't surprise Baudrillard a bit.

Media coverage vacillates between promoting Karma events as the "ultimate parties" or as last-ditch attempts to squeeze profits out of Hefner's faded empire. Truthfully, they are probably neither. Although rumors of Playboy's financial demise have spanned decades, it remains one of the most recognized brands in the world. The logo, a black bunny in a bow tie, can be found on almost any imaginable consumer product from limited edition wines to expensive duvet sets to pencil cases. *Something* about Playboy still speaks to the "cool kids"—even if some of them are in elementary school.

Is this what happens when revolutions are won? Or lost?

THE ORIGINAL PLAYBOY

Si Non Oscillas, Noli Tintinnare
"If you don't swing, don't ring."
  —Latin inscription on the door of the Chicago Playboy Mansion

Any book on group sex would be incomplete without a discussion of Hugh Hefner and *Playboy*. Hefner built his business and persona on a vision of a hedonistic lifestyle. He identified as part of the sexual revolution, standing up for the First Amendment and gay and lesbian rights. But his wars were waged on satin sheets rather than in dirty back rooms, and Hefner is more renowned for his consumption habits—lavish parties, beautiful women, and silk pajamas—than his politics. As Peter O'Toole supposedly commented after visiting the Playboy Mansion: "This is what God would have done if He'd had the money."

Hefner created *Playboy* magazine in 1953, featuring a nude pinup of Marilyn Monroe in the first issue. After the first year, *Playboy* began using noncelebrities as centerfolds (one of whom Hefner claimed to have found in his own copy room). These "girls next door" were not only beautiful but also supposedly sexually liberated; their risqué photographs appeared alongside work by established literary figures. As an upscale men's magazine, *Playboy* hit a cultural nerve. Circulation grew quickly and exponentially, reaching seven million readers by the early 1970s. Hefner expanded his business interests, developing merchandise and becoming a media personality. The first Playboy Club opened in Chicago in 1960, featuring scantily clad women and offering upscale masculine entertainment—a posh atmosphere, steak, liquor, and pornography.

As he turned "pleasure-seeking into an art form," Hefner's lifestyle became mythologized.[24] He dated his centerfolds and was publicly linked to multiple girlfriends at a time. Hefner's private plane, the *Big Bunny*, was painted black, sported the bunny logo on its tail, and employed eight "jet bunnies," beautiful stewardesses wearing miniskirts and knee-high boots. The rear of the plane was designated Hefner's private quarters, housing "a six-by-eight-foot elliptical bed complete with special seat belts and a Tasmanian opossum spread, a stereo and videotape system, a motorized swivel chair, and a shower with two nozzles."[25]

Hefner admits to consciously reinventing himself in line with his boyhood dreams. "You are handed a life," he reflects, "and if you're lucky enough and smart enough, you become the person you want to be."[26] Hefner was both. He portrayed himself as a modern rebel, resisting a puritanical upbringing and questing after personal and social freedom. He criticized the institution of marriage and openly rejected monogamy. This vision resonated with Americans of the time. As biographer Steven Watts claims, Hefner's creation of a fantasy life in *Playboy* magazine and through his persona, adventures, and series of essays, "The Playboy Philosophy," captured "two powerful trends in postwar American culture: sexual liberation and consumer abundance." *Playboy* addressed a "simmering male identity crisis," offering a "reassuring model of stylish consumer" to men who were confused by a changing economy and society. In popularizing leisure culture, "Hefner helped make consumer abundance an emblem of America throughout the world."[27]

Rumors abounded about his weekly parties at the Playboy Mansion as "sexual phantasmagoria": "conga lines of nude bodies snaking from floor to floor, hookers imported by the dozen, horses and other stud animals delivered in the dark of the night, SM dungeons, lesbian orgies, men sleeping with children."[28] Some insiders disputed the stories, while others confirmed them (or at least parts of them). Either way, the legend grew. Tales of celebrity indulgences added to the mystique of the Playboy mansions. In 1972, the

Rolling Stones blew through the Chicago Playboy Mansion in true rock star form, engaging in a "nonstop, four-day orgy of sex, drugs, and partying" that included group sex under the dining room table and in Hef's bathroom.[29]

In 1974, Hefner began living full-time in his Los Angeles mansion, fashioning it as a "Disneyland for adults" and hosting parties and photo shoots to promote this image. After a 1977 photo shoot where he ended up naked with seven playmates in the grotto, according to Watts, Hefner became "the center of a group-sex scene." Even though he'd slept with multiple women before and often slept with many women consecutively on the same night, he now positioned himself in his legendary spot as the only man in the middle of a posse of women. "Instead of having to choose one girl over another on any given evening," Hefner said, "I simply chose them all—and the more the merrier."[30] But there were no other men allowed. *Ever.*

Hef, apparently, is not motivated by sperm competition syndrome.

Group sex became the norm at the Los Angeles mansion and became symbolic, in Hefner's personal life and in the folklore surrounding him, of freedom and wealth. Wednesday nights became known as "orgy night," frequented by an inner circle of partiers that included Linda Lovelace, Clint Eastwood, Elizabeth Taylor, and Warren Beatty.[31] Breaking free of inhibitions was celebrated: "We were all enjoying the sowing of wild oats—men and women alike . . . with absolutely no strings attached"; "old rules didn't apply . . . it was like going to some infant's paradise where you could eat all the candy you wanted and you wouldn't get fat."[32] Hefner was not a favorite among 1970s feminists, as many believed that *Playboy* promoted objectification and that women participating in such a sexual culture were degraded. But Hefner's female companions expressed enthusiasm about the opportunities available at the mansion, calling the parties "a once in a lifetime opportunity to act out the fantasies we all have" and "a dream world" granting "the freedom to express ourselves in every way that felt good to us, without being labeled evil or promiscuous." One of Hefner's lovers recalls being overwhelmed by sexual energy during her first group sex experience in his bedroom, expressing feelings of euphoria, intense aliveness, and spiritual awakening: "I didn't even know what I was doing. I wasn't even aware of myself as being separate from the others. . . . It was the most amazing sex I've ever had. But the most amazing thing about it was that it wasn't really about sex. It was about life." Several of the women described their relationship with Hefner and the other women as being part of "a big happy family."[33]

Of course, nothing lasts forever—especially a dream.

During the 1980s and 1990s, Playboy Enterprises was shaken by scandals and continued criticism from both conservative and liberal groups for its representations of women and glorification of consumption. *Playboy* faced competition, first from publications like *Penthouse* and *Hustler* that featured more explicit images and then from easy-access Internet porn. As in gay communities, sexual experimentation began to seem foolish rather than cutting-edge in light of the AIDS epidemic. When Hefner married Kimberly Conrad in 1989, many commentators pronounced the fall of his empire.

The marriage lasted a decade. *Playboy* hung on. And America continued to change.

Hefner reentered the party scene after separating from Conrad in 1998, moving her into a house nearby and once again assembling a revolving "blondetourage." A few years later, he filmed for a reality show, *Hef's World*, but producers shifted the focus to his girlfriends. This turned out to be a smart move. The resulting hit series, *The Girls Next Door*, debuted on E! Entertainment Television in 2005.

In her memoir, *Bunny Tales: Behind Closed Doors at the Playboy Mansion*, Izabella St. James recounts her two-year tenure as one of Hefner's seven girlfriends. St. James met Hefner in a Hollywood club in 2000 and was quickly charmed by him; by 2002, she had moved into the mansion. "There was something about the Mansion that just lured you in," she writes. "It's not Hef himself. It's not the house. It's this enchanting feeling, this aura. There is a spirit to that place that makes your skin tingle, your mind relax. It makes you lose your inhibitions."[34] She received a weekly allowance, additional funds for "beauty maintenance," money toward a car, and other perks. Along with the other girlfriends, St. James accompanied Hefner to Hollywood parties and hot spots, hosted events with him at the mansion, and provided him with company in the evenings.

The enchantment didn't last, however, and overall St. James paints a less-than-flattering portrait of Hefner's regime. She whines about the boredom of being eye candy. (Having accepted this role as often as possible in my youth, I can attest to the occasional frustrations of being beholden to another's whims. But had she taken up another form of youthful labor instead—say, waitressing or scooping ice cream—she might have had fewer complaints about sipping champagne in Hollywood nightclubs.) Once ensconced in the mansion, St. James started to notice the dirty carpets and dated furnishings more than the aura. She was not fond of Holly Madison's dogs, which she insinuates are poorly housebroken. (One gets the feeling she wasn't enamored with Holly, either). The girlfriends, she alleges, dealt with curfews and internal bickering, punctuated by ritualistic and unfulfilling group sex. "I guarantee more scandalous and wild things happen at college parties than in Hef's bedroom," she writes.[35]

To prove her point, St. James divulges the details. Upon returning to the mansion after their evening excursion, usually to a nightclub or party, the girls would change into more comfortable attire. Hef passed out Quaaludes "to put the girls in the mood for sex"; he relied on Viagra. The head girl-friend would prepare Hef's bedroom, where other men were still never allowed, gathering "paraphernalia on the bed—toys, handcuffs, lubricants, whatever he had asked for or might come in handy." Porn played on two screens—"never unconventional or gay porn." Then Hef would lie on his back while the girls got stoned or drank Dom Perignon. He covered himself with baby oil and his main girlfriend, often Holly, would fellate him until he was erect. One by one, the girls would take turns lowering themselves onto his erection while he remained supine; eventually Holly would have sex with him in whichever position he desired. To finish, he always masturbated, with the girls gathered around him. The entire ritual, according to St. James, was mechanical and brief: "It is all an illusion; an illusion that he is still a swinger, a man with many women in his bed, a crazy orgiastic experience. It is just not so in reality."[36]

Yet despite St. James's blasé reports, many heterosexual men would likely still trade almost anything for a weekend in Hef's pajamas, even if left finishing themselves off while a bevy of busty blondes got baked in bed. After all, the seven naked women weren't exactly an "illusion," even if they were bored or bitter.

But *something* has changed.

More recent bunnies have also spilled their carrots about what happens in Hef's chambers. Their stories resonate more with St. James's descriptions than with those of his 1970s lovers, with their reports of out-of-body experiences and orgasmic bliss. In a scathing description that landed on dozens of blogs and websites, including The Huffington Post, for example, former mansion girl Jill Anne Spaulding claims: "Hef just lies there with his Viagra erection. It's just a fake erection, and each girl gets on top of him for two minutes while the girls in the background try to keep him excited. They'll yell things like, 'fuck her daddy, fuckk her daddaddy!' There's a lot of cheerleader going on! The main girlfriend wipes off his [uncondomed] penis. She's the girl who actually shares the bed with him. . . . She's around 22 years old." Based on Spaulding's report, only the order of the girlfriends has really changed: "When it first gets started his main girlfriend gives him [oral sex], then she has sex with him. She's the first to go because that's the safest for her. No protection and no testing. He doesn't care."

Kendra Wilkinson, from *The Girls Next Door*, described her first group experience at the mansion at eighteen years old:

> One of the girls asked me if I wanted to go upstairs to Hef's room. . . . It seemed like every other girl was going, and if I didn't it would be weird. One by one, each girl hopped on Hef and had sex with him . . . for about a minute. I studied their every move. Then it was my turn . . . it was very weird. I wasn't thinking about how much older Hef was—all the body parts worked the same. I wanted to be there.[37]

Weird.

When Hefner's ex-fiancée Crystal Harris began talking to the tabloids, claiming they only had sex once "for two seconds,"[38] it seemed like Spaulding and Wilkinson had perhaps been exaggerating in their claims that he performed for a minute or two with each girl.

Like many others, St. James suggests that Playboy's association with the sexual avant-garde is long over. As for the myths of the grotto, St. James writes that its "finest memories come from the swinging '70s, and thankfully the water has been changed since then." "Not much happened in the Grotto during the two and a half years I was at the mansion," she writes, although during the parties, a "bunch of naked guys would get in and hope for the girls to follow." Hef only ventured into the grotto himself three times while she lived at the mansion, possibly because of his heart condition.[39] (After the grotto was linked to an outbreak of Legionnaire's disease in early 2011 affecting hundreds of visitors, avoiding the steamy whirlpool is probably advisable for anyone.) Though the mansion remains a hangout for celebrities, musicians, and beautiful girls who turn heads even in a city as jaded as Los Angeles, it has been described as squalid, crumbling, and dated. And, while Hefner remains a retro icon, drawing crowds wherever he goes, he is also portrayed as pathetically past his prime. A blogger from the *Guardian*, writing about a masquerade party in early 2012, likens him to "a 176-year-old Galapagos tortoise wrapped in a dressing-gown."[40]

Who still hands out Quaaludes anyway?

Hefner disputes much of St. James's account, including the part about the Quaaludes. "Despite what she writes," he asserts, she was asked to leave the mansion "because she didn't get along with some of the other girls." Her exposé, according to Hefner, was just an attempt to exploit the publicity generated by his engagement to Harris. Hefner also stressed that he doesn't need to hold women hostage or drug them in order to get sex: "The strange reality is that I'm more of a target today than probably at any other time in my life in terms of attention from young women. . . . I think it has to with the curious nature of iconic celebrity."[41]

I tend to side with Hef on that one. Even if gorgeous eighteen-year-olds the likes of Kendra Wilkinson are mounting him for only a minute or less, whether out of peer pressure or youthful inquisitiveness, the truth is that there would be a line of such women outside his bedroom door any night he requested it. Just for the experience—or the fame. Weird or not.

Well, it makes a good story.

Watts writes, "The *Playboy* ethos has become mainstream, with its powerful current pulling along many, perhaps most, modern Americans toward a common destination: self-fulfillment in every way imaginable in a world with few restraints."[42] The fact that young women like St. James, Spaulding, and Wilkinson can write and talk openly about their group sex exploits, pursued for the sake of adventure and a few material perks, is evidence of changed times. People around the country have online access to hard-core porn, college students plan threesomes on Wednesdays after class, and eighth-grade girls carry purses emblazoned with the Playboy bunny logo because "it's cute." As Hefner once declared, "The fantasy in *Playboy* became a reality for society."[43] And that reality extends further than *Playboy* intended: the girl next door isn't just coyly posing for pictures nowadays but marketing her own sex tapes. In an e-mail to one of her biographers in 2009, the original gang bang queen, Annabel Chong, writes,

> The problem with the mainstreamization of porn is that now everybody is a pornstar—Kim Kardashian, those soldiers at Abu Ghraib, Verne Troyer. It makes performing sex for the camera common and banal. . . . Remember a decade ago . . . porn was the new rock & roll, since rock no longer has the power to shock—it has been co-opted into the mainstream. Well, I see the same thing happening to porn. It's no longer as taboo as it used to be. It's just what people do. And they do it all the time.[44]

The avant-garde moved on from the mansion, without a forwarding address.

But maybe it's more fun to be a rock star than a revolutionary, anyway?

PICKING UP WHERE HEF LEFT OFF

Las Vegas, 2004

Picture one of those diagrams of the United States they use on television during presidential elections—you know, the kind where the states turn red or blue when all the votes are counted? Except on this map, the color coding is neon pink, pinpointing swinger populations instead of political leanings. California, Texas, and Florida are almost solidly pink neon—swinging might even be called mainstream in those states, as every major event seems dominated by couples from those locales. Large cities along the coasts would be densely speckled with neon, with small pepperings of color along the rest of the coastline—humans tend to mate near water. The rest of the country would be darker—except for Vegas, which, despite its lack of ocean and its decidedly uncosmopolitan vibe, is the glowing exception to the rule, a blinding neon beacon on the swinger map.

The heart of the beast.

But even Las Vegas, where supposedly anything goes, exhibits some amount of shock during the annual Lifestyles Convention week. The convention attendees descend on the desert oasis lugging suitcases stuffed with "pimp and ho" outfits, laser star machines to decorate their hotel rooms, iPods and speakers, cases of Red Bull, bottles of Viagra, and enough Trojans to conquer any other city.

Walking around the convention hotel, there is no need to even check for the neon wristbands that signal one is with the lifestyle group—you can usually guess. The usual rules of social engagement are suspended for four days, becoming exceptionally clear during elevator rides where, instead of staring at the walls, people flirt: Where are you from, sexy? Any good parties last night? Stop by Suite 256, our door is always open! Occasionally hapless tourists end up in the elevator as well, looking at each other with apprehension, or a single guy gets on and after checking out the women—who might be kissing, holding hands, or wearing see-through clothing—asks eagerly, "How do I get one of those wristbands?" Vanilla guys are always mystified when they learn tickets can be purchased only as a couple.

You really do need to bring sand to this desert.[45]

> ### The Playcouple™ Philosophy
>
> Adult men and women are sexual beings. . . . Many in our society, such as the religious and political right wing, proselytize that open sexual expression is sinful and worthy of condemnation, while the political left wing seeks to inhibit and restrict sincere and honest expression. Others seem to resent or are threatened that somewhere there are men and women who are fully enjoying their life and sexuality. By contrast, the *Playcouple* supports both freedom of expression and tolerance towards the private lives of others. . . . They are comfortable with their sexuality and willingly explore new ways to heighten their sensuality. They believe that romance is one of life's greatest adventures just as love is one of life's greatest joys. From sharing erotic fantasies to traveling exotic paths, the *Playcouple* places the highest value on the intimacy they share with each other and those around them. —Lifestyles Organization materials

Layered onto the meanings of group sex in the United States is not just decadence, à la the Romans, or the revolutionary potential of either hippie free love or the "show hard" sexual excess of gay bathhouses, but also contemporary rock star, playboy indulgence. Like Hefner, other wealthy and powerful men surround themselves with female entourages; some openly state preferences for group sex. In the 1980s and 1990s, Prince Jefri Bolkiah of Brunei was as well known for his harem as his lavish spending habits, although he seems to have preferred sex with the women individually.[46] Media reports of upscale sex parties with hookers and groupies abound, from Europe to South America, cropping up almost anywhere you find business-men, athletes, musicians, or politicians congregating. Dominique Strauss-Kahn, the sixty-three-year-old former head of the International Monetary Fund, was accused of knowingly having sex with prostitutes in France and Belgium. Although he admitted to partaking in an "uninhibited lifestyle" and having sex with multiple women at parties arranged for him by friends, he denied the women were prostitutes. "Swinging parties are about having free and consensual sex," he explained. Strauss-Kahn never asked whether the women were paid to attend the parties—the question *does* seem rude—adding that he often had sex with very young women and that six girls at once "does not seem to me to be a considerable number." His lawyer defended him, saying, "At these parties, people were not necessarily dressed, and I defy you to tell the difference between a naked prostitute and any other naked woman."[47]

Especially if you're not the one picking up the tab.

Thomas Kramer is a German land developer who lives at 5 Star Island in Miami, Florida. After a string of lawsuits against him alleging sexual misconduct—none of which were successful—Kramer installed twenty-four-hour security cameras in his bedroom and posted a sign warning women that they would be filmed if they entered. Women who venture in are now asked to read the sign aloud, on camera. "If I don't show this to you I get accused of invasion of privacy," Kramer told a local journalist. "But with the cameras on you can't f--- with me and say what we did was not consensual." The cameras don't have much impact on what is rumored to be an eventful sex life for Kramer—girls arriving at his estate "by the limo-full," late-night parties in the hot tub, and kinky paraphernalia such as whips and riding crops decorating his lair. Girls who dare to enter take home a souvenir, a T-shirt that reads: "Good girls go to heaven. Bad girls go to 5 Star Island" on the front; "And all I got was this lousy T-shirt" on the back.[48]

Sir Ivan is a recording artist, peace advocate, and playboy who resides every summer in his medieval-style castle in the Hamptons. Described as the "Playboy Mansion of the East," "Sir Ivan's Castle" is a fifteen-thousand-square-foot estate designed as both "the ultimate party palace" and "the sexiest home in the world." The castle has huge gates, a moat and draw-bridge, a dungeon (for authenticity, not kink), and stone towers that guests can climb to watch the sunset. Dragons, gargoyles, and griffins perch along the stone walls. The centerpiece of the property is a sculpture rising out of the infinity pool—a naked woman morphing into a dragon. Sir Ivan commissioned the piece in honor of his long-time companion, Japanese model Mina. At night, the golden statue is illuminated in color and with fiery torches.

Sir Ivan throws several elaborately themed costume balls at the castle each year, donating the proceeds to charities. He also hosts more low-key, "go with the flow" parties almost every weekend during the summer season. These informal gatherings aren't reserved solely for the wealthy, the "inner-circle," or single females. They are, however, organized around one signature rule—"sarong or be gone." All guests arriving at the castle are required to remove all of their clothing, to stash their cell phones and cameras, and if they don't want to mingle in the buff, to don a Bali-patterned sarong. No underwear. No shoes. No exceptions.

On my first visit, like so many other new female guests, I was angst-ridden at the idea of padding barefoot around the pool. *Didn't he realize girls needed high heels at parties, especially if they are naked?* But I quickly acclimated. After all, Sir Ivan is also known as "Peaceman," a pop-dance singer known for his remakes of 1960s songs, and his "hippie" aesthetic is as much a part of the castle experience as the Roman, Asian, Egyptian, Balinese, and Moroccan-themed guest rooms or the "tribal" loincloths. Shedding the Louboutins or Jimmy Choos—this *is* the Hamptons—lends a democratic air to the gatherings. There is also a practical side to the rule. As Sir Ivan explains, "I don't want a spiked heel through my foot on the dance floor or through my balls in bed."

It's hard to argue with that one.

As castle guests for an entire weekend, my friends and I were allowed to lounge in bikinis or take photos of each other when there weren't parties going on. When Mina wandered out to the pool to greet us, clad only in teeny-weeny bikini bottoms and Ugg boots and cradling Sir Ivan's chihuahua in her arms, any lingering hang-ups evaporated. This wasn't going to be the kind of weekend where the guys eye each other competitively and the girls secretly size up each other's flaws. This was going to be the kind of party where Mina makes everyone feel as gorgeous as she is, swaps stories and laughs unpretentiously at your jokes, and then gives you a tour of the castle—she prefers the "Asian" room, she jokes—after making sure you have fresh-squeezed orange juice for your mimosas. How could you *not* feel comfortable in your own skin when the princess of the castle—your new best friend—is so comfortable in hers?

When other visitors arrived at the gates, we were alerted over a loudspeaker system—"Guests are arriving at the castle. Put away your cell phones and cameras. Time to get naked! The party is starting!" We would obediently strip down, store our valuables in our rooms, and make our way downstairs to greet them in sarongs, like carefree natives greeting a new boatload of nervous explorers. Sometimes the new arrivals were regulars at the castle; other times, they were tourists who had met Sir Ivan at South Pointe, 75 Main, or one of the other nightclubs in Southampton. You couldn't always guess how someone would respond to the new environment; even the most intrepid sensation seekers were often out of their element at first. Some newbies giggled a lot, tied their sarongs so low their knees were covered, and grasped their drinks with white knuckles. A college guy who'd boasted that nothing intimidated him would try to hide in the changing room or slip out the back door without his friends noticing. Then a young woman, who had arrived at the castle dressed for a society garden party, might be the first to shed her conservative sheath and dive naked into the pool.

Although he often steps out with a harem of young women befitting an Arab sheik, Sir Ivan's female fans are more tight-lipped than Hefner's—and he wants it that way. Reporters and regular guests are allowed to penetrate only so far inside the castle walls, and rumor has it that there is a secret passageway leading to the inner rooms, which have never been photographed. The temptation, of course, when contemplating a castle full of seminude revelers, is to focus on sex. But again, perhaps we should think about *sexy* first. Sir Ivan aims to envelop guests in a more extensive realm of hedonistic pleasures—the balmy pool (always kept at ninety-five degrees), platters of fresh fruit, bottomless glasses of champagne, twenty-four-hour butler service, and the freedom of abandoning the rules. "There is an erotic ambience to the environment I create," he says, "but to focus only on sex is to completely miss the point." The castle, he explains, is meant to encapsulate the opulence of St. Tropez, the twenty-four–seven party atmosphere of Ibiza, and the creative, hopeful spirit of Burning Man.

Not everyone has friends like Strauss-Kahn's to plan their sex parties, with or without hookers, and not everyone can host erotic galas, whether elaborate or low-key, at home. But there are other ways to live the "good life," at least when it comes to sexual consumption. If residing at the Playboy Mansion is what God would have done if he'd had the money, perhaps going to Vegas for a lifestyle convention is what the rest of us can do if we don't.

In 1999, anthropologist Hal Rothman declared that Las Vegas "surpassed Mecca as the most visited place on earth." Las Vegas is a place of glitz, glitter, and reinvention, even as it also promises "a luxury experience for a middle-class price." Las Vegas reflects the abundance that baby boomers take for granted as well as "the hedonistic libertarianism that is the legacy of the American cultural revolution of the 1960s."[49] While cities like San Francisco and Amsterdam are also linked with sexuality, the sexual indulgences associated with Las Vegas are heteronormative in comparison: bachelor and bachelorette parties, guys' weekends, strip clubs, brothels, and other opportunities to cheat on the spouse back home. The sexual side of sanctioned deviance is alluded to in the tourist slogan: "What happens in Vegas stays in Vegas." Rather than challenging the status quo, Las Vegas beats to the pulse of the masses.

For many American swingers, a pilgrimage to the annual Lifestyles Convention in Las Vegas, Nevada, was *de rigueur* until 2007, when it was held for the final time.

Robert and Geri McGinley founded the Lifestyles Organization (LSO) in 1969 in Anaheim, California. A few years earlier, while Robert McGinley was working as a contractor with the US Air Force, he had answered an ad in a swingers' magazine and started an erotic correspondence with a sergeant's wife. When his superiors found out, his security clearance was revoked for "sexual deviance" and he lost his job. During his hearing, McGinley was told that he was one of fifty thousand swingers who were being investigated and discharged because "swinging leads to blackmail by Communists, ruined lives, marriage breakups, suicides, and lost jobs."[50] He was struck by the hypocrisy and prejudice. Although he eventually won his appeal against the air force, he had already started down a different career path. He earned his PhD in counseling psychology and continued to work toward legitimizing and organizing swingers' groups.

What had begun as a small group associated with their on-premises swing club, Club Wide World, eventually encompassed around thirty-five thousand association members worldwide and offered a variety of leisure choices: parties in Southern California, houseboat getaways on Lake Mead, international cruises, trips ranging from a week to a month long at resorts in Jamaica and Mexico, and the annual convention. In 1980, McGinley helped found the North American Swing Club Association (NASCA), a trade organization now listing swing clubs in twenty-six countries.[51] First held in 1973, the annual convention continued for thirty-four years, settling in Las Vegas during its heyday and attracting thousands of couples. It included an erotic art show, a marketplace for purchasing sex toys and costumes, workshops, daytime pool parties, and evening dances. The workshops covered topics like jealousy, safety and STDs, sexual techniques, using the Internet to meet couples, legal issues, and the business of swing clubs.

My first trip to the convention was in 2003, when it was held at the Aladdin in Las Vegas. As an academic, I couldn't help feeling obligated to attend panels, regardless of how many empty chairs there were. But within hours I was lounging poolside in the only slice of shade I could find, wide-eyed and slightly drowning in a sea of neon thongs. At all the conventions I attended, I found the rowdy poolside parties—which included contests such as "edible bikini" or "best buns"—and the evening dances more crowded than the workshops. The daytime seminars certainly helped legitimize the lifestyle through the testimony of experts and provided useful information for newcomers. But most of the already-initiated members of the tribe knew that the annual gathering lasted only four days, and many had begun their ceremonial preparations months ahead of time. Connections made on the first day could set the tone of whole event.

At night, the hotel became a series of party rooms, some sponsored by Lifestyles Resorts and others hosted by couples from around the country. You might walk into a suite and find two women oil wrestling in a baby pool, nervous newbies sitting in a circle talking about their boundaries, or a full-blown orgy on the beds while other people mixed drinks and talked sports near the minibar (the hallways, I suppose, were enough of an "exploration zone" for some attendees). Everyone, everywhere, every evening was welcoming. Because the social dynamics and aims were so different from everyday life, it was easy to meet people. Women commented favorably on each other's outfits and talked up their husbands ("My husband gives great foot rubs; I can't wait for you to meet him"). Men struck up conversations with each other at the bar, offering to introduce each other to their wives ("My wife has a killer body and spends more time in the gym than I do"). Compliments flowed in a way that felt genuine; there might have been an ulterior motive, but there was no hidden game.

The LSO focused on the lifestyle as recreation, not revolution, an approach that resonated with enough couples to support the organization over three decades. Gilbert Bartell, who published a study of swinging in 1971 titled *Group Sex Among the Mid-Americans*, argued that the media affected the hopes and fears of both swingers and other couples from suburbia, giving rise to "boredom with marriage." Male swingers, he suggested, "want to see themselves as—and many groups actually call themselves—international Jet Setters, the Cosmopolitans, the Travellers, the Beautiful people."[52] But instead of having to "sit in silence and look at television," swinging couples "have a better relationship, both socially and sexually":

> These people are replaying a mating game. They can relive their youth and for many it is advantageous. They can get dressed up, go out together, and attempt a seduction. . . . If they do prove to be a fairly 'popular' couple and be in demand, they can now feel that they are both beautiful or handsome and desirable. . . . They may now feel that they are doing what the 'in' people are doing and living up to their playboy image.[53]

In fact, Bartell argued that swinging was not deviant behavior but rather a way to embrace both the ideal of marital commitment and the *Playboy* fantasy simultaneously.

A lot of change has occurred in the ten years since my first convention. The LSO was the first major player in the US organized lifestyle scene. Although the organization filed for Chapter 11 bankruptcy in California in 2007, this was not because swinging disappeared. In fact, throughout the 1990s, the number of lifestyle businesses—swingers' clubs, travel agencies, erotic couples' groups, and so on—increased rapidly. By the time the LSO began to struggle, the erotic couples market had grown highly competitive and niche-marketed. These days, one can attend lifestyle events almost every weekend in metropolitan areas like Miami, Los Angeles, New York, or Las Vegas, as well as in major cities across the globe. Organized events provide couples with "on-premise" sexual opportunities: hotels or cruise ships, for example, prohibit sexual activity in public areas, but guest rooms can be used for parties. Some groups strive for complete "takeovers"—booking every room in a hotel or every space at an all-inclusive resort, for example—to offer privacy. Many couples, of course, also still attend house parties, smaller-scale bar meets, and happy hours. As in other industries, market segmentation, differentiation, and upscaling theoretically supplement existing choices rather than replace them, although some argue that small, local businesses suffer in such a competitive market as much as an organization like the LSO.

Mainstreaming is a process; legal battles are still being fought by lifestyle groups and venues faced with community opposition. Still, the special needs of lifestylers for discretion, continually meeting new partners, and venues to engage in recreational sex have been readily harnessed for financial profit.

Some growth was spurred by the Internet; many websites now cater specifically to lifestylers. A couple who has been in the lifestyle for several decades told me that before the Internet, they loitered in the sexuality section of local bookstores, hoping to run into like-minded individuals, or placed advertisements in print newspapers. Online profiles allow for more discreet exchanges and a greater selection of potential partners. Webcams, instant messaging, and chat have been incorporated as erotic practices; for some couples, online interactions are an important part of their lifestyle experience.

As in other enclaves built around recreational sex, attractiveness often trumps other qualities in selecting partners. While there is probably more intergenerational interaction at open lifestyle events or clubs than you would find in a regular bar—you may see grandparents on the dance floor dressed in skimpy attire and laughing with younger couples—there is still a great deal of segregation at play parties. Some invitation-only events require couples to submit photos, provide references, or be hand-selected by the organizers. The more "exclusive" the event, the more participants are expected to adhere to mainstream ideals of attractiveness. Some lifestylers spend thousands of dollars on cosmetic surgery, expensive costumes, and professional photographs for their online profiles. Women bear the brunt of such expectations, although men in the lifestyle are also expected to attend to their appearance through tanning, working out, dressing well, and shaving their bodies or undergoing laser hair removal.

Lifestylers often wear revealing or ostentatious attire that would be inappropriate anywhere else. Themes for some events are advertised months in advance, and couples can spend as much time preparing their bodies and costumes. Themes range widely—from "Arabian Nights" to "Pajama Party," "Red, White, and Blue" to "Glitter and Glow," "*Eyes Wide Shut*" to "*9 1/2 Weeks.*" Some themes are perfect targets for feminist analysis: "Pirates and Wenches," "Pimps N Hos," "Sexy Schoolgirls." Residual guilt from my undergraduate women's studies years inevitably arose when I donned kneesocks, spike heels, and a school*girl* skirt. Somehow, though, the guilt made it even more rebellious. How can you anger your priest, parents, and professors all at once? Give in to sin, impropriety, and patriarchy at the same party. The 2004 LSO convention featured a Saturday night grand finale event with the theme "Hollywood Glitz and Glamour." In promotional materials, participants were invited to "take a stroll down Saturday night's Red Carpet into a lust filled night of Hollywood Glamour & Glitz dressed like one of your favorite movie stars or characters." Although I didn't spot many celebrity impersonations—outside of a few Marilyn Monroes—there was a cornucopia of long velvet gowns, boas, pearls, and elbow-length gloves, along with hats and suits on the men. Some of the more "artsy" lifestyle parties avoid costume themes in favor of lingerie or fetish attire, but one important feature remains the same—*where else can you dress like this*?

Contemporary lifestyle events present opportunities for sexual activity, but they also offer social worlds. Lifestyle parties provide a *relatively* safe space for women to dress or behave provocatively—the only "gang bangs" are those arranged by the women themselves. (This isn't to say that power and hierarchy don't come into play in some relationships or situations; the emphasis on couples invokes an element of male protection, if not ownership. Single women, even though highly sought after, sometimes narrate quite different experiences in the lifestyle than partnered women). For some couples, part of the appeal of events is the opportunity for grandiose self-expression, to live out fantasies of wealth, glamour, and sexiness. The parties provide opportunities to see oneself and one's partner in a new light, as both desiring and desired by others. These fantasies infiltrate everyday life, possibly for months ahead of the event and afterward. Photos taken at the event will be posted to couples' online profiles (It's not just teens who use social networking to develop reputations and gauge popularity.) The competitive elements of the lifestyle—displaying attractiveness, developing networks, building a reputation, and so on—appeal to some individuals and are draining to others.

During the years I attended lifestyle events, I shopped not only for micro-minis but also for glitter bikinis, floor-length gowns, and Moulin Rouge burlesque outfits—not your average "mom" clothes. The ex-stripper in me loved the porn-star fashion as well as the fact that porn-star fashion changes at a glacial pace compared with regular trends. The game hadn't changed since I'd quit stripping. Thong bikinis with rhinestone belts? Of course. In *neon* colors? Totally hot. Cheesy accessories? Bring on the arm bangles, anklets, dangly earrings, chokers, and belly chains. Lingerie peeking out of your clothes? How about *just* lingerie? Nipple peek, visible thongs, or butt cleavage? Sure, at the right party. Satin, lace, leather? Daisy dukes? Mesh shirts? Thigh-high stockings with boots? Yes. Just wait for the right theme.

My partner and I were almost always preparing for the next big event by working out, eating healthfully, making connections with new couples online, and staying in contact with the friends we'd already made. We weren't afraid of the morality police, although we sometimes had difficulty explaining to vanilla friends why we were *again* headed to Las Vegas or Miami—and why we never invited them to join us.

In a time when much of the media seems focused on celebrity—think of the popularity of the E! Entertainment channel, the fascination with the love and sex lives of the stars, the increase in "reality TV" programming where average Joes compete for a shot at stardom (and sometimes, as with ABC's

The Bachelor, live out a harem fantasy)—it makes sense that individuals with the means to do so would find ways to "play" at fame, capture the excitement of the lives of television and movie stars, and experience themselves as deserving of red-carpet attention.

Swingers and other openly nonmonogamous individuals have even started becoming celebrities themselves, for no other reason than their alternative lifestyles. Forget jumping into crocodile-infested swamps to win the attention of one available guy—how about a reality show where you live out fantasies about partner swapping and group sex, with no imposed scarcity? On *Swing*, served up on Playboy TV, there's no need for misattribution or sublimation. Group sex is expected in each episode, and producers get what they want. Every week, a new couple is invited to the "swing house" (a mansion that also housed *American Idol* finalists) to play with veteran swingers and discuss their experiences afterward with a sexologist. There are tears, breakups, drama, and orgies in the red-themed playroom. Being a committed couple isn't necessary: also on Playboy TV you can find *Foursome*, for example. In each episode, whether in Los Angeles or New York City, two single guys and two single girls reveal their fantasies, desires, and multiple tattoos and then uncork the champagne and get down to business. There are girl-on-girl scenes, BDSM "lite," and group sex—it's like an after-party that you can order up at home (and that doesn't start at 6:00 a.m.). In 2012, Showtime rolled out *Polyamory: Married & Dating*, which similarly intersperses group sex scenes with realistic, dramatic but unscripted moments of jealousy and negotiation. These shows aren't porn, although they are considered "adult" and appear on subscription channels, and the "stars" aren't *just* New Age hippies or refugees from the countercultural fringe—or at least they aren't as readily typed that way as in previous depictions. Group sex has appeared in mainstream films in the past, and swinging has certainly been a staple in amateur pornography, but the turn to reality-style, docudrama programming indicates an intriguing shift in the reception of nonmonogamy. Instead of lasciviousness, sexy parties are increasingly spelling luxury. Sir Ivan has filmed a sizzle reel with Lionsgate for his own reality show, although it remains to be seen whether the focus will be on his erotic soirees or the other aspects of his eccentric lifestyle.

Gary Rosenson, senior vice president and general manager of domestic television for Playboy, suggested in an interview about the success of *Swing*, "[Swinging] exists everywhere. People are interested in it. There are people that you probably know who may not have told you that they are swingers, but it's out there. . . . It just is a fact of America."[54] They might not consider themselves swingers or even "in the lifestyle." Sex partying is young, hip, and trendy as long as you don't try to label anyone.

Playboys. Playmates. Playcouples. *Partiers*.

In August 2012, Prince Harry was secretly photographed while partying at the Wynn in Las Vegas. The blurry pictures of him that appeared online, naked and cupping his genitals with his hands, caused "acute embarrassment" for palace officials. Although allegations of cocaine use—which, reporters remind us, *is* still illegal, even in Las Vegas—hookers, and a possible sex tape associated with the party remain unconfirmed, Harry found public support in London and the United States: "He's a lad, for God's sake." Sure, he was chastised by an ABC News public relations consultant for being careless—"Everybody knows better than to party naked in a room full of strangers without confiscating the cellphones. That's just Hollywood 101"— but few commentators expressed surprise that he'd hosted a nude billiards game in the first place. Such a lapse in judgment certainly made for a good story—just ask TMZ, *People Magazine*, or the girls who stripped down with the prince and his entourage in the VIP suite that fateful evening. One of the girls claimed it "was not like an orgy going on, it was just sexy naked."[55]

In the aftermath of the incident, Steve Wynn comped Prince Harry's tab, estimated at £30,000, but has thus far resisted naming the suite in honor of the infamous royal romp. Vivid Entertainment reportedly offered the prince $10 million to shoot a porn film, competing with bids from Playgirl and Chippendales for photos or onstage peeks at the royal family jewels. The Las Vegas Convention and Visitors' Authority responded to the scandal with an advertising campaign criticizing the photo leak as infringing on the ethos of "what happens in Vegas stays in Vegas": "We are asking for a shun on these exploiters of Prince Harry. We shall boycott partying of any kind with them. No bottle service. No bikini clad girls. No Bucatini from Butali. In other words, we will not play with them anymore."[56] Another advertisement read: "Keep calm Harry, and carry on; #knowthecode." The publicity generated from Harry's escapades has been valued at $23 million in revenue for the city.[57]

Perhaps Prince Harry should visit Sir Ivan in the Hamptons on his next transatlantic jaunt, where the colorful sarongs allow merrymakers to keep their hands free and the cell phone ban is rigorously enforced. What happens at the castle really *does* stay at the castle.

OF HOOLIGANS AND NUDE REVOLUTIONARIES

Ma Yaohai, a fifty-three-year-old college professor from Nanjing, China, was an accidental orgiast. After two divorces, he decided to try meeting women online. He began dating a twenty-three-year-old woman who used the screen name Passionate Fiery Phoenix and identified as a swinger. They went to their first swinging party together on New Year's Day in 2004. Although Ma suffered from performance anxiety that time, he soon became accustomed enough to group sex—his largest party was four couples—to begin offering advice to others online.[58] For the next two years, he also recruited participants online for sex parties, using the screen name "bighornyfire" (or, depending on the translation, "Roaring Virile Fire"). He organized eighteen orgies, some of which were supposedly held in the apartment he shares with his Alzheimer's disease–stricken mother.[59]

Ma's adventures took a sour turn in 2010 when he was charged with "group licentiousness" under China's Criminal Law 301. Twenty-one other participants at his parties were also charged.[60] "Group licentiousness" was originally a subclause under "hooliganism," which included all extramarital sexual behavior and treated offenders harshly, potentially with the death penalty. In 1997, the hooliganism statute was repealed in China, meaning that extramarital sex was no longer illegal; "three or more people having sex," however, remains a criminal offense, as does being a "ringleader."

In early 2010, Ma Yaohai was sentenced to three and a half years in prison.

Debate over Ma's conviction was heated. One commentator, Ming Haoyue, insisted that group sex is "decadent behavior" that challenges social morality and adversely affects "the normal social order, thus hindering the pursuit of the majority of people for good behaviors." Haoyue further observed, "Chaotic, indulgent sexual activities may fuel other evils."[61] A blogger charged Ma with inciting "social chaos": "You led a 22-person orgy. You have destroyed ethics and morality."[62] Chinese sexologist and activist Li Yinhe protested the verdict in the media, however, arguing that criminal laws against "group licentiousness, prostitution, and obscene products (pornography)," all victimless sexual crimes, were draconian remnants of the Cultural Revolution.[63] Experts estimate that fewer than one hundred thousand Chinese participate in group sex, although a chat forum dedicated to swinging on the website "Happy Village" has more than 380,000 registered members.[64] Citizens increasingly seek out porn, buy sex toys, and visit brothels. Consensual sexual behavior between adults, Li Yinhe maintained, is a "private matter." Ma Yaohai agreed, although some believe his sentence might have been lighter if he'd shown remorse instead of defending his actions in the press: "Marriage is like water: you have to drink it. Swinging is like a glass of fine wine: you can choose to drink it or not," he stated. "What we did, we did for our own happiness. People chose to do it of their own free will and they knew they could stop at any time. We disturbed no one."[65]

In August 2012, another sex scandal rocked China when "orgy" photos supposedly featuring several high-ranking government officials were posted online. Couples have been arrested, tortured, and imprisoned in Egypt and Iran for organizing sex parties. Gay men have been arrested and sentenced to death for group sex across the Middle East; at times, the accusation of orgy hosting is used as a justification for police raids on homes and businesses.[66]

Even attempting to educate about or conduct research on sexual behavior can put an individual at risk. Since Mahdavi's ethnography was published in 2009, she has received e-mail every week from around the world thanking her for writing honestly about contemporary Iran. She has paid a high price for her work, however. In addition to praise, she receives hate mail, faces hostile audiences, and has been accused of everything from sexual impropriety to falsifying her data by Iranian critics. More significantly, even though she took extreme measures to conceal the identity of her informants and protect them from government retaliation, she was unable to shield herself from political scrutiny. Mahdavi is no longer allowed to visit Iran for either personal or professional reasons. Still, she considers herself "one of the lucky ones"; another scholar she knew was incarcerated and spent time in solitary confinement for her research and political views.

Western swingers don't risk hard labor in prison, death by hanging, or exile. Perhaps this is part of the reason swingers have a reputation for being fairly politically conservative. Outside of radical utopian communities, early social science literature on swinging in the United States found participants to hold "general white suburban attitudes."[67] Modern American lifestylers are believed to be more interested in staying under the radar and maintaining the status quo than contesting it. One writer suggests, "The point of swinging is not to challenge gender roles, nor to question heterosexuality. People in the lifestyle enjoy being married or partnered and simply want to supplement their sex life by including intimacies with other couples like themselves."[68] In 1999 and 2000, Bergstrand and Sinski revisited the issue with a survey of approximately 1,100 self-identified swingers. By including questions taken from the General Social Survey, or GSS, they could compare swingers with the general population. As in previous studies, the majority of their respondents were in their thirties and forties, primarily white and college educated. They placed a high importance on marriage and marital satisfaction, valuing companionship more highly than personal freedom, the same as the general population. But swingers were also "more likely to favor gay marriage, less likely to condemn premarital or teen sex (fourteen- to sixteen-year-olds), more likely to reject traditional sex roles in their relationships," and "were less racist, less sexist, and less heterosexist than the general population."[69]

While Western lifestylers may not currently be rallying around an identity or political issue, there may be a time when they do, despite their relatively privileged social positions. Bergstrand and Sinski note that there have been fourteen legal cases challenging the closing of swingers' clubs in the United States, not counting clubs that closed because the owners didn't have the finances or ability to fight. Courts have consistently *not* found such establishments to be protected under the First and Fourteenth Amendments, which secure "constitutional rights to privacy, free speech or association." Free speech doesn't protect "purely physical conduct that lacks any corresponding expressive element," and swingers' clubs have been considered public places. These decisions, Bergstrand and Sinski maintain, are "part of an elaborate moral architecture of monogamy that has been constructed by the Supreme Court over the past century and a half." The stage has been set for this particular vision of sexual, emotional, and practical monogamy to affect legal decisions pertaining to sexuality, obscenity, and "a wide range of behaviors having to do with how we view community, public and private spheres of activity, and the construction of personal meaning in our lives."[70]

Highly publicized busts of swing clubs have occurred in the United States and Canada, and photos of "outed" couples have appeared in newspapers. Four of seven people featured in the documentary *Sex with Strangers* lost their jobs when employers learned of their practices.[71] In 2010, a couple was fired from their jobs at a theater in Spokane after being outed as swingers when an anonymous source sent copies of e-mails they'd exchanged with couples on Craigslist.[72] The couples from *Swing* have been more insulated— if you're going to openly deviate from mainstream norms, it helps to run your own business (even more if it's a lifestyle website). Perhaps writing political slogans on your body before visiting a swingers' club would be a good idea, or maybe it's easier to just follow the trend toward private or temporary venues. Will there even be a need for identity politics or a "community" if "sexy naked" parties are just part of a regular weekend for many groups of young adults?

Sexual practices have been linked to ideals of personal and social transformation in societies throughout history. Sex, as play, can become a way of learning about oneself and others. It can become a way of reimagining oneself. In certain contexts, sexual practice can also become a way of reimagining the world, sparking revolutionary hopes. As group sex involves relations of witnessing and being witnessed, it is uniquely and powerfully positioned to serve such purposes. Group sex is ripe as transgression and often promises transcendence—although it does not always deliver either. Is congregating for an orgy in a dry swimming pool, in a country where wearing open-toed shoes might land one in jail (and a miniskirt might earn lashes with a whip) more revolutionary than entering a "sexy buns" contest at a lifestyle event in Las Vegas? Perhaps it depends on whether you work at a conservative banking firm and your superiors are now asking for your resignation after seeing pictures on Facebook—perhaps you'd take the whipping if you could keep your salary? Participants in these events are obviously positioned differently in global networks of privilege—social class, ethnicity, religion, gender, labor, and so on. In terms of subjective feelings of jeopardy, however, there may be something commensurable about their experiences, at least some of the time. Just consider: If a twenty-two-person orgy can "destroy" the ethics and morality of a country with a population of more than a billion, it's a

powerful weapon of social change. Or, at least, it *feels* like one to some
people.

In a political address on Iranian state television from 2005, the supreme
leader Ayatollah Ali Khamenei warned of the conceivable success of a "velvet" revolution:

> More than Iran's enemies need artillery, guns, and so forth, they need to spread
> cultural values that lead to moral corruption . . . a senior official in an impor-
> tant American political center said: 'Instead of bombs, send them miniskirts.'
> He is right. If they arouse sexual desires in any given country, if they spread
> unrestrained mixing of men and women, and if they lead youth to behavior to
> which they are naturally inclined by instincts, there will no longer be any need
> for artillery and guns against that nation. [73]

Conservative fears that desires for greater sexual freedom among a populace
will beget desires for other social changes are not completely unfounded.
Mahdavi, for example, traces the emergence of Iran's Green Revolution of
2009 to the social and sexual changes she witnessed during her fieldwork.
Youth who had begun rebelling by sneaking out of their homes wearing
makeup, listening to illegal music, and throwing sex parties eventually became more explicitly critical of repression. They began organizing and ac-
tively challenging their leaders. The Green Revolution erupted after the election of Mahmoud Ahmadinejad, with protestors literally taking to the streets.
Sexual experimentation alone, Mahdavi cautions, does not automatically
transform society. But the disenchantment that had been building in Iran,
along with the fact that people had begun stealing moments of freedom and
pleasure, created changes in their thoughts and actions—not just around sex,
but toward everyday life more generally—that *did* spread to the political
realm.

The Arab Spring—a wave of political demonstrations spreading over the
Arab world— officially began on December 18, 2010, the day that a twenty-
six-year-old Tunisian street vendor named Mohamed Bouazizi set himself on
fire in front of the governor's office in Sidi Bouzid to protest mistreatment
and corruption. Bouazizi's action sparked other protests throughout the country; news of the situation spread rapidly around the world through reports on
Facebook and other websites. Although police attempted to squash the demonstrations, unrest grew. Within weeks, the Tunisian president fled the country after twenty-three years in office. [74] Protests and uprisings have since
followed in other nations, including Egypt, Libya, Syria, Morocco, and Ye-
men. Each of these political movements is unique, with its own history and
complexities, and the outcomes have varied. Scholars see common threads
across the uprisings, though, such as slow escalations of discontent, marginalized youth, and the multifaceted use of social media sites and the Internet.
Beyond kindling new visions and desires, the Internet allows for rapid infor-

mation flows and international connections never before possible. A 2011 study found that nine out of ten Egyptians and Tunisians reported using Facebook to organize protests or disseminate information during recent political struggles.[75] Whether increasing openness about sexuality is best seen a precursor to the Arab Spring or a consequence of the ensuing regime changes is debated, but sexuality is linked to visions of change put forth on both sides of the struggles.

In November 2011, a twenty-year-old Egyptian woman, Aliaa al-Mahdy (or Elmahdy), posted a nude photo of herself on Facebook. After Facebook removed the image, she allowed a friend to repost it on Twitter, using the hashtag #nudephotorevolutionary.

Al-Mahdy took the photo at her parents' home, using a self-timer on her camera. The image is black and white, although her flat shoes and the flower in her hair are red. Except for black thigh-high stockings and the flats, she is naked. There is no arched back, centerfold makeup, or pursed lips; she looks straight into the camera without smiling. Whether her gaze is interpreted as innocent or defiant depends on one's perspective; she does not, however, appear ashamed.

The photo, she claims, was taken and posted online to protest sexual discrimination, harassment, and inequality.

Since then, the young activist and blogger has been called deviant, mentally ill, and destructive; even liberal groups have distanced themselves from al-Mahdy and her boyfriend, another controversial blogger, out of fear that she damaged their cause by going too far. Despite receiving death threats and being accused of prostitution, al-Mahdy has vowed to remain in Egypt. In an interview with CNN, she stated, "I am a believer of every word I say and I am willing to live in danger under the many threats I receive in order to obtain the real freedom all Egyptians are fighting and dying for daily."[76]

For International Women's Day in 2012, feminist activists posed nude for a calendar in honor of Elmahdy, titled *Nude Photo Revolutionaries*. "Free thought in a free body," one of the captions reads. "Our naked body is our challenge to patriarchy, dictatorship, and violence. Smart people we inspire, dictators are horrified. Women all over the world—come, undress, win," reads another. Critics see the calendar and al-Mahdy's approach as subjecting women to even more objectification. Supporters claim the issue is about freedom of expression and that "nudity is the antithesis of veiling"—"when a tool of oppression can be turned into an assertion of power, it is a beautiful thing."

Because it involves the use of the body, nudity has been compared to self-immolation and hunger strikes. The revolutionary impact of nudity, sex, and transgression can be quite a slippery matter, however.

Instead of finishing her final year at Moscow State University studying philosophy, twenty-three-year-old Nadezhda Tolokonnikova will potentially spend the next two years in prison. In February 2012, the punk-rock activist group Pussy Riot staged a performance at the Cathedral of Christ the Saviour in Moscow. Donning colorful dresses, mismatched tights, and balaclavas—woven facemasks that are practical in Russia because of the cold but that also work well for guerrilla activists—a group of women stormed the stage near the altar. First they bowed as if in prayer and then began singing and dancing, "air karate" style. Their performance was brief, as security guards escorted them outside shortly after they appealed to the Virgin Mary to take up feminism and oust Prime Minister Vladimir Putin. No one was actually arrested until after a video of the performance appeared on YouTube, titled "Punk Prayer—Mother of God, Chase Putin Away."

Were the women's actions art? Crime? Political speech?

Tolokonnikova and two other known members of Pussy Riot, Yekaterina Samutsevich and Maria Alyokhina, were charged with hooliganism—"deliberate behavior that violates public order and expresses explicit disrespect toward society." The other members fled into hiding. The trial began in July 2012. Pussy Riot defended their performance as dissident art and political action, while Putin compared it to a "witches Sabbath."[77] Witnesses called by the prosecution accused the women of "sacrilege and 'devilish dances'" in the church. In August 2012, the women were found guilty of "hooliganism motivated by religious hatred," believed to stem from their feminist beliefs, and sentenced to two years in prison.

Although there was no sex or nudity in "Punk Prayer"—blasphemy was enough—Tolokonnikova already had an activist history. In February 2008, as part of another radical group called Voina, Tolokonnikova participated in an orgy at the Timiriazev State Biology Museum in Moscow that was photographed and filmed. The orgy, held to protest the "farcical and pornographic" election of Dmitry Medvedev, was called "Fuck for the Heir Puppy Bear!" The root of Medvedev means "bear" in Russian. Blogger and Voina member Alexei Plutser-Sarno claimed that the orgy denoted how "in Russia everyone fucks each other and the little president looks at it with delight." In the video, available online, participants quickly undress near a taxidermic bear. Four couples, including Tolokonnikova, visibly pregnant and on her knees with her underwear pulled down, begin having sex doggie style. A fifth couple has oral sex. Several of the men appear to have performance issues—not surprising, as group sex is intimidating enough without visions of Siberian labor camp flashing before one's eyes. In the background, a bearded Plutser-Sarno in a tuxedo and top hat holds a banner reading "fuck for the heir-bear." Tolokonnikova gave birth just a few days after the orgy, a detail rarely left out of Western media reports.

In a 2010 Voina performance, "Dick Captured by KGB," the artists painted a sixty-five-meter long, twenty-seven-meter wide outline of a penis on a drawbridge in St. Petersburg. When the bridge was raised, the penis appeared erect. The bridge, incidentally, led to the headquarters of the Federal Security Service (FSB), the successor to the KGB and the agency that sent twenty-five to thirty "men in suits with guns" to arrest Tolokonnikova and her husband after Pussy Riot's "Punk Prayer" hit the Internet.[78]

The Pussy Riot trial attracted international attention as a case about government infringement on freedom of expression and the suppression of political speech. Protests were held in numerous countries, and musicians such as Madonna, Sting, the Red Hot Chili Peppers, and Paul McCartney offered public support. British and American officials claimed the sentences were "disproportionate" and urged the Russian government to reconsider.[79] Within Russia, though, polls suggested far less support for the band members, whose actions were seen as hateful, disgusting, shocking, and without political merit. Ironically, Medvedev—the namesake of the 2008 museum orgy—called for the women's release in mid-September, possibly in response to international pressure.[80] In October 2012, Yekaterina Samutsevich's sentence was suspended because she had been prevented from actually dancing on the altar by a security guard, but Tolokonnikova and Alyokhina were sent to labor camps. On November 1, 2012, Medvedev again suggested the women should be freed.

Some bloggers claimed that the focus in the Western media on defending the women's right to "freedom of expression" was a self-serving contortion of Pussy Riot's message, which is more radical than most Americans or British would swallow if they truly understood it: the need to overthrow "patriarchal" society, "including capitalism, religion, moral norms, inequality of all forms, and the corporate state system." The women in Pussy Riot, one writer argues, have "more in common with insurrectionary anarchists than with the bland pop-culture 'icons' who so vocally support them."[81] On the cartoon show *South Park*, Jesus appears to a community wearing a "Free Pussy Riot" T-shirt under his robe; the episode critiques American tendencies to jump on a popular bandwagon without excavating the entire issue.

In terms of accumulating American supporters, Tolokonnikova is probably lucky that she landed in jail for challenging the intermingling of church and state with Pussy Riot rather than for her Voina museum capers. Although "Punk Prayer" and "Fuck for the Heir Puppy Bear" might indeed be protected speech in the United States, performers could still have initially faced arrest and charges for trespassing or lewd conduct. When Al Gore lost the presidency to George W. Bush despite winning the popular vote, his supporters protested, but a staged and videotaped orgy in the United States Botanic Gardens in Washington, DC probably wouldn't have gone over so well. Freemuse.org tracks the torture and imprisonment of artists in countries around the world. Few gain an international spotlight like Pussy Riot did, and doing so has as much to do with the political moment and the message being delivered as with people's commitment to abstract concepts such as "freedom." Certainly, it helped that these women were pretty, had young children, and had chosen a band name like "Pussy Riot." Who doesn't want to talk about "Pussy Riot" while waiting in line at Starbucks? Suddenly, people who'd never even said the word "pussy" could toss it out brazenly in public. But more importantly, it is far easier to defend transgression when it isn't *your* cherished beliefs being transgressed. The performance in the cathedral wasn't emotionally upsetting to Americans or Brits who already believe in— or at least give lip service to—the separation of church and state. The message of "Punk Prayer" made *sense*, even if the singing was dreadful. And if evidence was sought that Russia hasn't really become a free, democratic nation after all, the government's defensive response to "Punk Prayer" served as a timely example.

But while the American public might stand behind photographer Spencer Tunick, who has been arrested numerous times for staging nude public photo shoots, it *is* fickle about transgressive sexual expression. A US adult film directed by Thomas Zupko titled *The Attic* makes a point similar to that of Voina with their orgy. In one scene, four male performers in masks—Bush, Reagan, another Bush, and a demon—"fuck" a woman painted like the Statue of Liberty. By the end of the scene, she has been thoroughly defiled; not only is she not recognizable as *Libertas*, but she is hard to look at onscreen. Throughout the film, other figures of state authority from cops to men dressed like Hitler also sexually brutalize immigrants, Native Americans, and a woman dressed as a Japanese geisha. The sex is very aggressive and coercive. In a last-minute, likely brilliant, decision during production, Zupko praised the First Amendment in the film: "This video was made as a tribute to America, not as an attack against it. It is meant as a grand celebration of the First Amendment and the freedom of artistic expression. That we can do this proves once again that America is not only the greatest country in the world today but also the greatest country in the history of civilization. God Bless America!" Zupko's political speech cannot be simplistically compared with Voina's, given contextual and historical differences. Still, the use of transgressive sex in art, politics, and porn raises complex issues—the most pressing is how to decide which is which.

Although Zupko was not prosecuted for obscenity under the Bush administration, many others in the adult entertainment industry were indeed indicted and sent to jail. Both Rob Black (Robert Zicari) and Lizzie Borden (Janet Romano), the husband husband-and-wife team behind Extreme Associates, were incarcerated for a year; another controversial pornographer, Max Hardcore (Paul Little), also did time. The films that made their way to the courts in these cases portrayed not just orgies but "rough sex," incest, extreme misogyny, rape, murder, and fantasized sex with underage girls. *Cocktails 2*, a series discussed in chapter 4, involved mixing and ingesting body fluids; *Ass Clowns 3* includes scenes of a woman raped by a gang led by Osama bin Laden and of Jesus having sex with an angel.

Let's just say that Madonna wasn't calling for leniency or wearing an Extreme Associates T-shirt onstage.

Zicari sold the films he was being prosecuted for as a package called *The Federal Five* to help with his legal fees. Pornographers generally do not protest capitalism, probably part of the reason why their products are stigmatized rather than celebrated. Americans have strong beliefs that art and sex should remain "free" in a market economy—although that is a topic for another book. But even if Madonna and Bjork had sold his films as they sell Pussy Riot merchandise to raise money for the women behind bars, Zicari might not have found public favor.

To many Americans, Zicari's films are hateful, disgusting, shocking, and without artistic or political merit, much like the way conservative Russians view Tolokonnikova's performances. What constitutes transgression, sexual or otherwise, varies. One person's art becomes another person's crime, porn, or politics—and back again. Transgression *can* shake things up, whether it's meant to be explicitly political or not—at least for a while. Just try painting a giant penis on public property. But transgression as politics will always have a limited range of efficacy. One has to hit the right moment, the right medium, the right locale, and the right intensity for an audience to receive the message. If a taboo is too deeply entrenched, the transgressor is simply deemed insane or criminal (though perhaps his ideas can be resurrected a century after the beheading). If, on the other hand, the taboo is already ready to crumble, transgression comes off as more silly than daring—at least by those who consider themselves cutting edge.

In a special episode of *Skins* that originally aired in 2007 on MySpace,[82] the teenagers sit on a hillside, high on drugs. One of the characters, Chris, is suddenly struck with an idea for a party based on the antics of a historical group he calls the "Diggers," who supposedly lived on that very hill they are tripping on. His friends do not need much arm twisting to help him prepare for the event. Posters of a cartoon clown are hung around the city; guests will follow the clown signs to the secret party location.

During the preparations, Chris hallucinates an old man who appears alternately in clothes and nude. The old man, who calls himself "the lord of the manor," claims to have thrown parties that "made history" at the same location—including "Diggers parties," "foam parties," and "naked orgies." His orgies, he boasts, featured a "four-poster bed" in the center of the room where "Napoleon sucked Brigitte Bardot's toes."

Chris looks impressed.

"What kind of party would *you* like to throw?" the lord asks.

The answer appears in the next montage of scenes: girls undressing; punch being spiked with drugs; girls kissing girls; boys kissing girls. Chris swigs from a champagne bottle, reacting as if it isn't just champagne. A girl sticks out her tongue, revealing an Ecstasy tab, and then pushes a skinny boy down on a bed in the center of the room. Chris sucks a woman's toes while wearing a Napoleon costume. The quickly flashing images become more disorienting, set to a repetitive indie rock song: A guest throws up. A young man applies lipstick and looks down at the corset he is wearing in confusion. The lord of the manor toasts a guest. A girl kisses one boy, then another on the bed. Teens dance in clown masks. A boy in a cropped red military jacket climbs on top of Jal, one of the regular female characters, who is wearing a frilly pink dress. He pulls down a coffin lid, shutting the two of them inside.

The final scene cuts to the aftermath of the party. It is daylight. Chris, still drinking from the champagne bottle, wanders away from the party, passing guests sleeping in the yard while Simon and Garfunkel's "Me and Julio Down by the Schoolyard" plays in the background. (In the 1970s song, a "mama" is so upset by seeing what two boys have done that she spits on the ground and reports them to the police. In an interview for *Rolling Stone*, Paul Simon was asked, "What is it that the mama saw? The whole world wants to know." Simon replied, "I have no idea. . . . Something sexual is what I imagine."[83] Guesses range from buying drugs to having sex with each other to hanging out with a drag queen—"Rosie, Queen of Corona." Simon later swore he would never tell—a smart move, given that specifics would have cast his lyrics into irrelevance.)

History collapses in the ten-minute episode. The music—from "The Clapping Song" (1965) to "Me and Julio" (1972) to "Hummer" (2007)—and the references—from the nineteenth-century French leader Napoleon to 1960s actress Brigitte Bardot to the "Diggers"—cut across centuries and continents. Reality blurs with fantasy. Many of the guests at the Diggers party were not actors but *Skins* fans that won a competition to attend a real "secret Skins party" and were then filmed. Chris "invents" the "Diggers" during his hallucination to justify his party, but "Diggers" was actually the name of both a British communist group from the seventeenth century and an anarchist group in San Francisco during the late 1960s. Both groups were associated with sexual licentiousness and revolutionary politics. The Diggers of 1649 believed that land ownership was immoral on biblical grounds. The San Francisco Diggers challenged capitalism, providing free food in their stores, along with free art, music, and even housing; sex and drugs were intertwined with a belief in the creation of a more peaceful and egalitarian society. Peter Coyote, an actor who was involved with the San Francisco Diggers, claimed he was "interested in two things: overthrowing the government and fucking. They went together seamlessly."[84]

As for the *Skins* teens of 2007 and the young partiers inspired by the show, the idealized sex of the 1960s is still present. So are the drugs. It is less clear where social critique comes into play, however, if at all—though the fact that Chris is inspired by the "lord of the manor" is perhaps best interpreted sardonically. In historical documents about the English Diggers, the first lord of the manor was a man named Francis Drake, who organized numerous attacks on the group, including beatings and arson. Some of the surviving Diggers moved to Little Heath in Surrey, where they encountered another lord of the manor, Parson Platt. Platt also systematically harassed the Diggers, burned their communal homes, and finally drove them from Little Heath. He is credited with destroying the movement.[85]

AFTER THE ORGY, PART 1: COMMODIFICATION

Sex has a degree of radical potential, as so many individuals and social movements throughout history have proclaimed. Participation in group sex can stimulate critiques of negative cultural attitudes that lead to shame, guilt, secrecy, hypocrisy, or inequality. Group erotics or sex can feel liberating to participants from very different backgrounds and contexts because it requires transgressing both psychological and social boundaries and norms. It can inspire feelings of belonging. Sometimes, these feelings of liberation and belonging lead to a reimagining of the everyday that bursts into reality. "Sexual adventurousness," Tim Dean writes, "gives birth to other forms of adventurousness—political, cultural, intellectual."[86] In certain times and places, witnessing and being witnessed in socially and psychologically transgressive activity becomes explicitly political.

But how far can this adventurousness reach? And although change is inevitable, is freedom the end result? Or do we simply submit to the new forms of social control that predictably arise?

Pussy Riot's colorful balaclavas are meant to render performers anonymous—the emphasis, the group insists, should be on the idea rather than the individuals expressing it. (Of course, anonymity also helps when the FSB comes knocking.) But when photographs of the women in everyday attire began appearing after their arrests, their aim of vanquishing capitalist patriarchy was less news- and blog-worthy than that Tolokonnikova had a "bangin' body" and "Angelina Jolie's lips." It is as easy to find the "Puppy Bear" performance by googling "sexy pregnant orgy photos" as "Voina political protest." "Free Pussy Riot" T-shirts are available on Café Press and Amazon.com.

Balaclavas are flying off the shelves.

Well, maybe we can't go *that* far. But there is already talk of a Hollywood film, and a battle over the Pussy Riot trademark has begun.

Classic sociologist Max Weber warned of the "iron cage" of capitalism, a process of increasing rationality and bureaucratic control that promises freedom but imprisons us instead. Like Khamenei, later theorists, contemplating how working classes around the world often welcomed capitalist expansion rather than revolting, suggested that perhaps the cage is "velvet" rather than iron. A velvet cage is comfy, comforting. It probably has a nice view. Even if we realize we are confined, we prefer that to trying something different.

"Revolutionaries don't take weekends," a colleague of mine is fond of saying.

Weekends, though, are when the best parties happen.

An online advertisement for the Renault Grand Scenic—a car offering "vast interior space" and seating for up to seven passengers—shows the vehicle parked on a moonlit beach, rocking. Crickets chirp. The rocking stops, and after a moment, there is a flash inside the car as a cigarette is lit. Six more cigarettes light up the darkness. Someone giggles.

Rebels become consumers. Rebellion becomes fashion.

The orgy is over; the sales are starting.

Chapter Nine

Upping the Ante or Over the Edge?

The Edge . . . there is no honest way to explain it because the only people who really know where it is are the ones who have gone over.
—Hunter S. Thompson

STAN COLLYMORE: FROM ATHLETE TO ADDICT?

Stan Collymore, a former English footballer recognized as much for his personal foibles as his athletic ability, knows a bit about scandal. When he struck his girlfriend, Ulrika Jonsson, in a Paris bar during the 1998 World Cup, an already tempestuous relationship splashed across the tabloids. In 2000, he was kicked out of a hotel at La Manga, a Spanish resort where he was staying with his teammates, for setting off a fire extinguisher in a "drunken fracas." After a series of additional public setbacks with his career, Collymore sank into depression. In March 2001, just a few weeks after signing with the Spanish football club Real Oviedo, he announced his retirement at the age of thirty. "Flattened" by personal and professional turmoil, he returned home and "slept for the next three years."

Well, not quite.

He also went "dogging."

Just before Christmas in 2001, Collymore received the news that Oviedo was suing him for breach of contract to the tune of £7 million. Since his retirement, financial troubles had plagued him. His relationship with his wife, Estelle, was strained. Their daughter, Mia, had been born in July, but he could barely get through each day, much less help care for a colicky infant. Without the "buzz" of playing football to occupy his mind and deflect his growing anxiety, he felt himself spiraling. The quest for a new adrenaline rush—a mix of "danger and excitement and a bizarre feeling of adventure"—

295

sent him driving to a Midlands parking lot one evening, on the road to his next big scandal.

Collymore had heard about "dogging"—supposedly England's newest sex craze—from a friend. Some commentators suggest that the term is derived from the way single men "dogged," or spied on, couples having sex on lovers' lanes. Other lore points to dogging as derived from the euphemism "walking the dog," an excuse supposedly given by straying spouses to explain their evening absences.[1] Either way, dogging now refers to public, often anonymous, multiperson sexual activity in parks or other outdoor locations. Doggers frequent known cruising spots, which may also be used by gay men, looking for sexual activity. Doggers also rely on modern communication technology—such as e-mail lists and news groups, websites and forums dedicated to dogging, and text messaging on cell phones—to make connections and arrange sexual encounters.

After surfing the Web for information, Collymore decided to check out Barr Beacon, a reputed dogging hotspot. He maneuvered his Range Rover up the hills to a parking lot known as the "Airport," a spot that offered panoramic views of the countryside during the day. In the dark of the night, the former aerodrome presented another unique perspective: dozens of car headlights winding slowly up the hill, each on a similar quest for sexual adventure.

He was intrigued.

He parked next to a car with two men in the front seat and two women in the back. "Suddenly," he writes in his memoirs, "a man came out of the shadows and the inside light went on in the car next to me." Later, he would learn that turning on the interior light was a way for couples in their cars to signal interest in someone who approached. That first night, however, he knew none of the etiquette; this was a "strange new world" he had never known existed. With his "heart in his mouth," Collymore peered through his car window as the single man advanced toward the other vehicle. The car door opened. When Collymore realized "the bloke" was "getting sucked off" by one of the women, his curiosity was piqued. He approached the car, too, and was invited in. While the husbands watched from the front seat, he "had a bit of a fiddle" with the other woman.

Dogging proved seductive for the former athlete. On nights when he felt anxious and overwhelmed by his troubles, he found himself drawn to the "midnight world" of Barr Beacon. He developed a routine. He would stop at McDonald's, picking up food and a large Diet Coke. He would drive up the hill to the lot. As he had a television in his car, he would eat French fries and watch live football. He would smoke cigarettes. And he would wait.

The sex, when it happened, was often "unfulfilling." But for Collymore, "the addictive nature of dogging was nothing to do with the promise of sex." Sex, after all, was easy for a footballer to find—even a former one. If he wanted sex, he could simply pick up a girl at a nightclub instead of driving to a remote location, waiting around for hours, and then maybe "shagging a bloke's wife." The thrill of dogging was in the cocktail of emotions he experienced over the course of an evening. There was anticipation: "Just imagining on the way up there what I might find gave me a buzz. I imagined I might find an orgy going on in a car. If I got there and there were no other cars there, I would tease myself with the thought that one would pitch up any minute." There was a sense of mystery, subterfuge, in being with strangers pursuing the same thrills: "Some of those car parks are like an underworld. . . a scene from a film noir. There are sometimes a couple of hundred cars. . . . There might be 40 or 50 couples looking for something to happen." There was anxiety about whether the other cars held doggers or police: "You are watching in your rear-view mirror and suddenly headlights will come on or a car will do a quick U-turn and other cars will be darting off all over the place." There was a sense of danger: "a combination of the fear of people recognizing me, and the fear of doing something that I shouldn't be doing." And then, finally, there was a payoff, an escape from his everyday worries: "A couple comes along and starts shagging and it takes your mind away from everything. You're buzzing and you're no longer in that weird, tortured zone where you are tormenting yourself with strange imaginings of the horrors that may lie ahead."

When dogging, he was also once again part of a team. Some of the excitement was "seeing couples and other blokes taking chances in this alien environment." Doggers weren't social outcasts, he found. They were professionals, driving Mercedes or Range Rovers. Most of the couples he met "appeared to be perfectly normal, unremarkable, down-to-earth people." He enjoyed the camaraderie among them, despite the anonymity of many exchanges. These were "businessmen by day," "heading for the hills in the evening because they don't feel they have another outlet for their urges that they can be open about."

Perhaps it was because of such feelings of amity that Collymore endeavored to initiate a nervous-looking couple into the culture of dogging one fateful evening. He shared with them what he knew: where the best locations were; how to signal interest using the car's interior lights or headlights; the options and procedures for joining in when people were having sex; the safety reasons that couples didn't usually exchange addresses or full names with strangers; and the basic principles of respect and consent. "You don't do anything you don't want to do," he assured the couple.

Or perhaps he was so forthcoming because the woman, who used the name Lucy, was young and attractive, and her "husband" indicated that he wanted to see her with another man. Either way, by the time Collymore discovered they weren't neophyte doggers but undercover reporters from *The*

Sun newspaper who were audiotaping and photographing their interactions with him, it didn't really matter why he'd been so candid. He was caught.

As the story broke, Collymore checked into the Priory Clinic, where he had spent time in the past, to be treated for depression. The BBC promptly dropped him from his position as a sports commentator on the radio show *Five Live*. Estelle left him, taking Mia with her. The tabloids kicked off a relentless assault: "Collymore Dogged by Sex Shame"; "Soccer Star's Sex Shame."

In the aftermath of the scandal, he used the language of addiction to make sense of his shattered life. He sent a text to his friends and family: "I have thought long and hard about it. I am a sex and love addict. I always have been and I always will be. I am going to face it. I am going to go through a 12-step programme to enable myself not to use again. As my friend, I'm pointing you towards Sex and Love Addicts Anonymous, which can be found on the Internet, so you can understand what it is, how it affects me and my friends and my family. It doesn't mean I'm bad, a freak, or morally corrupt, just an addict, plain and simple."[2]

Plain and simple.

Yet, in *Tackling My Demons* (2004), his autobiographical account of the emotional rollercoaster of his twenties and early thirties, Collymore is more ambivalent about dogging than in his apologetic text blast. He admits to using sexual encounters with women as a way to deal with stress, a habit that actually increased his anxiety after providing momentary release. He also admits that "hanging out in car parks at night wasn't really what I wanted to be doing, and it certainly wasn't going to help me raise my children or protect them from ignominy and comment." Still, he emphasizes, he did not deserve "the disgust" aimed at him by the media.[3] Nor did the doggers, who were also being denigrated in the press: while *he* had been cheating, he points out, the dogging couples he had met "at least knew what the other was doing." He writes:

> Was having sex in a car park with other consenting adults such a terrible sin? Forgive me, but I thought that people had been having sex in cars in car parks and country lanes ever since cars started driving down country lanes. I hadn't done anything illegal and, apart from the huge distress I had caused my own wife, I hadn't hurt any of the strangers I had become involved with. But we are still in deep denial about sex and deceit in England.[4]

Other celebrities who engaged in infidelities might make the news, he pointed out, but not many were treated with such contempt. His dogging scandal led to an "ecstasy of sanctimony," a phrase borrowed from Philip Roth that he found ideal to "describe the scared, trembling little minds who rush to judgment when they catch somebody doing something they, the self-appointed moral arbiters of our society, have decided is a threat to the lie that there is some norm of behavior out there that the silent majority adhere to."[5]

Undoubtedly, dogging can present a nuisance for communities. Puttenham, a small town about an hour south of London, features a rest stop that has long been known as a dogging destination. Residents complain about the litter (used condoms, pages ripped from porn magazines) and the disruption caused by "half-dressed men who materialize from the shrubbery and theatrically pretend to be foraging for nuts and berries." One can imagine that parents dropping their kids at the nearby nursery school dislike seeing gay men "sunbathing" in "tight little white underpants" or explaining why "two blokes" are nonchalantly watching a couple writhing in the grass. But while dogging might make some people uncomfortable, it is relatively victimless. Some residents of Puttenham are even supportive of the doggers: "I think we should just let them get on with it," one woman told reporters. The police have been reluctant to close the rest stop completely, which would jeopardize business for the owner of the Hog's Back café on site; they instead erected a sign warning against engaging in "activities of an unacceptable nature."[6]

Stan Collymore, sneaking French fries in his Range Rover while hoping to score with a horny English housewife, was certainly doing things that made him feel guilty. After all, he had a wife at home who knew nothing of his whereabouts. And who doesn't feel guilty about eating food from McDonald's? Public sex, anonymous partners, infidelity, ingesting fast food full of "pink slime" and empty calories—all of these things can also dredge up strong emotional reactions. But is Collymore a "sex addict"? Were his dogging adventures—perhaps fifteen excursions in two years, he estimates—excessive? Was his foray into dogging related to his diagnosis with borderline personality disorder or his struggles with depression? Is his mind really a "mess of tangled wires," as he claims in his memoirs, such that seeking sex became a "fucked up coping mechanism" for dealing with stress of any sort?[7] Or was he yet another sacrifice of the "trembling little minds" he invokes in the same book, those who publicly condemn any deviation from sexual norms (but might themselves harbor secret desires or practices)?

Collymore doesn't seem sure.

As we have already seen, sex readily becomes a form of play, and even adventure, for some people. This chapter delves into how people raise the stakes of their play with group sex—finding additional ways to heighten arousal, intensify sensation, delay satisfaction, and fulfill aims beyond reproduction or physical pleasure. Group sex, being already psychologically and socially transgressive, is uniquely positioned for such experiments. The practices discussed in this chapter—the pursuit of anonymous sex on Craigslist, "barebacking" and "bugchasing," and BDSM—are examples of how intensity can be generated by increasing physical, emotional, or social jeopardy. Exploring such "edgy" sexual behavior, wherever it occurs, necessarily

raises questions of pathology. Is there a difference between indulging alternative sexual desires, toying with the erotics of transgression to increase
arousal or pleasure, and displaying symptoms of a psychological disorder? Is
the desire to heighten one's arousal, perhaps because a certain activity or
scenario makes one feel *alive* or perhaps after becoming desensitized to
sexual scenarios that were once exciting, the same as an unhealthy compul-
sion to escalate one's behaviors? Is it possible to play with transgressive
sexuality, perhaps even straying into "dangerous" territory, and then to find
one's way back?

What are the dangers, anyway?

And where, exactly, *is* the edge?

Despite posing the above questions, my aim here is not to establish
whether sexual addiction *really* exists, as plenty of qualified psychologists
and psychiatrists are already battling over the issue. Instead, my interest is in
the interactions between individual psychologies, cultural norms and beliefs,
and sexual practices. Are some people more likely to explore the edges of
acceptable social behavior, occasionally in ways that cause distress for themselves and others? Or are "sex addicts" created through restrictive social
mores, existing power structures, and the cultural and psychological processes by which people manage fear, anxiety, and uncertainty around sex?

For my purposes here, the answer to both questions is yes.

RISK TAKING AND THE SEXUAL ADVENTURER

Some amount of risk is unavoidable. Sometimes, risks are taken as a matter
of convenience. People compensate for increased safety by taking more risks,
for example: driving faster when using seatbelts, having equal numbers of
accidents with antilock braking systems, incurring more neck and spine injuries in football when helmets are used to decrease head injuries, and so on. [8]
Personal histories, relationships, physical capabilities, social positions, and
current situations influence which activities are deemed risky and which risks
are believed to be "worth" taking. Risk calculations fluctuate as people assess what they think they have to lose and what they care about losing at each
moment. An American college student who always wears a seat belt at home
may find herself bouncing over mountain roads on a Guatemalan "chicken
bus," repeatedly pitching forward onto an irritated goat swaying in the aisle.
Whether she is cursing her decision to visit the countryside or counting her
lucky stars that she caught the only ride out of town that day might depend on
why she is on the bus in the first place. Her assessment of the immediate risk
of plunging over a cliff depends on whether she knows that another bus, on
this same road, plunged over a cliff last week. And while her parents may
initially be horrified to hear the story, their perception may change if they

learn that she was en route to an urban hospital after a grueling week of fever, chills, and nausea and that a doctor diagnosed her with leptospirosis— a bacterial infection possibly caught while posing for pictures with another irritated goat in a small town now three bumpy hours away.

Notions of risk are also cultural and historical. If your grandparents lived in Romania, chances are they will chastise you for opening a window on a hot summer day. That cooling breeze isn't viewed as a gift from the gods but as a hazardous stream of *curent* (pronounced "coo-rent") blamed for numerous ailments from toothaches to death. It is tempting to dismiss fears of *curent* as rooted in antiquated folk beliefs. After all, we now know that toothaches are caused by decay or infection rather than air current, right? But if you're an American homeowner recently diagnosed with a "fungal sinus infection," which started with a toothache and was caused by toxic black mold, you might be highly aware of the risks of airborne pathogens. The situation grows more complicated as you learn that "fresh air" and air circulation techniques can direct the mold spores outside your home *or* disseminate them throughout every room. Most likely, you'll spend the next several months alternately venting and sealing up rooms, waging war on invisible assailants. Your grandmother can insist *curent* was to blame; you can trot out the statistics about black mold. You can argue over the "facts," but decisions about risk taking often involve weighing options in the context of conflicting or incomplete information. If you live in Beijing, China, or Atlanta, Georgia, for example, you might be accustomed to periodic warnings to stay indoors due to toxic levels of air pollutants outside—see, *curent* can kill you. What if you also have a black mold problem?

Oh my.

The examples above, quite purposely, are not about sex. Many readers probably grew up in or currently live in societies where sex is so shrouded in discourses of risk that it is difficult to think of it otherwise. Which brings me to my third point about the social construction of risk: our notions of risk are often deeply entangled with emotions. Emotions, in fact, sometimes trump other considerations in our responses to risk.

After a series of sensationalist news stories about "pink slime," for example, people who'd been cheerfully eating hamburgers made with "lean, finely textured beef" (LFTB) for over a decade were suddenly hysterically calling for boycotts, worried about health risks. In 2011, due to public pressure, McDonald's discontinued use of the product. By then, Collymore had probably already ingested a great deal of LFTB in his Big Macs, as back in 2001 it was still considered a boon for the processed food industry. LFTB was made up of scraps of lean meat salvaged through complicated mechanical and chemical processes. Not only could the additive increase the ratio of lean beef to fat, but the sterilization process protected consumers from deadly bacteria. The ammonium hydroxide used to make the beef scraps in LFTB safe for human consumption was FDA approved and is found in other processed foods from Wonder Bread to Chef Boyardee Mini Ravioli.

So why was there a cultural panic attack?

Certainly, meat products could be labeled more accurately. But the truth, sadly, is that banning or avoiding pink slime won't do a thing about the fact that processed meat needs to be treated with chemicals such as ammonia for a real public health reason—it's *dirty*. Eldon Roth, the inventor of LFTB, has actually dedicated his career to making industrially produced meat safer for consumers.[9] Because factory farms and slaughterhouses are cesspools of bacteria, he fights an uphill battle. Despite technological advances, the Centers for Disease Control and Prevention estimates that one in six Americans, or forty-eight million people, get sick from foodborne illnesses each year, and around three thousand die.[10] Consumer advocates admit that LFTB sounds "disgusting," especially when referred to as "pink slime," but it has not been tied to outbreaks of illness and may in fact be preventing them. LFTB may also just be the "tip of the iceberg" as far as the nasty chemicals, bacteria, and antibiotics found in processed meat, not to mention other random substances from insect parts to rodent hair.[11] But pink slime scares Americans because it hits a cultural nerve. Many of us are completely dependent on others for our food and ignorant of how it is produced. We must trust thousands of strangers to protect our health, a scary prospect. There is also a real danger underlying the panic, as evidence is growing that many autoimmune disorders, cancers, and other illnesses can be caused by modern diets. We may need to completely rethink what we eat, how we produce our food, and even how we live in modern societies.

That's a big problem.

And pink slime is an easy target.

Like some forms of alternative sexuality discussed in this book, pink slime also has what some therapists and writers call the "squick" factor—it causes a knee-jerk experience of revulsion that makes it difficult to evaluate the facts. With forty-eight million people sick from foodborne illnesses each year, should you worry more about ingesting ammonia or bacteria in your burgers? With around nineteen million cases of new STDs each year when gonorrhea, syphilis, and chlamydia are combined[12] and around fifty thousand new cases of HIV each year,[13] should you be worried about your food supply, lesbians fisting at the local sex club, or dogging in the United Kingdom? I'll admit to not having the math skills or enough confidence in the data to answer this question. But that is precisely my point—when we do not have the expertise or information to assess the risks of situations we find ourselves in, our emotional responses tend to fill in those gaps.

So, enough about microscopic threats to your health and journalists, family members, and government officials with strong opinions about what's going to kill you and what you should do about it.

On to risks and sex.

Sometimes people take risks because they *want* to, for the sheer thrill of doing so. As discussed in earlier chapters, some people seek more novelty or higher levels of sensation than others. Almost all of us, though—sensation seekers or not—court some amount of risk in everyday life, as risk taking is essential for survival, fun, and "rewarded intrinsically, as well as by society."[14] Australian social scientists John Tulloch and Deborah Lupton found that people associated everyday feelings of risk with uncertainty, insecurity, fear, and loss of control over the future, but also with adventure, excitement, enjoyment, and "the opportunity to engage in self-actualization and self-improvement." Risk taking, they argue, generates "a heightened degree of emotional intensity that is pleasurable in its ability to take us out of the here-and-now, the mundane, everyday nature of life."[15] These pleasurable states of arousal provide "a powerful incentive for searching out situations that can give us this feeling again."[16]

There are, of course, ultimate human limits—insanity and death—beyond which neither escalation nor play is possible. At these ultimate limits, individual and social edges merge. Yet somewhere before that point, the line between life-enhancing and self-destructive risk-taking behaviors grows fuzzy. Who decides where that line is drawn? The very things that make one individual feel intensely alive—whether skydiving, having affairs, or traveling in war-torn countries—can make others shake their heads in disbelief. When it comes to sexual choices, head shaking can quickly turn to outright condemnation. Sexual adventurers often see their activities as life enhancing; others, however, may deem them self-destructive symptoms of psychological illnesses. But if sexuality already draws energy from emotional ambivalence (such as fear or anxiety), preexisting wounds, prohibitions, and power differentials, do any of us really know when our explorations drift into dangerous territory?

ORCHESTRATING ANONYMOUS SEX (INTERVIEW, SERGIO)

I used to have this fuck buddy. He was great. He was twenty-five. He was in a really good headspace and thought sex was for fun: let's play with it and have a good time. I still wanted group sex more than any other kind of sex. But luckily, he wanted group sex, too. We lived in a small town and there was nowhere to go, so I had to do it in my house. We really liked to get these random guys from Craigslist to walk in on us while we were sixty-nining. Usually we would set up threesomes because arranging more than that is so complicated. My bedroom is on the second floor. When the guy arrived, I wanted to be already going at it up in the bedroom. This is going to sound so weird, but the sound of the front door opening—it was such an erotic charge for me I just about lost my mind. First, the sound of the door opening. Then hearing this stranger walk up the stairs, hearing the floorboards creaking. That was such an erotic charge. I always orchestrated it so that I was on the bottom in the sixty-nine, that's the position I like best, and so that my fuck buddy's head and my feet were toward the door. So I couldn't see the new guy even when he came in. I would hear him walk in . . . I know he's in the bedroom at that point and then he starts to undress and I can hear him undressing. There was something about that too. I mean, eventually, after a minute or two of him being there, I'd look. But that initial period of not seeing him, but hearing him and knowing he was in the bedroom with us . . . it was exciting. There was none of this bullshit talk before we had sex. This was a way of orchestrating it so that you walk in, you strip, you jump in. I'm fine with getting to know someone afterwards, but I'm not here to talk about your dreams and aspirations. Afterwards, maybe, but now I'm not here to talk, I'm here to have sex.

Another level of it was knowing how excited these guys were, thinking about what an experience it must be for them, too, with their hearts beating in their chests, scared, not knowing where they were going in this strange house, looking for the bedroom. And then they walk in and see us sixty-nining on the bed. It must have been crazy, the sexual excitement mixed with the nervousness. So they'd strip their clothes off right away and then jump right in, and if you're the new guy, you're jumping in with two people who are already there. Incredible. Incredible erotic charge for me. And we did that as much as we possibly could. It wasn't a lot. But we'd laugh and say we did pretty well for ourselves in such a small town.

CRAIGSLIST AND THE PURSUIT OF NSA

Craigslist, the great purveyor of random sexual encounters, began in 1995 when Craig Newmark set up an e-mail distribution list to inform friends about events in the San Francisco Bay area. Soon, however, the list grew beyond friends. People began posting employment and housing opportunities. Newmark designed a Web interface, turning his "list" into a free, self-service, online classified advertising website. Craigslist has since spread to over five hundred metropolitan areas in fifty countries, from Acapulco to Zamboanga, although the bulk of its coverage is within the United States. The site works like a constantly updating electronic bulletin board, allowing users to sublet apartments, sell furniture, offer piano lessons, and organize carpools.

Or find sex partners.

Volumes could be written on Craigslist as a contemporary cultural phenomenon, as it has served as an example of the best and the worst potentials of the Internet, from the benefits of open access and democratization to the perils of deception and violence. Craigslist was denounced in the media after a few high-profile murders drew attention to the risks of meeting strangers online. Craigslist has also been linked with "sex addiction" in the popular imagination, as some experts argue that the ease and anonymity of seeking sex online creates opportunities for already troubled individuals to lose control: "In the '80s, you had gateways. You could go to Plato's Retreat in New York and meet other people who did 'swinging.' Now the Internet isn't a gateway, it's a floodgate." [17]

Although there are dating sections on Craigslist, the Casual Encounters section is far more infamous. Casual Encounters is where people of any sexual orientation seek one-night stands, "friends with benefits," "no strings attached" (NSA) sex, or similar types of arrangements. Unlike websites that require users to create profiles, such as Adult Friend Finder (AFF), Swinger's Date Club, or Man Hunt, the bar to entry is lower on Craigslist. You don't have to come up with a brilliant and original user name, like LOOKN4SEX69. There is no need to explain that you're "just as comfortable at an orgy" as "having sex at home." You can post an ad using a dummy e-mail address, giving out only your phone number for verification. No credit card necessary, no real name. Later, you can delete the post with a click of a mouse.

Casual Encounters, Newmark explains, offers an "inside look at how people like to connect these days." Users, he believes, appreciate the opportunity "to be both candid and, initially, anonymous" about the sex they are seeking. [18] Individuals who would not, or could not, risk being seen publicly at a sex club or lifestyle party sometimes feel safer if they are personally able to prescreen potential partners through e-mails—at least in countries where e-mail is not monitored by authorities. Some people find the thrill of the unknown erotically appealing; even when photos are exchanged, meeting sex partners online involves an element of mystery. For individuals who feel the need to constantly escalate the frequency or intensity of their sexual behaviors, or who wish to "up the ante" in terms of arousal through the pursuit of anonymous or random encounters, Casual Encounters offers intoxicating novelty and easy access.

Some people posting ads on Casual Encounters are truly looking to meet others for sexual activity. Some intend to meet but "flake." Some are spammers or escorts. In keeping with what one writer calls the "male sex deficit," [19] there are far more men on Casual Encounters than women. Single women are a gold standard of sorts (given that an ad that appears written by a woman might be authored by a single man hoping to get a foot in the door of your cheap hotel or turn out to be a clever scam directing you to a webcam site costing $19.99 a minute). But it isn't just the "beautiful 18 year old w4mmm" who might not be *real*, if real means desiring more than online interaction. Some people enjoy fantasizing about finding partners online, and posting ads provides enough excitement without ever having to leave their computer. Some individuals create fake ads for kicks, "research," or with malicious intent. Henry Russell, a Los Angeles lawyer, posted outlandish ads and published a book about the responses he received. Although he admits he is "probably going to hell" for "having fun at the expense of so many people," he protected the identities of the people who wrote to him (almost all were men).[20] Jason Fortuny, on the other hand, pretended to be a female submissive looking for a dominant man, collected 178 replies in twenty-four hours, and then posted the responses online without any such courtesy. Many of the respondents, surprisingly, had provided him with real names, e-mail addresses, phone numbers, and even pictures of their genitals (with their faces included).[21]

In a 2010 incident, men responded to a post reading: "Married West Hartford soccer mom . . . looking for group sex . . . I want to please as many as I can before going to work!" The ad, which included a nude photo and an address, was actually posted by Philip James Conran of West Hartford, Connecticut, as revenge after a dispute with his neighbor. Around a dozen aspiring orgiasts knocked on the door or drove by the house before the "soccer mom" alerted police. One of the hopefuls, Richard Zeh, even assaulted an eighteen-year-old neighbor of the soccer mom—he is dyslexic and went to the wrong address, he later explained to police. Although the young woman who answered the door seemed "nervous," Zeh assumed it was "sexual tension" and forced his way into the house. Apparently, he simultaneously had a serious wardrobe malfunction. According to the Smoking Gun website: "He acknowledged that the button on his shorts had 'fallen off' and that his 'pubic hair and his erect penis could have been sticking out of his pants' when he walked into the teenager's residence."[22]

But let's not rant about the vengeful evils of technology. This sort of "revenge" is at least as old as the telephone—how many people dialed "867-5309" in the 1980s? The number was relayed in a song by Tommy Tutone, *867-5309/Jenny*: "I know you think I'm like the others before, Who saw your name and number on the wall . . . For a good time, call . . ." Mrs. Lorene Burns, an Alabama resident who was unlucky enough to have "Jenny's" phone number, disconnected her phone after receiving more than two dozen calls a day, starting after school let out and continuing until 2:00 or 3:00 in the morning. Her husband, who was hard of hearing, often thought the calls were for their son, "Jimmy." As for Tommy Tutone, Mrs. Burns said, "I'd like to get a hold of his neck and choke him."[23]

One can only imagine how some of those ancient hieroglyphs were intended.

Casual Encounters offers a variety of search combinations for those interested in group sex, such as mw4mw (man and woman for man and woman), m4mw, w4mw, and more. Ten minutes on the Los Angeles Casual Encounters screen turns up an assortment of posts from those seeking group sex: a sixty-two-year-old couple wanting to full swap with another couple; some supposed "newbie" couples looking for group gropes or "girl-girl" play; couples seeking transsexuals; couples offering photos, videos, and a pharmacy full of drugs; a man with a "small cock" looking to submit to a married couple with a "cruel" wife; black couples seeking white partners; white couples seeking black partners ("girlfriend wants to go BLACK while I watch"); and a "pansexual" couple looking for bisexuals interested in "games, kink, porn, soft swap, anal, strap on play, same sex swap, or even just socializing." A couple advertise "kinks & fetishes" and invite someone to "bring a canine." (Such a request is rare even in the fantasy world of Craigslist, but if you're going to see something like this on Casual Encounters, you're probably going to be in LA). There are ads for swingers' parties. Exhibitionists seek voyeurs. Dominants seek submissives. Some men just offer sexual pleasure as a reward for responding to their posts; others offer "ro$e$." One man presents two photographic lures: his erect penis and a quart-sized Ziploc bag stuffed full of weed.

Casual Encounters has a local flavor. One might still turn to Craigslist if seeking group sex in Washington, DC, for example, although one couldn't always expect such a robust showing. Despite one posting from "wild fuckbirds," my first ten-minute surf turned up more subdued taglines than in Los Angeles: "hot white couple, real" or "Normal prof. couple seeking Same."[24] Follow up browses revealed more colorful language and variety in requests, but "educated," "clean," and "military" seem to have more cache on the Washington, DC, list than offers of illicit substances (though those still appear). One polite poster even proposes his hotel room for an "orgy, party, etc.":

> Hello everyone. I have a hotel room available near Arlington VA for tonight. It has two beds and pretty nice room and location. If any couples want to use it, feel free or if there are swingers who want to have a party there, more the merrier. I will be there, but you can stay till around 1am if you like.

One can imagine him climbing into bed in his pajamas at 1:15 a.m. after graciously bidding his party guests good night.

Another man on the Washington, DC, list employs an intriguing bait and switch, possibly hoping a couple will be so thrilled with the qualities he claims to embody—or, perhaps, so bored—that they will fail to read through to the end of his "screed" (which I edited for length):

We are a happily married couple who are seeking a sharing of our sexualities with a like married couple. We are healthy, D/D free, non smokers who are affable, sociable, easy to get to know, virile, attractive couple, in shape and wanting some extra curricular excitement. Hubby has been an enlisted man in the Navy and Marine Corps, attended Annapolis and retired from the military and subsequently retired from his Professional career. Hubby speaks French and a smattering of German. We have traveled extensively in E and W Europe and the Far East (Japan, Taiwan, SVN, etc.) and enjoyed meeting the people of these various cultures. . . . Discretion is paramount. It would be nice if you have had the fortune of having climbed to the upper rungs of the socio-economic ladder but this is not all important—what is is desire, character and values similar to ours. . . . We would like for us to develop a friendship in and out of the bedroom where we have a relationship into the future and especially satiate each other orally and otherwise for your sexual joy is ours. ADDENDUM: Due to last minute circumstances after the publication of the above I was informed that my Lady does not desire to re-enter the Life Style (rather than re-writing the screed above I use this addendum) thus, I am only able to bring to the party myself hoping to find a couple as described above who desire to bring into their happy marriage a second male for their satiation as desired.

Online sex seekers, not surprisingly, are more likely to appear in Western countries and larger metropolitan areas. Casual Encounters on the Sydney, Australia, website fell somewhere between Los Angeles and Washington, DC, in terms of numbers of posts, as did Copenhagen. In Morocco, however, there were only four Casual Encounters posts in the previous two months, and none at all in Tunisia.

Sergio, the interviewee quoted earlier, used Casual Encounters to add a pinch of danger to his threesomes, a dash of anticipation and anxiety. He did not experience his sexual desires as unwelcome compulsions or shameful secrets; still, because he and his regular partner lived in a small community, they were careful to be discreet. Could he have been killed during one of his adventures? Possibly, though it is statistically unlikely. Knowing that there was danger involved, however, was part of the thrill.

Eric, another interviewee, pushed the limits further. He once made a spreadsheet of his sexual conquests, listing over one hundred women, what they looked like, where he met them, whether there were drugs involved when they hooked up, and details of the sex they had. About sixty of the women on the spreadsheet were from Craigslist. Like Collymore, Eric realized he could pursue sex in more efficient ways. He was young, attractive, well educated, and had a professional, high-paying job. He had a beautiful girlfriend and a roster of women he could sleep with if he so desired; his regular girl on the side even occasionally went to swingers' parties with him. If he was just looking to get laid, why spend four to five hours at the computer, posting and e-mailing with strangers, when the outcome was uncertain?

Because Craigslist held him in thrall.

Some of the "hottest" sexual experiences of his life had been with people he'd met on Casual Encounters. Those memories lured him back time and again even though *most* nights failed to compare to the peaks.

He loved the mystery. The randomness. The unknowns. Who would respond to his posts? Would the person he met, if it got that far, look like the pictures he'd seen? What kind of sex would they have?

The juxtapositions between his professional day job and his nighttime excursions were exciting. He enjoyed the incongruity of pulling up at a crack den in his BMW to have sex with a girl he wouldn't normally even take to dinner.

He also appreciated the simplicity of sexual pursuit. In everyday life, one had to be polite, considerate, and engage in endless social rituals—especially if one hoped to have sex. Even at swingers' parties, Eric found the codes of conduct stifling. The couples were often a tight-knit group, so he had to be careful not to offend anyone. If a more alluring situation presented itself, he couldn't just leave a gathering without explanation. If he wanted to flirt with a woman, he also had to interact with her husband or boyfriend. Then there was the possibility that his own date would get jealous and even cause a scene. On Craigslist, there were fewer expectations. He could play solo. Sure, people sometimes misrepresented themselves, stood each other up, or didn't follow through on plans. But how else was it possible to arrange a sexual encounter without ever speaking a word to anyone face to face and with no expectations afterward? He could e-mail or text right up to the final moment, even walk into a room where people were already having sex, and "bolt" when the mood struck. No one owed each other anything.

The lying required to pull off a casual encounter—to his girlfriends, friends, and family—added another layer of complexity and excitement. He invented overnight work trips and business meetings. He pretended to visit family members out of state. Making up excuses for being late or breaking plans became second nature. He recalled the sheer craziness of one such incident: while his girlfriend was waiting for him at their favorite restaurant, he decided instead that he would pick up a woman he'd been talking to on Craigslist and take her to a party. He faked a car accident as an excuse to his girlfriend for his absence and called her from the road, pretending to be distracted by filling out a police report while actually texting with the other woman.

On Casual Encounters, Eric knew the ropes. He could tell which ads were fronts for webcam girls or posted by professional escorts. He understood how people used slang—referring to "skiing" (cocaine), meeting at 4:20 (marijuana), or bringing along "friends"—"Tina"(meth), "Molly" (MDMA), or "Emily" (Ecstasy). Some posters used slang to evade law enforcement, though Eric doubted the LAPD believed that the dozens of men "seeking ski bunnies" in July were interested in hitting the slopes. But the codes were useful in another way, as Eric realized that some people were looking for drugs as much as sex. He preferred cocaine, but it was good to have other options on hand in case he found a late-night "party girl" who was looking for something specific. It wasn't exactly a trade. It was more like bait, something he could toss out to distinguish himself from the pack.

Unfortunately, Eric began "chasing the high" to extremes, sometimes staying awake for days to do so. He snorted lines of cocaine alone, forgetting to eat or drink, while he sifted through responses at his computer. The anticipation would build as he traded photos, e-mails, and eventually phone numbers with someone online, rising even more as he plugged an unfamiliar address into his car's navigation system and set off into the night.

> Most of my craigslist adventures started out with the same post. I just placed the same ad over and over. I would sit at my computer, doing lines of coke and emailing people. The ritual always started out the same, but then it was what it turned into, whatever else came up, that made it exciting. As the night progressed and drugs got heavier in my system, my willingness to explore things progressed too. I always started out as a guy looking for a girl, or maybe a couple, to see where that would go. But then I would end up at random sex parties, crack dens with strangers, or even with guys. It was like, it's 3 in the morning, at least this is better than jerking off. A lot of my experiences were just going with the flow . . . I was in the pursuit of maximizing the moment. And at the right moment, with the right amount of drugs and the right sexy vibes, someone could have brought in a fucking donkey. Well, maybe not a donkey. [laughs] But there's not much I would have said no to after a certain point.

But strangely, shortly after he arrived somewhere, a private home or dim hotel room, to claim his payoff, even before or during the sex, his arousal began dissipating. He would start plotting the next, bigger adventure—posting ads, sending e-mails, trading pictures, and searching for additional partners. Eric's quest was not for sexual pleasure or physical release. He craved the chase itself—an experience producing its own physiological and emotional "high."

But a peak becomes a cliff if you haven't prepared for the descent.

After a particularly crazy weekend binge that cost him his job, Eric ended up in rehab for his cocaine addiction. By the end of his stay, he had compiled the spreadsheet of Craigslist conquests, shared it with his therapists, faced the wrath of his girlfriend *and* the girl he was cheating on her with, and acquired another diagnosis.

Sex addict.

THE SEX ADDICTION MODEL

According to popular news reports, the United States is facing an "epidemic" of sex addiction (although around the same percentages of individuals are afflicted with ADHD, social phobias, or Alzheimer's disease). The Society for the Advancement of Sexual Health defines sex addiction as "engaging in persistent and escalating patterns of sexual behavior acted out despite increasing negative consequences to self and others." Patrick Carnes, the author of numerous books on the topic, estimates that 3–6 percent of Americans are sex addicts. Like those suffering from chemical addictions to substances such as alcohol or cocaine, sex addicts are said to exhibit obsession, denial, loss of control, compulsive behavior, continuation of behavior despite adverse consequences, and escalation of behaviors over time. Sexual addiction thus follows what some see as a destructive cycle similar to other addictions: A person uses a sexual behavior to fulfill emotional needs, but the degree to which that behavior satisfies those needs declines with repetition. The addict must then escalate the intensity or frequency of the sexual pursuits and in this process "engage in behavior that is increasingly risky to their well being."[25]

Whether or not behavioral addictions are comparable to chemical addictions is subject to professional controversy. Lab research on animals indicates that pleasure centers in the brain may be related, as scientists have managed to "swap out" chemical and sexual addictions. Researchers have also been able to create sexually voracious leeches, rats, and other creatures through conditioning and by altering regions of the brain. In *The Myth of Sex Addiction*, psychologist David Ley counters that even though sexual behavior can become problematic, sex is not comparable to drugs or alcohol because people do not build a tolerance for it or experience withdrawal. Debate also arises around whether sex addiction should be included in the *Diagnostic and Statistical Manual of Mental Disorders* or whether it is best to treat problematic sexual behaviors as manifestations of other disorders, such as depression or OCD. But even as sexual addiction remains an unofficial diagnosis, many psychologists, therapists, researchers, and self-proclaimed sex addicts use the term and believe that sexual thoughts and behaviors can be excessive, inappropriate, destructive, and in need of treatment.

Curious about how the lines between pathological and normal sexual behavior might be drawn, I self-administered the Sexual Addiction Screening Test (SAST), available online through the International Institute of Trauma and Addiction Professionals, an organization founded by Carnes. The SAST is an initial screening instrument, designed to help individuals determine whether they should seek professional help for their sexual behaviors.[26]

Although I started out confidently on the test, checking "female" on the first page of questions, I almost immediately began struggling with my answers. The questions, meant to be answered "yes" or "no," were far from straightforward. Should I should check "yes" to the question "I feel my sexual behavior is not normal," I wondered, because I've seen and done things that many people haven't, often while writing this book? Or should I check "no" because through these investigations, I learned that I prefer one-on-one encounters and now feel painfully vanilla at times? Was the question asking me to consider whether my current sexual behavior is "normal" in relation to my own life history or in relation to the sexual behavior of others around me? And who decides what "normal" is, anyway?

After some deliberation, I invoked the "Trident method"—four out of five people surveyed, most likely, would feel that my sexual behavior is not normal. I checked "yes."

"Are any of your sexual activities against the law?" I hesitated again. Oral sex is illegal in many states, and in Washington, DC, where I was at the time, the only legal sexual position is missionary style. Guessing that they weren't interested in my knowledge of such archaic (and usually unenforced) sodomy laws, I checked "no." "Do you hide some of your sexual behaviors from others?" Yes, of course. *What happens in Vegas* . . . "Have you ever been at risk of arrest for lewd conduct?" After a Google search on the definition of lewd conduct, I learned that even wearing a bikini could be considered lewd in some places if it exposed the portion of the buttocks legally considered "genitalia"—

> [the] one third of the buttocks centered over the cleavage of the buttocks for the length of the cleavage . . . more particularly described as that portion of the buttocks which lies between the top and bottom of the buttocks, and between two imaginary straight lines, one on each side of the anus and each line being located one third of the distance from the anus to the outside perpendicular line defining the buttocks, and each line being perpendicular to the ground and to the horizontal lines defining the buttocks—[27]

Hmm. I checked "yes." Although the mental imagery required was tricky, I concluded that a thong could potentially violate the law.

Several questions focused on what *others* thought of my sexual behavior, making me grateful to socialize with other sex researchers and anthropologists. Having different kinks from those of a spouse seemed like asking for trouble on the SAST. Based on my undergraduate college days, I answered yes to questions about *ever* feeling degraded or depressed after sex. I also checked "yes" to "Is sex almost all you think about?" Writing a book on group sex could either be motivated by omnipresent thoughts of sex or be the cause of them—either way, I had to admit that I thought about sex as much as a bonobo lately, even if those thoughts were more analytic than erotic. On the other hand, I answered "no" to questions about whether I felt out of control or had tried to curb certain behaviors and failed. A few questions were pleasantly clear cut, such as those about whether I was monogamous, visited strip clubs or sex clubs, or ever used the Internet to look at pornography or meet sexual partners.

I scored a 10. The accompanying report suggested that one might be concerned about sex addiction with a score of 6. Wondering how others might score who weren't presenting for treatment or conveying concern about their sexual behavior, I posted the test on my Facebook page. Thirty friends agreed to take the test and report their scores to me. Almost all scored in the "sex addict" range, between 6 and 15 (with only three falling in the nonaddict range, one of whom had worked in the porn industry). These folks were by no means a random sample, but their test results betrayed the serious side to this unscientific Facebook fun: it's not that difficult to earn an unofficial label of sex addict, even if you don't necessarily experience your behavior as problematic or uncontrollable. If you *do* feel that your sexual activity is shameful, wrong, or deviant—or if your spouse, friends, or family do—then it is even easier.

Now, of course, not every psychologist who believes in and treats sex addiction would use a measure like the SAST, and those who do would likely use it only in combination with a clinical evaluation. Carnes points out that it is a mistake to think that sex addiction is about the sex; it is "really about pain . . . or escaping or anxiety reduction." Sex addicts use sex as a "solution" to other problems or as a way to deal with painful emotions.[28] Yet while a conscientious therapist wouldn't diagnose a swinger as a sex addict on the basis of nonmonogamy alone, neighbors, colleagues, or spouses might. Adulterers are readily diagnosed in the press as sex addicts, with very little supporting information. Potential employers may not yet require the SAST before deciding on a hire, as some do the Myers Briggs personality test, but it is easy to see how such labeling could potentially get political and personal in workplaces, courts, and troubled marriages.

Some critics deem the concept of sex addiction a moralistic social construction: "nymphomania" becomes "hypersexuality"; "hypersexuality" becomes "sex addiction." When sexuality is believed to be a dangerous and unruly force, the "invention of new sexual diseases and identities" becomes a way to regulate it.[29] The sexual activities and desires considered excessive, pathological, or destructive change with the times—as do the psychological diagnoses and treatments associated with them. Women are no longer diagnosed with "hysteria," for example, although a quarter of the women in the United States were thought to suffer from it in 1859. And any contemporary psychiatrist who treats patients with genital massage, as was then customary, will see his name in a lawsuit before seeing it in an edition of *America's Top Doctors*. Perhaps there is a silver lining to some of the ways that medicine changes over time—after all, we wouldn't have the modern vibrator if we hadn't first had doctors attempting to cure "hysteria" with orgasms. But we don't need to mine the medical lore of the 1800s to find examples of "truths" being overturned, and unfortunately, we are sometimes left with the painful legacy of the frontal lobotomy rather than the Hitachi Magic Wand.

Sex addiction, from this perspective, describes sexual behavior that brings someone too close to the edge of *social* acceptability—not just those who plunge over their own precipices. During the 1970s and throughout the 1980s, Janice Irvine argues, the term "addict" became widely used in the United States to designate people doing anything excessively in the eyes of others, whether shopping, eating, or loving. The popularity of the concept of sex addiction is related to demographic shifts occurring during those years, such as changes in patterns of marriage and child rearing, and to attitudinal and behavioral changes affecting the dominant system of sexual meanings.[30] These social transformations produced anxieties and counterreactions, including calls for a return to traditional sexual morality. The sex addiction model draws on a "rhetoric of danger and chaos" and "was fashioned during this larger cultural moment of competing sexual ideologies."[31] It is also shaped by dominant ideas about male and female sexuality, such as beliefs that male sexuality is uncontrollable and victimizes women. Through the language of addiction, Irvine argues, sexuality could be judged healthy or pathological; "dangerous sexuality," such as "masturbation, nonmonogamy, pornography, sadomasochism, and, for some in the more restrictive groups, lesbian and gay sexuality," was denounced as unhealthy.[32]

One of the supposed benefits of addiction models, according to Irvine, was the presumed neutrality of medicine. An addict is viewed as dealing with a sickness, in need of understanding and treatment rather than condemnation as "bad" or sinful.[33] The readiness with which celebrities and athletes—Rob Lowe, David Duchovny, Tiger Woods, Stan Collymore—declare themselves sex addicts and enter costly treatment centers is in part because the path to salvation is so clearly marked. Even noncelebrities sometimes need a quick trip down redemption road: for someone trying to rescue a marriage or career, embracing the addiction model can be like grasping a life preserver regardless of whether the person ever felt out of control sexually.

Some individuals, of course, need redemption more than others. It wasn't exactly a scandal, after all, when Mötley Crüe members published their joint autobiography and admitted to—*gasp*—having a lot of group sex. Maybe fans didn't actually *know* that Tommy Lee once inserted a telephone inside a groupie's vagina and then ordered room service with Nikki Sixx and Vince Neil, but the revelation shocked the public far less than when President Bill Clinton inserted a cigar into his young intern's vagina. Rock stars are expected to have scandalous sex lives. (In fact, it was more outrageous that the band members wrote so little about their sexcapades and instead about broken hearts, money troubles, and weight gain.) Except when under pressure to gain favor with "good girls" like Heather Locklear, the naked women peeing into cat boxes during their backstage breaks and servicing them *en masse* after concerts were simply job perks.

Excessive sexual behavior, after all, is contingent on what is considered "normal" sexual behavior at any given time, in any given place, and for any given person. Whether a man's pursuits of extramarital affairs, prostitutes, or "underage" women are accepted as natural male desires or viewed as symptoms of sex addiction depend not only on whether he is a rock star but on whether he lives in Cartagena, Colombia, or Carthegena, Ohio. A young woman who attends sex parties with "shaking bones" might be seen as a political rebel or feminist crusader if she lives in Iran but as suffering from low self-esteem if she hails from Indiana. The contemporary "epidemic" of sex addiction, then, might be seen as a reflection of ongoing cultural struggles over the meaning and regulation of sex, often coupled with a fear of technological change. Sure, "seeking sex partners online" seems pathological to someone who asked out his high-school sweetheart *in person*, but what about to those who grew up dating on Match.com? A friend's teenage son sent ten thousand text messages in one month, primarily conversing with girls, and his generation will likely use an iPhone app to accept or reject prom dates. Will it be any weirder—or more risky—for them to seek sex partners online than it was for their parents to "hook up" after getting drunk at a local bar?

The etiology of sex addiction, from this angle, is rooted in our social worlds as much as in the chemistry of our brains. Yes, rats can be created that copulate to death, forgoing food or sleep. Addiction—as it is operationalized in lab research—precedes death but denotes that a creature is approaching its physical limits. But lab research and real life part ways, for both ethical and practical reasons. There are many people who do not pursue chemical dependencies to the point of suicide but whom are still judged as going too far (sometimes because the substance they prefer is illegal). When it comes to sex, the addict label is usually applied long before such physical or ultimate limits are in sight.

This doesn't mean that the concept of sex addiction is useless. There are indeed individuals who feel out of control in the face of their sexual desires or activities and who cause themselves and their families a great deal of suffering. Some individuals compulsively engage in illegal sexual behaviors, a clearly self-destructive pattern. Someone who masturbates fifteen times a day or spends five hours a night looking at porn online may not be breaking the law but might still be unable to succeed at work or in relationships. Compulsive sexual behavior, such as continually seeking anonymous partners, may be physically or emotionally risky for some individuals. In addition to causing feelings of shame or self-hatred, an inability to control one's sexual urges can be financially devastating. A therapist told me of a client who spent tens of thousands of dollars on Internet porn in a single weekend while his wife was out of town. During the years when his behavior was most compulsive, Eric racked up debts in the hundreds of thousands, ruined relationships with friends and lovers, and sabotaged his career. The destruction he left in his wake is "daunting" for him to reflect on. Taking on the identity of "sex addict" can be a relief for individuals, offering an explanation for their distress (addiction), procedures to follow (confession; therapy; twelve-step programs), and the possibility of recovery. Sexual "sobriety," occasionally pursued to the point of attempting to eliminate sexual fantasies, can be a welcome promise after a person has experienced intense sexual preoccupations. A diagnosis of sex addiction can also help friends and family understand and forgive transgressions.

But a contextual view raises important questions. When does sexual behavior become so risky to someone's well-being that it should be treated as pathological? What risks are involved? Not having a monogamous marriage? Not being a productive member of society? Debt? Physical danger? Hurting others or breaking the law? We are no longer talking about shots of lithium chloride, and these very different negative consequences are often lumped together as if one begets the next. Further, the labels used to discern between acceptable and unacceptable behaviors and healthy or unhealthy individuals can quickly proliferate. Is Eric a sensation seeker? A sexual adventurer? A sex addict? Someone who, apparently unlike Sergio, lacked the psychological resources to shield himself from the negative consequences of his sexual explorations? Did his behavior become problematic the first time he posted on Casual Encounters, the hundredth time, when his girlfriend decided it was a problem, or when he could no longer hold down a job? What if he'd stuck with Diet Coke instead of cocaine, like Collymore?

Regardless of which constructs researchers measure or the labels used, some people do appear more prone to needing a "buzz," thrills, or adventure than others; some people are also more likely to seek those thrills through sex. But the picture is far more complicated, and our exploration cannot stop at the individual level. The edges of social acceptability, after all, beckon to rebels, revolutionaries, troublemakers, explorers, and all sorts of transgressors.

AFTER THE ORGY, PART 2: BOREDOM

Hugh Hefner may have been in the trenches of the sexual revolution, but there were times he seemed indifferent to both sex and revolution. Even during the heyday of the Playboy Mansion in Los Angeles, some insiders reported that he seemed "more interested in backgammon than sex, sometimes playing for up to twenty four hours at a time."[34] Hard rocker Nikki Sixx admits he didn't know what to do with himself after realizing his ambitions with *Shout at the Devil* and reaping the benefits of fame: "It was the orgy of success, girls and drugs I had always wanted. But, now, I was confronted with a new problem: What do you do after the orgy? The only thing I could think to do after the orgy was to have another one, a bigger one, so that I didn't have to deal with the consequences of the last one."[35]

Eric spoke similarly:

I've been in therapy for several years now, and I don't use Craigslist anymore. I have better relationships. I don't have a coke problem. But I have less desire for sex.

Even if I see an ideal girl, pursuing her doesn't excite me. It's like I'm a former alcoholic who's working in a brewery. I would drink my ass off before if I had the opportunity but now I have the keys to the plant. I almost don't have any interest. Sometimes it bothers me. It's good because I have control of my life, but then I wonder where it all went, all that crazy desire. I'm just not interested.

Regular sex is boring. I have sex with somebody twice and I'm bored. A friend of mine has watched this carousel of girls go through my life and he's shocked that I'm leaving them all behind. But it's boredom; it's lack of desire. Indifference. I've already played the scenario out in my head and there's nothing interesting there. I guess it's the shamefulness that makes it interesting for me, that's the fuel. And the chase—the elation you feel from the chase becomes a drug itself, and then wondering how far can you go, how can you take it to the limit or the next level. I miss the intensity. Even though that period of my life was painful, there are days when I think, "Wow, that was a lot of fun."

Sometimes I wonder if I came upon a group of girls now who were beautiful, getting it on, and I could jump in, would I? I don't know. It wouldn't be as fun for me. The desire isn't there, that pure, animalistic pursuit, the addictive piece of it. I'd have fun and cum and I'd be done. Before, I could fuck hard and shoot my load across the room; as soon as I'd finish, I'd be energized and want more sex.

Now I would just want to go to bed.

Well, that sounds boring.

The reality is that even transgressive sex can lose its allure. The edge is rarely the edge forever. And what do you do then?[36]

FROM BAREBACKING TO BUGCHASING

"Riding bareback" means riding a horse without a saddle. Since the 1990s, however, the term has also been used as slang, primarily in publications for gay and HIV-positive men, for the intentional decision to have sex without a condom. The term is also used in heterosexual swinging as well as referring to a popular genre of gay pornography[37] and a specialized, often more expensive, service offered by some escorts or prostitutes.

Public health researchers, when initially faced with evidence that people were not always practicing safe sex with casual partners, often assumed that this was due to a lack of education. Not using a condom, given the risk of contracting HIV/AIDS or other STDs, they reasoned, must be a mistake. The answer would therefore be *more* education, *more* outreach programs, *more* materials to distribute focused on the dangers of unprotected sex.

But is barebacking a mistake or a decision? Could these very strategies backfire?

As with any human sexual behavior, the complexity of motivations belies a singular answer. Most barebackers, whether gay or straight, do not *want* to contract HIV or other sexually transmitted diseases but decide that the increased physical pleasure or intimate connection with partners is worth the risk involved. Some barebackers attempt to reduce their risks—for example, by avoiding partners considered "high risk" or engaging in regular STD testing, sharing the results, and having unprotected sex only with others who test similarly. Among gay male barebackers, "serosorting" is relatively common, which limits unprotected sex to partners of the same HIV status.[38] Barebackers may also reframe the debate by arguing that actual risks of unprotected sex are exaggerated or unknown. Among lifestylers, I have heard arguments that individuals who have had over a certain number of sexual partners have most likely already been exposed to herpes or HPV and that other common STDs are easily treatable. HIV is often dismissed as highly unlikely among the middle-class, primarily white, heterosexuals who make up the bulk of lifestyle participants—even by those who do not bareback.[39] Barebackers sometimes also express concern that important information about HIV has been withheld because of homophobia or sex negativity. Some even argue that HIV is not the true cause of AIDS and that this myth is propagated through either conspiracy or ignorance.

Another approach to justifying barebacking is to compare its risks with other outcomes or activities. HIV infection is sometimes likened to living with a manageable disease such as diabetes, given the availability of retroviral drug therapies. Or, as in this post from a lifestyle discussion forum: "Some of you are freaked out about getting AIDS, but think nothing of lighting up, driving after a few drinks, not wearing a motorcycle helmet, or jumping out of a perfectly good airplane! We are all going to die sometime, we just don't know when, where, or from what. Some activities are riskier than others. What you do is your choice . . ."[40]

Despite attempts to manage or downplay the dangers of barebacking, the discourse of risk adds to its erotics, whether consciously or not. Before HIV/AIDS and the push for "safe sex" in the United States and Western Europe, there was no "barebacking." Sure, people had sex without condoms—but the meaning of doing so was different. Condoms provided birth control, and, in fact, wearing them was transgressive for some heterosexuals, given that the

Catholic Church prohibited contraception. Tim Dean, who writes on barebacking among gay men, argues that "before gay men in San Francisco or
New York started fetishizing the virus, U.S. scientists and public health
experts did so—whether as the ultimate object of high-prestige research or as
the phobic object of sex-education campaigns."[41] In the mid- to late 1990s,
Dean maintains, there was a rise in barebacking websites catering to gay men
in San Francisco. Self-identified barebackers developed a subculture, in the
sense of forming their own vocabulary, rituals, etiquette, institutions, and
iconography.[42] Although barebacking subculture has spread to cities like
Berlin or London, it would make little sense to discuss barebacking in other
cultural contexts, such as in the "African AIDS" crisis, even if some men in
Africa consciously shun condoms. It is the discourse of safety versus danger
that makes barebacking far more than "condomless sex."

Barebacking, once labeled, becomes a source of controversy; reactions
contribute to its dangerous aura. Larry Kramer, an American writer and
LGBT activist known for being outspoken about gay men's sexual practices,
argued that not using condoms "is tantamount to murder."[43] Metaphors of
death abound in discussions of barebacking in forums for gay men, as it is
compared to being "like smoking . . . you know it is going to kill you,"
"putting a bullet to someone's head," or "playing Russian Roulette."[44] Similar proclamations arise in lifestyle forums: "Of course, bareback is better.
Duh. But I want to live, thank you very much." Perceptions of danger, of
course, generate not only desires for protection but also desires to "skate
close to the edge." As one researcher writes, "Danger can be erotic, even the
threat of contracting a deadly disease."[45] Discourses of risk thus interact with
other beliefs, fantasies, and needs as well as contextual factors in complicated ways.

The "Three or More Study" (TOMS) of Australian men who had group
sex with other men found that most participants planned on using condoms
for anal intercourse at sex parties but did not always follow through (HIV-
positive men were more likely than others to engage in unprotected anal
intercourse). The men expressed a "tension between desires and norms,"
claiming to be committed to safe sex and knowledgeable about HIV transmission but having desires to forgo condoms as well. A TOMS interviewee
found barebacking appealing because of the "naughtiness." "That illicit
thing, something that you really shouldn't be doing. That makes it a bit more
special, to be honest. The forbidden element."[46] He enjoyed watching others
have unsafe sex, in porn or at sex parties, because it was "raunchy." Another
TOMS interviewee discussed his desire push the limits:

> Lately, I've been feeling compelled? I've been feeling the urge. Or need. Or
> something, to start off any fucking by . . . even if . . . we have sex with a
> condom, which is my rule, I find that I want to put it in just for a minute or

two, at first, without a condom. . . . Look, I know I shouldn't. But I do. I
usually, at least for a few strokes, just stick my cock in. Or let him, whoever
I'm having sex with, I let him do it. Just for a bit. I feel almost compelled, at
first. Especially the first time I have sex with someone. . . . And I don't know
why. . . . We all think condoms are a hassle, and a necessary evil . . . we all
wear them, all of us. But I often do . . . [pauses] what I told you before. Just for
a minute. Especially in the heat of the first time I'm having sex with someone.

In some contexts, being willing to take such a risk, with or for someone
specific, can become a route to increased intimacy or a way to prove commitment. For heterosexuals, the possibility of pregnancy can add another layer
of meaning onto the choice not to wear a condom, both as perilous—"the real
risk isn't STIs, but 18 years or more of bills and being responsible forever for
a life"—or as intimate. Even in situations where one's partners are casual or
even anonymous, barebacking can foster a sense of shared trust or connection, something mentioned by TOMS interviewees. One man explained, "I
think there's a wholesome, spiritual connection that happens when you have
sex, especially without condoms. And that's magnified in the group environment."[47] Barebackers may thus also be motivated "by a desire for certain
emotional sensations, particularly the symbolic significance attached to experiences of vulnerability and risk."[48] Unsafe sex, one commentator suggests, can "disrupt time" and rationality, bringing one fully "into the moment."[49] Humans quest after intensity and aliveness in a variety of ways; sex,
especially edgy sex, is a route to such experiences that becomes more or less
salient in different contexts and time periods.

Despite the fact that barebacking has some shared meanings across
groups, it has not been taken up as an identity among American lifestylers as
it has among gay men. Both the straight press and some gay writers and
activists tend to interpret gay men's sexual practices and desires as the pathological result of low self-esteem, shame, or internalized homophobia. Yet, as
one writer argues about barebacking, it is useful to "locate in gay men's
social world, rather than in our psyches, the springs for what might appear to
be incomprehensible or self-destructive behavior."[50] To fully understand
barebacking in either enclave—gay men and lifestylers—requires a detailed
analysis of social, cultural, political, economic, legal, and historical factors.
Here, I want to briefly focus just on the significance of witnesses to barebacking and identity in each group sex setting.

Among lifestylers, unprotected sex with one's own spouse or primary
partner is *not* considered barebacking and is *de rigueur* at clubs, events, and
parties. Swingers' clubs often post rules requiring condom use for intercourse, although condoms are not expected for oral sex or between committed partners. Barebacking with extradyadic partners is highly stigmatized;
although it happens, barebacking conflicts strongly enough with ethical and
behavioral norms that relatively few lifestylers openly admit to it. When

outsiders report observing barebacking in swing clubs, it could stem from a misunderstanding about what "playing without a condom" means for committed partners. An outsider may not be able to tell whether he is witnessing "barebacking" or condomless sex unless he is aware of the relationship between the individuals involved or understands the difference. In visits to swingers' clubs on several continents, I never observed barebacking; extremely rarely, I have noticed it at private parties. Some parties specifically cater to barebackers, who are usually closeted to "mainstream" lifestyle acquaintances. Barebacking also occurs in separate-room play. Separate-room play is sometimes considered edgier than group play, which provides an interesting twist on normative expectations of sexual privacy and points to another layer of significance to witnesses. Recreational sex, some lifestyle couples believe, is safe as long as emotional monogamy is maintained. Separate rooms, one-on-one dates, late-night phone calls, or other behaviors that could lead to emotional connections with outside partners potentially challenge the primary bond. Condomless sex, because it is expected among primary partners, demonstrates the uniqueness of a couple's bond to everyone present. Regardless of the meanings barebacking carries for an individual or a couple, then, it can be interpreted by other lifestylers as reflecting a lack of commitment to one's primary partner. As there is an emphasis in the lifestyle on presenting as a strong couple, even couples that allow unprotected sex with outside partners often still prefer to manage the possibility of witnesses.

There are certainly gay men who are "fluid bonded" or for whom condomless sex similarly signifies dyadic commitment, or transgression, if it occurs with an outside partner. For some, barebacking remains a relatively private activity. But public sexuality has long been important for some groups of gay men as a form of political resistance and sign of solidarity; sex *witnessed* by others challenges the public/private divide that many view as essential to heteronormative power relations. Barebacking continues this tradition of engaging in public or group sexual activity as a challenge to mainstream morality, especially if one believes that the meaning of sex and safety has been hijacked by homophobic and sex-negative discourses. San Francisco, the city Dean pinpoints as the ground zero of bareback subculture, has a long history of attracting sexual outlaws; many of them eventually stake claims to alternative identities. Thus, even though many gay men refuse to bareback or criticize those who do, a visible barebacking "subculture" does not necessarily conflict with more widely shared ideals.

Dean argues that some men who participate in bareback culture claim an amplified masculinity, representing themselves "as uber-men—as sexual professionals, experts in eros, and as outlaws, pioneers of the avant-garde."[51] Bareback group sex parties sometimes advertise using the military phrase "don't ask, don't tell," which means that discussion of one's serostatus and condom use is prohibited.[52] In bareback subculture, according to Dean, "witnessing is central." The gang bang becomes the "paradigmatic sexual form" because it "guarantees the presence of witnesses."[53] A pig, in bareback sub-culture, is "a man who wants as much sex as he can get with as many different men as possible, often in the form of group sex that includes bare-backing, water sports, fisting, and SM ('pig pile' is a long-established term for a gay orgy or gang bang)." "Being a pig entails committing oneself to sexual excess, to pushing beyond boundaries of propriety and corporeal in-tegrity." Some men use tattoos, T-shirts, or other means of advertising their pig status.[54]

What could be more excessive than a bareback pig pile?

Bug chasing.

"Bug chasing" is the purposeful pursuit of HIV infection, a practice oc-curring only among a small subset of Western gay male barebackers. Grego-ry Freeman's 2003 *Rolling Stone* article is often given the honors of having sparked the panic about bug chasing; like the episode of Oprah that stirred hysteria about "rainbow parties" among teens, much of the "evidence" pro-vided in the original piece was later retracted. Bug chasing, however, was here to stay. Freeman's primary informant, a man using the pseudonym Carlos, endorses bug chasing in the article as "the ultimate taboo, the most extreme sex act left on the planet." Bug chasers seek "freedom": "What else can happen to us after this? You can fuck whoever you want, fuck as much as you want, and nothing worse can happen to you. Nothing bad can happen after you get HIV." Carlos also claims that the moment he contracts HIV will be "the most erotic thing I can imagine."[55]

Clearly, if bug chasing didn't exist before Freeman's article, someone would have had to invent it.

Men can become "bug brothers" one on one or "at special marathon group sex parties" held "for the purpose of seroconverting as many HIV-negative participants as possible."[56] In a twist on the view of unprotected sex as murder, HIV-positive men who participate are called "gift givers." If barebacking is controversial both within and outside the gay community, bug chasing is usually seen as fully pathological. Still, Dean argues, bug chasers have complex motivations, such as desires for deeper intimacy with positive partners, desires to conquer fears of becoming infected, and loneliness. Some men see becoming bug brothers as an act of unity; others view it as a political statement against homophobia or dominant cultural values.[57] Risk is both eroticized and dramatized at group sex events for bug chasers, such as in the following ad for a "roulette party":

> B[irth]day fuck fest at my hotel in SOMA just off Harrison [Street]. I have a few neg bottoms lined up to take some Neg and Poz loads. Here is the party format. Everyone will arrive around 9:00 pm at my hotel room. When you arrive you will write down your hiv status on a card. You will be the only one

to see this card. It will have a fake name on it but one that you will be known as. Once we are all done fucking and the tops leave[,] the bottoms will reveal the cards and see who took what. The tops can remain for round two if they like or you can bail if this freaks you out. No one will discuss status until every one is done with the breeding. If this sounds hot to you email me with a current chest and cock shot, face if you like, and I will get back in touch with you close to the date of the party. This will be my 37 b[irth]day and I want a gift to keep on giving. [58]

Dean likens viral exchange to the development of kinship networks; the erotics of "breeding" is a metaphorical impregnation with HIV. [59] This argument brings us back to a view of dyadic, unprotected sex as reproductive and to the use of condoms as a comment on both the status of the partner and the purpose of the relationship, especially when witnessed.

At the individual level, barebacking and bug chasing may be associated with other risk-taking behaviors and personality traits. Researchers found gay male barebackers to be more likely than nonbarebackers to use alcohol in sexual contexts, use the Internet to meet sex partners, engage in any unsafe sex, and report higher degrees of sexual sensation seeking. [60] And when compared with barebackers, bug chasers ranked higher on behavioral and psychological measures of sex addiction. [61]

Comparisons like this should be taken with a grain of salt, however. Or perhaps a whole shaker.

With only a handful of academic studies presenting data on bug chasing, along with a few clearly sensationalist articles by journalists, the paucity of evidence has led some to declare bug chasing an urban legend. Methods used to study bug chasers (and often barebackers) are questionable. Recruiting subjects from online communities—or worse, simply analyzing ads posted on barebacking websites—is problematic. Some of the desire to become "poz" explored by researchers in Web-based projects may in fact be fantasy play, as some individuals never intend to pursue physical encounters. On the other hand, when a practice comes to represent the extreme edge, it automatically appeals to some individuals. When even barebackers distinguish themselves from bug chasers, it pretty much guarantees that at least a few people are going to side with the outlaws—or decide to *be* the outlaws.

The demonization of bug chasers in the media might be considered alongside other practices where individuals take risks for political, aesthetic, or community ideals; because sex is involved, the level of panic may be out of proportion to the real public health danger. Bug chasing might also be considered alongside other phenomena that took on new life after being "discovered" and given a catchy name by the media—a powerful combination. (Just ask the people who are trying to get "pink slime" called "lean finely textured beef" again.) After all, before journalists and social scientists identified bug chasers as an at-risk group to study, these men were arguably just "lonely, troubled outliers."[62] Yet once named, the minority of individuals engaged in such activities can be invoked to scare mainstream constituencies, potentially becoming lucrative symbols in a competitive funding environment. Are there also heterosexuals who wish to become infected with HIV? Probably. But at this point in time, heterosexuals who pursue sex with HIV-positive partners are still considered isolated weirdoes, not nearly as scary as bug chasers. There have always been individuals who fetishize a certain medical condition or type of death—just as there have always been teens who have oral sex with multiple partners, want to get pregnant, or experiment tragically with autoasphyxiation. But when does hysteria break out? It breaks out when teenagers start attending "rainbow parties," making "pregnancy pacts," or playing the "choking game"—and when these activities resonate with the cultural fears of the moment. The process of naming is powerful and moti-vated; while things that are named may indeed exist, they must do *more* than exist to be worth naming at a given moment in history.

Barebacking and bug chasing are controversial because of how they relate to contemporary cultural understandings of sexual risk, regardless of whether the risk taking involved is experienced as life enhancing or self-destructive for any given individual. They are also examples of how the edge looks different depending on one's perspective: some people insist all barebackers are crazy; some barebackers swear that bug chasers are the truly nutty ones.

Let's turn to the case of contemporary BDSM. Participants have histori-cally been considered sick, troubled, and even insane. Today, however, one might attend a BDSM convention at a Ramada Inn, purchase a flogger at a sex toy party, or take part in a discussion of "cock and ball torture" at a coffee shop. While some outsiders still respond to BDSM with fear and pathologize an interest in "kink," ongoing attempts by the BDSM community to foster an acceptance of sexual variation have had some effect on public perceptions. BDSM provides an interesting example of how sexual "out-laws" can become civilized—kicking and screaming all the way—and raises another question about the very nature of the edge.

Are we looking at a cliff? Or a series of rolling hills?

DOMESTICATED OUTLAWS: BDSM AND PLAYING WITH POWER

"I do some knife play, but I don't really slice anybody up. I'll cut a couple layers of epidermis and then blood will pool up on the cut."[63]

An important role of BDSM organizations has been to provide outreach education about BDSM to the general public as well as to community mem-bers. The National Coalition for Sexual Freedom (NCSF), for example, is a US organization working toward protecting rights for consenting adults involved in a variety of alternative sexual practices—BDSM/leather/fetish, swinging, and polyamory. Mediating the relationship between BDSM practitioners and the general public has been crucial because of the history of pathologization in the United States and Europe. "Sexual sadism" and "sexual masochism"—both defined as paraphilias—were long considered disorders, even within consenting relationships. Such a history, as social theorists point out, can stimulate the creation of resistant identities. The label "homosexual," for example, both was used to pathologize people with same sex-desires and became an identity from which to resist the definitions of the medical and psychiatric establishments. In 1973, homosexuality was removed from the *Diagnostic and Statistical Manual of Mental Disorders*, in part due to pressure from emerging gay and lesbian rights groups. BDSM has undergone similar processes. In 1994, the *DSM* was changed so that engaging in a paraphilia was no longer inherently seen as symptomatic of mental illness. Suggested revisions for the *DSM-V*, to be published in 2013, specify the difference between "benign paraphilias" and a paraphilic disorder, which exists only when a paraphilia "is currently causing distress or impairment to the individual" or its "satisfaction has entailed personal harm, or risk of harm, to others in the past."[64] While this solution does not please everyone, some activists see it as a positive step. Similar moves to free BDSM from its association with mental illness have been made in Denmark, Sweden, Norway, and Finland.

In contrast to Craigslist sex seekers and to a greater extent than barebackers, BDSM practitioners have developed a sense of identity and community around their sexual practices. Although fighting a history of pathologization is part of the reason, other contextual, structural and interpersonal factors also contribute. One social theorist suggests that a large SM subculture "will develop in a society that has an unequal power distribution, that has enough affluence for the development of leisure and recreational activities, and that values imagination and creativity."[65] BDSM mixes well with capitalism. While it would be tough to figure out what to sell to the folks on Craigslist Casual Encounters to enhance their experience—and, let's face it, the ability to buy stuff makes a group as real as naming does—the possibilities for commercialization are vast with BDSM. Players can purchase fetish clothing, sex toys, dungeon equipment, and "how-to" manuals; they attend workshops on technique. There is also the issue of scale. BDSM clubs create environments conducive to the experiences sought—often dark and gothic, with themed play areas such as prison cells or stables, and out of hearing range of the neighbors. Many clubs also provide specialized equipment. The St Andrew's cross, for example, is an X-shaped cross allowing for various positions and types of restraint—probably an excellent conversation starter in the living room, but highly impractical. Because the atmosphere provided by a club is not reproducible in most homes and on most budgets, community venues meet the needs of a critical mass of players.

On an interpersonal level, additional factors contribute to the development of community: for example, the tendency to take on identities within scenes that are relatively enduring, such as top/bottom/switch or dominant/submissive, and the need to manage risk through competence while also creating *authentic* experiences of power exchange. Although players negotiate scenes beforehand, setting "safe words" and discussing limits, the aim is to create "as total and as authentic a sense of power imbalance as possible within the confines of consent."[66] Anonymity is not prized under such conditions. The presence of witnesses is crucial to demonstrating skill, developing a reputation, and displaying status. Tops gain status for being demanding, skillful, and trustworthy, bottoms by being expressive during scenes (through screaming, moaning, writhing, etc.) or "edgy" in their activities or in how much they can endure.[67] Highly skilled tops, according to sociologist Staci Newmahr, will have the most opportunities to play. This means being proficient with the equipment—whips, crops, ropes, bondage, and so on—but also in terms of interaction, pushing the limits of the bottom physically and emotionally without going too far.

The transmission of skills and knowledge spawns hierarchies based on experience and dedication; these hierarchies are dependent on community recognition. BDSM practitioners have developed an art form out of heightening arousal, intensifying sensation, and delaying satisfaction. Floggers, canes, and paddles, for example, each create distinct sensations and arguably should be chosen based on the area of the body selected (back, buttocks, or legs) and the desired effect (sharp stings or heavy thuds). Blindfolds, hoods, and restraints distort time and block some sensory input while increasing awareness of other stimuli. Experts regularly offer classes on technique, negotiation, communication, and "aftercare," or how to treat partners after scenes. Knives or electricity, used negligently, can cause irreversible physical damage. Even incorrectly tying a person's limbs could result in adverse consequences. Practitioners thus spend money on equipment; they also spend time acquiring the skills and knowledge necessary to use their gear (and bodies) safely and effectively. Some types of play, like spanking, may not leave lasting marks but involve potential psychological risks. "The physical, emotional, and psychological intensity of SM," Newmahr writes, "combined with its marginalized status," generates intense emotional responses.[68] If a person reworks past trauma in a scene, skilled players can create an environment conducive to healing rather than reopening old wounds.

But players want more than therapy, or they would be reclining on a couch instead of strapped to a St. Andrew's cross.

Sociologist Stephen Lyng developed the concept of "edgework," borrowing the phrase from gonzo journalist Hunter S. Thompson, to describe the "voluntary pursuit of activities that involve a high potential for death, serious physical injury, or psychic harm."[69] The edgework model has been applied to extreme sports such as mountaineering and rock climbing, crime, stock market trading, and dangerous occupations such as wilderness rescue or firefighting. Edgework goes beyond voluntary risk taking as a self-conscious refinement of how boundaries—such as order and disorder, life or death, or other significant human limits—are approached: "Edgeworkers of all stripes ultimately seek to get as close to this critical line as possible without actually crossing it."[70] Doing so requires managing risks and developing skills in conditions of uncertainty; part of the allure of edgework, then, is the need for creative responses. "Participants are seduced," Lyng writes, "by the transcendent and intensely authentic nature of the experience."[71] Mountaineers, for example, claim that their activities lead to "a heightened psychological and physical experience" where participants gain "permanent knowledge of what it is to feel so totally 'wired' or 'alive.'"[72]

Like some extreme sports, BDSM involves a variety of risks, from the physical to the psychological, and requires commitment and specialization to manage them. Many organizations and practitioners uphold the standard of "safe, sane, and consensual" (SSC), a phrase now associated with the organized BDSM scene. Still, participants want to push and be pushed against the limits that have been imposed. BDSM is thus a form of "collaborative edgework," according to Newmahr—it is not just the bottom who is engaged in edgework because of the bodily or emotional risk; rather, participants need each other.[73] And although not every activity is equally physically dangerous, she argues that all SM is "emotional edgework," exploring the "line between emotional chaos and emotional order, between emotional form and formlessness, between the self and the obliteration of the self."[74]

Acceptable and desirable types of play are defined, debated, developed, and displayed through interactions with others. In a sizable community, knowledge can no longer be passed simply from master to disciple; community organizations, rules, and standards can take on some of the responsibility. Authority structures and hierarchies create forms of policing. In San Francisco, for example, the Dungeon Monitors Association, or DMA, trains "dungeon monitors" in safety, first aid, CPR, and acceptable play. Many of the practitioners that anthropologist Margot Weiss interviewed during her fieldwork expressed ambivalence about the DMA and other attempts at policing scenes. As the community became "almost obsessed with rules and order, safety and security," some players believed it was losing its "allure of the clandestine, outlaw, or dangerous."[75] Similarly, as with any boundaries, the SSC guideline breeds both controversy and desires for transgression. Some dissenters dislike the value judgments implied in SSC—who, after all, decides what counts as "sane"? Some practitioners prefer RACK, or "risk-aware consensual kink," as a guiding principle; others stress individual responsibility and ethics. As one practitioner explains in a critique of SSC: "For me the whole beauty of SM play is that it doesn't always make sense, that it does take us outside our 'safety-zone,' that it is frightening; it taps into the purest essence of sex which is ultimately chaotic, chthonic, exhilarating, exuberant, a dizzying abyss, an electrifying scream."[76]

As I learned the hard way by letting a friend zap me on the arm with her "violet wand," individual differences in pain tolerance contribute to interpretations of bodily sensation as gratifying or insufferable. While I didn't produce an "electrifying" scream, I did let out a pathetic shriek; she merely giggled when I turned it back on her. But BDSM, ideally, involves far more than the triggering of nerve endings. Players make sense of their relationship to "pain" in a variety of ways. Newmahr discovered that instead of using the word "hurt," for example, both tops and bottoms preferred the phrases "giving pain" or "receiving pain" to highlight their voluntary participation. Players point out that heightened levels of arousal can also literally transform physical sensations into pleasure or alter their sensitivity levels, as anyone who has been surprised to discover painful bruises after a steamy sex session can attest. Some players approach pain as a sacrifice, something endured as a gift of devotion to the top. Still others, like athletes, view pain as "an investment toward a greater reward"—pushing through pain eventually leads to intensely desirable levels of experience. Only a minority of players, Newmahr found, claimed to want pain for its own sake and its own ends. A few bottoms, for example, claimed that pain was pleasurable to them; it "hurts," but "they like it *anyway*."[77]

As mentioned in chapter 5, BDSM is sometimes compared with traditional practices where altered states of consciousness are created through tests of physical endurance. Some players maintain that processing pain allows for an intense mental focus that generates self-knowledge, personal growth, and experiences of transcendence. An interviewee in Weiss's ethnography explains that pain "becomes meditative for me just as a test to see how much I can handle, how much I can take, what hurts, what doesn't, how much it takes to mark, and so it becomes for me an exploration of my body: its tolerances, its abilities to not be injured." Another participant describes her experience during a flogging:

> She put me in a chair and started to flog me and flogged the skin off my back. . . . We channel energy on purpose . . . there was actually a feedback, consciously flying between us. I need that so I can process that level of pain. . . . I'll be in certain positions with my palms flat to the ground, and I'm running energy through my body [and] breathing and [finding] the rhythmic way to flow with it.[78]

Giving community or spiritual meaning to a desire for intense bodily sensation can temper the interpretations of outsiders. The "anorexia" of saints is received differently from that of college coeds; the wounded flesh of a sun dancer is treated distinctly from the skin of someone who "cuts" to release anxiety. Descriptions of transcendent experience cannot be reduced to bids for legitimacy, however.

Some BDSM players seek erotic humiliation through being displayed in submissive poses or "forced" into degrading situations, such as being trained as a pony, sold as a slave, or serving as a human toilet. While not necessarily involving pain, these scenes can still facilitate shifts in consciousness associated with submission. Subspace can also be created by activating emotional memories. I learned this the hard way as well, after volunteering to go on-stage as a submissive during a demonstration. My exchange with the male top involved little more than my refusing to submit to the first things he asked and then his pinning me against the wall, one hand on my throat, while whispering something inaudible in my ear. I felt a brief second of fear (only later did I consciously recognize the memory triggered by the sensation of his finger pressing on my necklace). When I struggled, he dropped his hand immediately. That was it. Still, it was like being drunk. I tripped leaving the stage and then gave him my phone number—my primary regret of the evening, given that he left a long, explicit message on my answering machine the next day that my more experienced roommates highly enjoyed.

Ah, life before cell phones.

"Edgeplay" is a term used to describe scenes that push community boundaries of acceptability. Newmahr found that edgeplay was associated with challenges to ethical boundaries, such as inflicting extreme pain, hitting a woman in the face, or invoking illegal fantasies in scenes, such as bestiality. It was also associated with severe risk, as in bondage leading to unconsciousness, permanent body modification, intense catharsis scenes (which risk dredging up or leaving psychological issues), potentially deadly types of play such as "breath control, blades, guns, blood, and fire," and—the most serious form—scenes that blur the boundary between consent and nonconsent.[79] Some practitioners argue that the "edge" is relative. One of Weiss's interviewees argues, for example, "If you have a phobia of needles, that's edge play. If you're freaked out because you're a woman and I don't want you to wear pink lingerie, that's edge play. Whatever makes you nervous and you don't want to go there, I want to go there 'cause that's where the exchange of power comes from."[80] Still, most practitioners express ambivalence about certain practices and seem to want to distinguish between pushing boundaries and going too far. They just aren't always sure how to do so.

Newmahr and Weiss didn't pass out the sensation-seeking scale to their interviewees. But labels are not necessary to ascertain that while the "borderlands" of sexuality appeal to many, the distant frontiers appeal to others. (Still others, of course, are perfectly content following established trade routes.) But these differences are not necessarily related to underlying pat-

terns of pathology. Recent studies have found few, if any, differences between BDSM players and control groups in terms of a history of sexual abuse
or a place along common psychometric measures.[81] An Australian study
found that although BDSM players were not more likely to be anxious or
depressed than the general population—in fact, men involved in BDSM
scored significantly lower on a scale of psychological distress—BDSM
players had engaged in more sexual practices.[82] Interestingly, these practices
were associated with "sexual adventurism," especially the "esoteric sex practices"—oral or anal sex, sex with multiple partners, group sex, use of online
porn or sex toys, and so on. People involved in BDSM, then, like to *do* some
of the same things as each other and as individuals in other alternative sexual
enclaves. But believing that doing those things automatically says something
about a person's psychological health is partly a result of how Westerners
think about sex as essentially and inherently connected to who we are. We
might find the same to be true of Craigslist sex seekers and barebackers if we
conducted similar studies—that is, *both* psychologically "normal" and
psychologically "abnormal" people could find those practices appealing.

   At the same time, people clearly desire different levels of intensity, in
their sex lives and more generally, and exhibit varying tendencies toward
escalation. Edgeplay—not the pink-lingerie-wearing kind but the kind that
just might send you to the emergency room—could be what some people
need to get *there*, to that headspace where they are "buzzing," "in the moment," "feeling alive," or experiencing the "dizzying abyss." If you achieve
personal growth through flogging and I prefer to read *Chicken Soup for the
Soul*, who's to judge the means to the end?

AFTER THE ORGY, PART 3: NORMALIZATION

Edgeplayers, because they threaten the image of BDSM that activists have
worked hard to shape, are controversial.[83] Yet edgeplayers also represent
valued outlaw qualities—qualities that some practitioners fear are being lost
with the commercialization and mainstreaming of BDSM. Weiss argues that
mainstream media representations of BDSM have "increased dramatically in
the last 20 years" in films, television, advertising, and fashion, and that this
increased visibility engenders issues of authenticity for both mainstream
viewers and players.[84] BDSM, she suggests, stands for sex that is dangerous
or taboo, but the images produced and consumed in pop culture are often
distinguished from "the really sick and twisted side" that supposedly hasn't
found its way into suburban living rooms.[85] But what exactly counts as really
sick and twisted? One need only consider the recent success of *Fifty Shades
of Grey*—an e-book that became a *New York Times* best seller for erotic
fiction—to realize that SM isn't just for perverts anymore. Experts are

quoted in the media claiming that "BDSM is part of a normative sexual experience that feels healthy and enjoyable to many people," and that hopefully *Fifty Shades of Grey* "will give some people a language to talk about sex, ask questions, explore different fantasies and know that those fantasies are okay."[86] Some days, even in small-town America, everyone seems to be dabbling in BDSM.

Hearing that one's fantasies are not dark and disturbing but actually "okay" might bring relief to some people. All the talk about BDSM as "healthy," "normal," and "enjoyable" sexuality might even get the paraphilias removed from the *DSM-V* more quickly. It might also send some practitioners running for the hills.

Or the next set of cliffs.

Chapter Ten

What Are You Doing *after* the Orgy?

For a long time, people said that procreation was the point of sex. Today people tend to think that the point of sex is pleasure, orgasm. But sincerely, I don't think there's any point to sex at all. People think there's some secret they'll discover in that black box of sex, which will help them to live better or make them happy. And in fact there's nothing, nothing, nothing there at all.
—Catherine Millet[1]

In the end, we are all just fucking ourselves anyway.
—Marco Vassi

LIVING IN THE MOMENT

In 2007 and 2008, Danish anthropologist Christian Groes-Green studied a group of young Mozambican men known as *moluwenes*. The word *moluwenes* means "wild" or "unruly," a description that fits many young males from eighteen to twenty-seven, although these men's struggles were particularly intense. *Moluwenes*, Groes-Green explains, were "hurting" in every area of their lives. They lived in Zona Verde, an impoverished area of Maputo, with no access to electricity or sanitary water. Some had grown up homeless, cast out when their families could not afford to feed them; often these men had the highest status in the group, given their familiarity with hardship and survival. Other young men left their families behind in smaller villages and traveled to Maputo hoping to find work, ending up on the streets instead. Those few who had families to turn to during crises, such as when they were wounded or arrested, were relatively privileged. Culturally marginalized and unable to find employment, *moluwenes* engaged in criminal behavior, violence, and unsafe sex. Sometimes, *moluwenes* fantasized about becoming rich; they also conceded "the impossibility of getting access to the riches,

333

fashionable brands and cars that the 'ladrões' and their middle-class peers possess and how poverty decreased their chances of 'catching' the city's beautiful girls."[2]

One thing that *moluwenes* had in abundance, however, was time. Faced with extreme poverty, boredom, joblessness, riots, and a devastating HIV epidemic, the men were uncertain about whether a "real future" with a home or family would ever be possible. *Moluwenes* thus used the slang phrase *curtir a vida*, meaning to celebrate and enjoy life, or to "live in the moment." Middle-class masculine ideals referenced a belief in the future through "disciplined planning," hard work, education, and the "reproduction of family traditions; the *moluwenes'* ideal of masculinity was "primitive," "organized around the here and now of bodily desires, erotic skills and spontaneous acts."[3] *Moluwenes* had complicated relationships with the women they partied with, called *curtidoras*. *Curtidoras* were also involved in the informal economy, exchanging sexual relationships with older men (*patrocinadores*, or sponsors) for gifts and money, and often supporting themselves, their families, and even their boyfriends through these "sugar daddy" relationships. During his time in Mozambique, Groes-Green accompanied the *moluwenes* on some of their "everyday journeys 'on the edge,'" such as "death racing" or *corridas de morte*—"sitting in the back seat of a car gunning through the city at a hundred miles per hour." Groes-Green also observed "unprotected sexual orgies, violent battles and excessive drug use." *Paulado* was the "high" that the men pursued through these activities, a state during which fear of death and pain disappeared.

Groes-Green describes one of the orgies he witnessed, which began around 2:00 a.m. when a group of young men he knew picked up four women. The women looked around eighteen years old; two of them had been walking along a boulevard where sex workers waited for clients. The group went to a house, where one of the men began playing loud music. A bottle of cheap whiskey was passed around. Another man laid out piles of *coca* while two of the women started a striptease. When the women had removed all of their clothing and two men began to have sex with them, Groes-Green moved to leave. One of his informants grabbed his wrist, saying, "Come and enjoy, nobody can get us now. We are getting *paulado* (high), everybody else is in their beds." Although Groes-Green left, the next day he asked one of his informants to tell him more about the sex party. The young man said: "So ok, you think I should use *camisinhas* [small shirts: slang for condoms]. Well, I knew that I could have broken the *gaja's* [derogatory slang for girls] asshole, but I kept banging, the *coca* was working. Clearly it is going to bleed if you are being hard on a girl and she is tight, but it is not often. Even if you smell that she's got the shit [period] you don't care (laughter). It is like if you are running to catch a wild animal. You don't stop. . . . Even though you know she can give you the disease of the century [AIDS]. I told you, it is about enjoying life."[4]

The men often refused condoms, even though they understood the risks of catching HIV. Unprotected sex was referred to as *sexo puro* and was linked to ancestral beliefs that interrupting the exchange of fluids could lead to insanity or impotence. The men also used the phrases *nhyama ni nhyama* (flesh against flesh) and *ku nyicana n'gati* (to mix blood with semen) to describe the sex they preferred. The risk made having unsafe sex even more of an example of "being in the moment": "If you just look at people you cannot see the difference between who use [condoms] and who do not, but the one who use will always feel more relaxed. But that is the thing, who wants to be at ease all the time? That is not life is it? And sex, sex is like, crazy, and I like to be in the crazy moment."

Groes-Green struggled with understanding why *moluwenes* continued to have unsafe sex despite understanding the risks of HIV transmission and having the power and knowledge to protect themselves. He sometimes felt guilty for observing their dangerous behavior so closely, yet knew that he could not intervene without being rejected by the community. Eventually, though, he began to grasp what *moluwenes* sought in their "crazy moments." He describes arriving at another party in an abandoned house, where he is supposed to meet a friend, a 23-year-old-man named Dolito:

> When I entered the house, most people were already naked and some were dancing to reggae music from Angola. I found Dolito in a small dark room lit only by two candles. He was lying on the couch with three young women, and another guy was standing in the corner commenting on the way he performed oral sex on one of the women. The guy in the corner handed me a glass of whisky and a chair. Placed right in front of the action, watching the moving silhouettes of lustful youth, smelling the sweat from their naked bodies and listening to the moaning sounds, triggered a combination of a sense of utter displacement and an almost dissociated state of mind where my ordinary desire for control and rational thinking was obliterated, not as a deliberate choice but as a direct bodily response to the erotic sensation.

It was in that kind of moment, Groes-Green writes, that he began to appreciate the "value of erotic transgression as momentary ecstasy."

"Excessive tendencies among marginalized young men," Groes-Green argues, "are observed in postcolonial cities around the world," especially in places with growing poverty, rising unemployment, and a collapse of traditional institutions.[5] Some social scientists focus on the desperation of everyday struggle in these urban environments, analyzing young men's criminal, addictive, or dangerous behavior as the internalization of frustrations and powerlessness. "Excessive" behavior is viewed as an ineffective form of resistance, an attempt at creating a new social order that often backfires, or as a "safety valve," releasing aggression without ultimately disturbing the status quo. Groes-Green is more interested in Bataille's understanding of transgression, however, with its focus on subjective experience. Death racing and orgies, he suggests, produce experiences of what Bataille calls "sovereignty," "a feeling of being in charge of the world which, far from being rooted in rational thinking and factual power, is rather an inner sacred state." For *moluwenes*, facing death directly by taking extreme risks gave them a *raison d'être* they were deprived of in their daily lives.[6] Their excesses represent a "creative violation of rules and norms," allowing the young men to subvert existing hierarchies, even if temporarily, and achieve "a sense of superiority based on and embedded in the transgressive experience." Taking refuge in sexual excess and momentary pleasures may not bring about social change in itself, but it does not preclude political engagement or the development of oppositional identities either.

Paulado.

WHEN SEX FAILS

For Marco Vassi, shattering cultural prohibitions was a powerful route to transcendence. In the philosophy that emerged through his essays and novels, group sex, anonymous encounters, and forbidden sexual acts became practices leading to self-fulfillment, liberation, and spiritual communion. "I don't really care what the other person's name is," he wrote. "I don't even care what my own name is. Ecstasy has no name."[7] Every lover, Vassi believed, was magical and unique; yet, at the same time, lovers were interchangeable. On his visit to a San Francisco bath, he almost immediately dove headfirst into a "writhing pile of bodies." "The next fifteen minutes had no description," he writes,

> simply because there were no discrete units of activity. It was all touch, all liquid, all sound, all excitement, all images. During that time, I went through every imaginable variation on the physical homosexual act imaginable. There was neither the chance nor the inclination to take any of them to their full conclusions. Rather, it was a sort of smorgasbord, with the joy coming in the many different flavors and sensations. It provided me with the single most glorious moment of total anonymity I had ever experienced in my life, and when I finally crawled out, I felt as though I had gone through a baptism of orgasm.[8]

Like Purusha, Vassi was concerned with transcending dualities—male or female, "good" or "bad," homosexual or heterosexual. Even bisexuality was a dead end, as he wanted to experience erotic life beyond gender and beyond identity. During a threesome with a man and a woman, he glimpsed such a possibility: "With a buzzing connection, the male and female inside me began to undulate in a series of sine waves. I lost my sexual *identity* and became a sexual *entity*."[9] And like Catherine Millet, who at one time found freedom and meaning in "debasement," Vassi challenged himself to overcome his own prejudices, fears, and experiences of disgust, shame, and guilt. After his sexual experiences in California, Vassi revisited the bathhouses in New York City, etched in his memory as "cesspools of lust" with "urine-caked hallways," "paint-peeling walls," and "dribbling old men," with a new perspective. He had learned "how to find sapphires in the mud, how it is possible to soar into the greatest ecstasy when one is at the depths of degeneracy."[10]

Eventually, however, Vassi became disillusioned. When he was diagnosed with HIV in the late 1980s, he continued traveling but changed his philosophy: "This time I cannot deceive myself into thinking that the trip has some destination, that there is some final act which will draw everything together into a bow of understanding. Never can I forget that everything I know, or do, or think, or feel, or create, or understand is but a brief poignant gesture into the supercilious face of the unknown."[11] The final words in his autobiography were austere: "There is only what is, and that is mute. *I have stopped searching.*"

After walking around snowy New York City, barely dressed, Vassi caught pneumonia. Instead of seeking treatment, he sequestered himself in a room, ignoring phone calls from friends for weeks. He died on January 14, 1989, at the age of fifty-one. [12]

Sex partying makes a young Tehranian woman "feel alive." An Egyptian couple escapes "marital boredom" by throwing secret orgies at their apartment. A young gay man, wanting to "be fabulous," dives into group sex at a bathhouse. *Curtir a vida.* A Playboy bunny enters "a dream world" where multiple sex partners bring joy rather than shame or censure. Young Russian activists strip down for sex on a cold museum floor for politics, not pleasure.

And then there's Kendra.

There's *Foursome*, group sex as late-night reality television.

Pretty soon, we'll be watching *Ass Clowns #51*, yawning.

Over time, regardless of where they are from, which type of play they engage in, and even why they do it, many participants come to find group sex mundane, even disappointing. They become desensitized to the nudity and habituated to the sex clubs or party rooms that once seemed daunting and exciting. The thrill of the chase fades as they become better at maneuvering through whichever enclave they've chosen, finding partners more easily. Commodification may make participation safer and easier. New sources of pleasure arise, as when an American swinger treasures his "rock star" weekends. Sex might become part of a more all-encompassing recreational experience, feeling less revolutionary and more like, well, a *lifestyle*. But dissatisfactions arise, too. If overcoming shame about the body or sexuality was part of the adventurousness of group sex, these scenes lose power when there is less shame to overcome. Or, patterns of shame and guilt can eventually permeate people's experiments with sexuality, tipping the balance too far in the other direction. Power dynamics and cultural beliefs may impose limits on one's sexual adventures that become less pleasurable to confront over time. Amanda Hughes, the young British football groupie, ultimately found herself cringing after each escapade rather than "buzzing."

Gay activist Stuart Norman, who also uses the name Cyrwyn/Leatherfae-rie Shaman, distinguishes between spirituality and religion, claiming that spirituality is "always seeking new understanding" and "always changing" while religion creates "fixed doctrine and dogma out of one individual's profound spiritual experience at a crucial point in a culture's development: Jesus, Mohammed, Buddha, and many others. That knowledge is then applied to everyone's lives, to mold the thinking process and form a cultural belief system."[13] Perhaps this is part of the problem when sexuality becomes championed as a path to spiritual growth, cultural change, or transcendence—the suggested practices become fixed around one person's experience. But maybe fisting doesn't lead all of us to that "ultimate" place, even if it did for Purusha or thousands of other men. Maybe now it's double penetration that leads to enlightenment, *satori*, or "continuous euphoric bliss." Maybe it's spanking, barebacking, dogging, or something we haven't even started doing yet. Maybe it's monogamy.

Or maybe nothing works for everyone.

And maybe nothing works forever.

THE POINT OF SEX

The debate over whether orgies are transcendent of the social order or regenerative of it will likely continue, as it does over other practices, sexual and otherwise. The orgy usually enters this conversation as a metaphor, or symbol of the edges of sociality. In some theories, "the orgy" becomes a descent into chaos—social and individual—that serves as a temporary rebellion, an ultimately conservative form of transgression. Other times, the orgy is imbued with the power to shatter the foundations of the social order—in such a scheme, prohibitions against group sex are not necessarily the first moral domino to topple, but once they do, other taboos fall swiftly. Whether one then should expect the downfall of society or its transformation depends on who makes the prediction. Or, modern life is contrasted with the "way things used to be," where ritual debauchery or sexual sharing was supposedly part of the social fabric—whether one then breathes a sigh of relief, thankful for the safety and decency of civilization, or mourns the loss of a possibly more "natural" sexuality, depends on the theorist's position.

The problem with using the orgy as a metaphor, of course, or of homogenizing the experiences of the group sex participants, is that what feels to the theorist, and sometimes his readers, to be an intriguing contrast—between nature and culture, primitive and civilized, order and chaos, self and other, individuality and communion, and so on—is a fantasy. Orgies become meaningful in social theory in ways that they may or may not be for actual participants.

One of the organizing themes of this book is that group sex derives symbolic and emotional potency in part through its positioning as a practice requiring transgression and, at least occasionally, promising transcendence. Yet as transgression intrinsically depends on taboos, it eventually fails as a strategy of escape, rebellion, or liberation. Transgressors may become disenchanted as there are increasingly fewer, or less enticing, rules to break, sacred objects to defile, or people to shock. Maybe nobody is watching. Or maybe there are no more orifices to fill; there is no more skin to flog off their backs. The ultimate limits—exile, insanity, or death—may be within reach.

And what about transcendence?

There *are* moments in both sex and group sex, for some individuals, when "the gulf between self and other—the source of psychological alienation and spiritual loneliness which has troubled philosophers throughout the ages—momentarily disappears."[14] For contemporary theorists writing against depth models of subjectivity—who argue that subjects are wholly produced within discourse, power, and so on—these experiences indicate the existence of particular social conditions and meanings rather than psychological capacities. But while there is variability in how sexual experience becomes meaningful, humans tread many similar pathways across space and time. Questing after transcendent experiences where the boundaries of the body, self, and other are radically altered is one of these well-trodden paths whether we draw on Bataille's understanding of sovereignty or (dis)continuity, psychoanalytic models of self, Maslow's concept of peak experience, or some other model to describe it. Some individuals seek these experiences more than others, of course, and some are more likely to seek through sex. At some historical junctures, sex takes on a heightened importance for entire groups. Yet it isn't only the privileged classes or only subalterns—rebels, "gangsters," hippies, and so on—who seek these subjective rewards. *Moluwenes* are perhaps as much like edgeplayers as thwarted insurgents, young men who want to feel "wired" or "alive," even if the routes by which they attain such states are limited. When privileged individuals seek such experiences through skydiving, rock climbing, or drag racing, they are often seen as adventurous. But when anyone, privileged or not, seeks such experiences through sex, their behavior can be taken as evidence of dysfunction, immorality, or coercion.

Of course, feelings of aliveness, escape, bliss, or spiritual communion are not guaranteed, nor does everyone have the same experience even at the very best orgies. One person may indeed be soaring beyond a sense of fixed identity, lost in a world of pure experience like Vassi in the bathhouse, while another participant strains to see the clock on the nightstand over a tangle of bodies, wondering how to slip out of the room without disturbing the others—the babysitter needs to be paid, the kids have an early soccer game in the morning, and sleep beckons. Transcendence, when it happens, also depends on the inevitable return to one's own body and life. Bliss or ecstasy is followed by the wreckage at the end of a party, the dirty sheets and comedown after a night of sex and cocaine, or heavy Goth makeup in the daylight. It is not surprising that orgies become imbued with power—for some people, group sex tracks persistently between the sacred and the profane.

And it is no wonder that libertines end up disillusioned. The edge looks different when one is actually standing on it.

Throughout this book I've presented firsthand accounts of group sex, scholarly research, and media representations, questioning which stories are told about group sex, by whom, and for what ends. Sex, or group sex specifically, does not have an ultimate transhistorical or transcultural meaning. Sexual practices unfold in particular contexts—men finding group sex partners on www.barebackrt.com, *moluwenes* seeking *sexo puro*, or Papua New Guinea men who sometimes have anal sex with each other during *singel fail* are all having group experiences without condoms, but the meanings and relationships involved are different in each instance. Group sex does not even have an ultimate or stable personal meaning, as bodily experiences become embedded in narratives and social worlds. *A "stingy" young woman is waylaid by a group of men, but later takes pleasure and pride in her sexual generosity. Another woman, in a another place and time, is "taught a lesson" for rejecting a man's advances; as his friends take turns having sex with her, she does not resist because she is naked, ashamed, and should have known better than to get caught alone. She never forgets the experience and never tells a soul. Still another woman revels in being the bukkake girl at a party, the center of attention in a room of hungry, desiring men. Years later, she recalls that someone said, "dirty slut" as he ejaculated. Why hadn't she noticed that she was degraded? Even later perhaps, revisiting the memory again, she delights in her bravery and willingness to take risks. She is a rebel, not a victim.*

Nevertheless, across time and place, sex has been and will remain important matter from which meaning can be shaped. Because sex involves the boundaries of the body and self, it becomes a significant repository for meaning, fantasy, hopes, and fears. Experiences of disgust, shame, and guilt that emerge during these boundary crossings animate our encounters and dramatize our relationships to others as well as to social norms. Group sex, even when it becomes meaningful in ways having little to do with erotics, pleasure, or sexual identity as those are understood in Western cultures, has symbolic and emotional power as potentially more rules are broken, boundaries are violated, and fears and fantasies are triggered.

But group sex participants are motivated by more than desires for transgression or transcendence, anyway. People have group sex for personal and social ends. Group sex can be a means of heightening arousal, increasing stimulation, gaining self-awareness, or experimenting with bodies, identities, or relationships. Whether consensual or violent, the practice and meaning of group sex becomes entangled with conflicting human desires for individuality and belonging, forging, dramatizing, and reinforcing relationships between individuals and between individuals and the group. Hierarchies can be shattered or reinforced; bonds can be created or destroyed. Occasionally, group sex becomes important in fostering identities, communities, or an entire cosmology. However, unlike the orgies of myth that degenerate into mass frenzy, participants come to actual group sex scenes with varying motives, perspectives, aims, and interpretations. Group sex, as it involves witnessing and being witnessed, can be a means of realizing desires for respect, status, and recognition. Witnesses can confirm one's desirability, sexual prowess, position of power or submission, or identity (as gay, straight, masculine, loved, "wild" or "unruly," etc.). Participants can experience feelings of affirmation; they can also face fear, shame, rejection, and coercion. For some participants, group sex generates feelings of liberation, however fleeting. For others, group sex is disappointing or silly. Occasionally, the same encounter generates multiple experiences: it depends on who you are, why you're there, and, probably, where you're going next.

One of the concerns raised over group sex is that unsuspecting individuals, especially children, could wander into scenes of decadence. It might be more realistic to consider how few times this actually happens: Have you ever stumbled upon an orgy? Barged in on a group of men masturbating in a restroom? Gone to a party in your neighborhood where you were unexpectedly asked to throw your keys in a bowl or strip down to a thong? Been walking your dog—really, just walking your dog—and waved over to a Renault Grand Scenic by a woman who wanted to have a "fiddle" with you while her husband watched? Most likely, if those things *did* happen to you, I'd wager that you were pleasantly surprised rather than horrified—most of the time, most people will read your subtle signals correctly even if you don't realize you are giving them. Group sex might be transgressive, but it isn't a free-for-all; group sex is ordered, from the places and times it occurs to the way that participants interact. Even violent group sex is structured, unfolding according to hierarchies, and symbolic, from the victims selected to the specific types of violence involved. And even individuals who fantasize about a revolving door of relatively anonymous partners don't necessarily want to include *just anyone* who walks into the bathroom. Hapless, unwanted intruders are more than a buzz-kill—they can also be dangerous.

If a lifestyle party looks like a Roman bacchanal, that's probably because someone planned it that way.

Group sex also sparks fears of disease. Sexually transmitted diseases and infections are indeed a serious issue, though not at all limited to people who engage in alternative sexuality (see appendix A). The *other* meanings of group sex, however—especially of the orgy as leading to the degeneration of civilization and individual morality—often overwhelm responses, causing panic rather than promoting judicious discussions of risk and intervention. The two brief case studies presented in this book—of the Marind-anim in Netherlands New Guinea in the early 1900s and of urban, gay male public sexual culture in the United States during the 1970s—focus on communities that were decimated when clusters of beliefs and practices led to outbreaks of disease, not just because of the diseases but because of the public response. We will never know what might have happened if either situation had provoked more imagination and less panic, but we can be absolutely certain that the future will present opportunities to confront our fears and possibly approach things differently.

If better ways to live, love, or have sex are to be found, they will be created in the future, not excavated from the past. Sex did not have some deep, authentic meaning "back then," whenever that was, which is now lost, or stolen, or co-opted by globalization, capitalism, Christianity, or whatever else. We *don't* actually live in a post-orgy world—literally or metaphorically—although some of us may indeed be searching for our underwear, pulling on our socks, and heading home to do something else. Sex, even transgressive sex, might sometimes be the answer—to boredom, or to desires for affirmation, feeling liberated, or connecting with others. But sex is not the only answer, the best answer, or a lifelong answer.

We should not put so many of our hopes in sex.

But neither should we put as many of our fears.

Appendix A

Group Sex and STDs

Inevitably, people inquire as to whether individuals who have group sex are at increased risk for sexuality transmitted diseases (STDs) or sexually transmitted infections (STIs, the abbreviation used here). This question always arises when I talk about nonmonogamy, although it rarely does so when I speak about infidelity or sexuality more generally. There are thus two important issues to address—the factual question and the underlying assumptions about people who have group sex.

Rates of STIs differ around the world, as does the quality of the data collected. The following information is from the United States; readers with an interest in a specific country or population are encouraged to consult the appropriate databases.

Given that we don't force STI testing on the general population in the United States, the only way we know how many individuals contract STIs each year and how they do so is from data collected from clinics or self-report data provided to researchers—both of which are limited sources. Physicians treating STIs usually do not collect detailed information about their patients' sex lives that would allow us to ascertain whether those individuals participated in group sex or not—and even if they did collect such information, it would not be readily available to researchers. Further, many people infected with STIs are asymptomatic. People reporting to a clinic are not representative of all those who have STIs, but only those who seek treatment. (As a man in the lifestyle told me of his commitment to regular testing, "People who like having sex do what it takes to keep themselves in the game.") People with alternative sexual lifestyles, including those who have group sex, may be more likely to notice the physical changes accompanying an STI and therefore more likely to seek medical attention (or to suggest it to someone else). Thus, while one high-profile study conducted in the Netherlands found "swingers" reporting to a clinic with higher STI rates than other heterosexuals, these individuals may have been more likely to visit a clinic in the first place.[1] Self-report data is problematic for the same reasons. Some groups of people are asked frequently about their sex lives and about STIs—gay men who use bathhouses or college students, for example—but it is difficult to make meaningful comparisons with the general public based on this data because questions remain about how many people even realize they are infected with various STIs.

Still, sex is a risk factor for sexually transmitted infections (even though some are transmitted in other ways as well). Studies have shown that *anyone* with more than one sexual partner in a given time period is more at risk for STIs than those who abstain from sex altogether or are 100 percent sexually exclusive with a partner and have tested negative. People who have group sex might have more partners than the "average" adult in any given year. They might, however, have fewer partners than the "average" college student or philanderer. Either way, *anyone* with more than one sexual partner has an increased risk of catching an STI. Having concurrent sex partners in rapid succession can theoretically promote the spread of STIs if even one individual is careless.

According to a 2013 CDC report, young people (ages fifteen to twenty-four) account for 50 percent of new STI infections, although they represent only 25 percent of the sexually active population.[2] Untreated STIs can increase one's chances of contracting HIV, create problems during pregnancy, and cause other complications. Treatment for most STIs is readily available, however, and effective if the infection is detected early. HPV, a virus that includes more than one hundred "types," and genital herpes (herpes simplex virus 2, or HSV-2) are viruses that cannot technically be "cured" but can be managed or suppressed (whether HPV is cleared, latent, or a mix of the two remains unclear). HPV and HSV-2 are also quite prevalent and often asymptomatic. Certain HPV types cause cervical cancer in women everywhere, but most women who get HPV do not develop cervical cancer. Regular screening with Papanicolaou ("Pap") tests is important; the FDA has also approved several vaccines to help protect against some of the more dangerous strains of HPV. The CDC claims that HPV is so common that at least 50 percent of sexually active men and women will acquire it at some point in their lives;[3] most will never even realize it, however, and in many cases, the body's natural immune system clears HPV within two years. The CDC also reports that one in six people aged fourteen to forty-nine years in the United States has genital HSV-2, or genital herpes.[4] This means HSV-2 is about as common as food allergies, "odontophobia" (a fear of visiting the dentist), or being overweight as a child, although all of these conditions affect some groups more than others. HSV-1, or oral herpes, is also quite prevalent and can be transmitted to the genitals through oral sex; if statistics for both HSV-1 and HSV-2 are combined, the frequency of occurrence is greater than one in six. HIV, the virus that causes AIDS, is also more prevalent in some groups than in others. Outside of sub-Saharan Africa, the risk of HIV is primarily within high-risk groups such as men who have sex with men, injection-drug users, and heterosexuals with risky practices such as unprotected sex with multiple or anonymous partners. Once thought of as a "death sentence," many medical professionals now recognize the possibility of managing HIV through the use of antiviral therapy, even though doing so is complicated, resulting in much longer life expectancy than in the earlier days of the AIDS epidemic. Despite warnings that HIV would sweep through the lifestyle population, very few cases have been reported among self-identified swingers. Gay men who have group sex in public venues or while "intensive sex partying" are still considered a high-risk group for HIV, although as discussed throughout this text, the sex practices of men who have sex with men can vary widely.

So are people who have group sex at a greater risk than other individuals who have more than one sexual partner in a given time period, such as those who are single and dating, sexually unfaithful, or consensually nonmonogamous? Not necessarily, as there are mitigating factors. Community norms influence sexual practices. Many people put themselves at risk, for example, because they believe that a careful choice of partner can protect against HIV and STIs. In many sex clubs for heterosexual swingers in the United States, however, condoms are mandatory and are expected with extradyadic partners (though not necessarily with committed couples). In the presence of witnesses, people may feel more pressure to conform to safety precautions—known "barebackers" can be stigmatized in many lifestyle enclaves. People are also more likely to engage in unsafe sex under the influence of drugs or alcohol. College students—who frequently report more than one sexual partner in a year and admit to the use of intoxicants before and during "hookups"—suffer high rates of STIs/STDs. The claim that as many as "an estimated one in four college students has a sexually transmitted disease"[5] is widely repeated; some experts believe this estimate to be low. While some group sex participants drink alcohol or use drugs before engaging in such activities, many venues and events discourage intoxication. Being part of a community can combat shame and promote discussion of sexual health. People with alternative sexual practices may also be more at ease negotiating for safe sex if they are more at ease with sex in general. A recent study comparing sexually unfaithful individuals and those in open relationships found that people who were secretly cheating were less likely to practice safe sex both in their primary relationship and in outside encounters. They were also less likely to be tested for STIs or to discuss safe sex with their partners.[6]

Educating about STI prevention is essential across the population regard-less of sexual practices, as is regular screening for individuals who are sexually active.

Appendix B

Researchers and Other Voyeurs

Researchers interested in sexual behavior must consider how to handle their own sexuality in the field; this decision is influenced by the scholar's discipline, theoretical orientation, and research questions.

Researchers can choose to use methods that do not implicate their own identities or sexual practices in the study. Sociologists Curtis Bergstrand and Jennifer Sinski conducted online survey research and interviews among American swingers, for example, but chose not to participate, claiming that "frankly, swinging is not for everyone and everyone is not ready for swinging."[1] Researchers in public health or related fields who study gay men's group sexual behavior often collect data from subjects during visits to medical clinics or after circuit parties or other public events.

Other researchers participate to various degrees, openly or covertly. When sociologist Laud Humphreys wanted to study men who utilized "tearooms," or public restrooms known for same-sex activity, he found that the layout of each facility and the reactions of participants to his presence affected his ability to *only* observe. The men worried about being arrested or observed accidentally, so one man often served as a lookout, or "watchqueen," alerting the others when someone was approaching. "The very fear and suspicion encountered in the restrooms produces a participant role," Humphreys argued, "the sexuality of which is optional." He initially pretended to be a straight man entering the restroom or to be "waiting" for a sexual partner, but the role of lookout worked better, as it allowed him to observe without being expected to join in.[2] Richard Tewksbury, also a sociologist, presented himself as a "potential participant" in his covert research on two gay male bathhouses. Spending several hours at each location, he

347

"circulated with and among patrons," carefully observing "their activities, movements, interactions and the use of the physical features of the environment." Periodically, he retreated to private areas to write notes.[3] In their research on women's bathhouse events, self-identified lesbian researchers Catherine Nash and Allison Bain presented themselves as both voyeurs and potential participants, although they avoided sexual activity.[4]

Sometimes a researcher's participation in a sexual community or practice precedes the researcher's academic interest. In 1972, anthropologists Charles and Rebecca Palson, a married couple, were involved in swinging before they decided to formally study it. In his research on gay leathermen in the Netherlands during the 1990s, Maurice Van Lieshout used an "opportunistic research strategy," suggesting that sociologists might take advantage of familiar social situations. As he had already participated in the Dutch gay leather scene, he gained rapid entry into the setting he wished to study and easily developed rapport with participants.[5] English professor Tim Dean admits to participating in unprotected sex in his book on barebacking. Dean does not consider his work to be ethnographic; he is not a social scientist and didn't conduct formal interviews. Barebacking, he claims, is an "underground sexual subculture" that "by its nature, tends to resist conventional research methods." But he had sexual experiences, and he listened to other men talk. "After uninhibited, multipartner sex," he writes, "men tend to speak more freely." Being in an "overtly sexual space" such as the back room of a gay bar helped "dissolve some of the barriers and pretensions that constrain verbal exchanges elsewhere."[6] Sociologist Russell Westhaver, who writes on gay male circuit parties, was a participant at events and also worked for a company involved in their production. He situates himself as an insider who has engaged in "sensuous scholarship," which he explains as ethnography "grounded in a commitment to seeing, hearing, feeling, smelling, and tasting the body through poetic processes of transcribing, revisiting, and elaborating bodily experiences and memories as fieldnotes."[7]

Although some social scientists believe that being or becoming *too* much of a participant in a community one is studying biases data collection or interpretation, many ethnographers argue that there is never an unbiased or objective position from which to conduct research. Each of us is a particular race, class, gender, and sexuality, for example; these social positions impact how we perceive and interact with others—and they with us. No matter how objective a researcher attempts to be, he also brings his own beliefs and experiences to bear on a topic.

Some researchers believe that sexual involvement with subjects should be avoided for ethical reasons, both to maintain confidentiality and ensure that subjects are not coerced into either sexual activity or participation in the project. But while the potential for abuse should always be considered, research carried out in naturalistic settings involves complex social relations.

Field sites are not necessarily distinguishable from one's everyday social world. Researchers may also have more or less privilege than their informants nowadays, especially when studying "at home." People who are written about can comment on or publicly reject a scholar's results. Although in 1969 Humphreys could claim that an observer in a tearoom is not yet "suspected as being a social scientist," this has not necessarily been the case in recent years. BDSM communities, for example, have been extensively studied in the past few decades and now often engage proactively with researchers.

Erotic entanglements may be inevitable in some situations. Anthropologist Ralph Bolton found that the line between his personal and professional lives blurred while he was studying gay bathhouses in Brussels. "In gay culture," he writes, "sex is where the action is."[8] His relationships with friends and lovers provided him with access to social events and experiences that would have been unlikely had he remained distant: "I became a player in the scene, reciprocating by introducing my tricks, friends, and lovers to others in my network. . . . By experiencing them, I came to learn of blow jobs from bartenders when the door was locked at closing time, of jacking off in cruising spots in a park near the Grand Place in partially public view, of sexual encounters in alleyways between someone headed home from the bars and someone on his way to work at dawn, of sexual action in the dunes along the coasts and on the piers in Ostende and in the backrooms of discos and in the bathrooms of ordinary bars."[9] Participation also informed his research in bathhouses and saunas. Although some sites where sex took place were relatively public, such as the steam room and the orgy room, he found that nonparticipants altered the flow of interaction and that the dim lighting presented difficulties with observation. And while interviewing could have been done in nonsexual areas of the sauna such as the bar area or television lounge, most conversation took the form of "post-coital sharing."[10] These conversations provided valuable information. He did not ask sexual partners to sign consent forms; some did not know he was conducting research on sex and AIDS. Still, Bolton "*never* engaged in sex for the purpose of collecting data," never coerced anyone into having sex with him, and protected people's confidentiality. He also stresses that his partners did not suffer physical or psychological harm from the encounters (beyond the emotional pain of relationships ending on their own).[11]

Sometimes, abstaining from participation can actually disrupt one's investigation. During his fieldwork in Mozambique among marginalized young men known as *moluwenes*, anthropologist Christian Groes-Green found that because of differences in gender, race, and status, his informants perceived him as "morally righteous" and were wary of discussing their sexual practices with him. Groes-Green slowly earned their trust by drinking with them, partying, "being wild," and "celebrating spontaneity, naughtiness, and excess."[12] But when he turned down a local woman's offer to participate in group sex one evening, he suddenly reverted back to being an outsider, even a "traitor," and realized his access to the community was at stake in such decisions. His awareness of his privileged position in relation to the community he was studying often led him to withdraw from lust-provoking situations and "create social boundaries and physical distance." Yet the social milieu also required managing his ambivalence. He continued to experience anxiety and guilt when confronted with scenes of unsafe sex, feeling "complicit" in their risky activity because he was unable to intervene without losing his ability to observe. Still, Groes-Green grasped that "delimited involvement"—by which he meant being in close proximity without including "direct sexual or carnal merging"—was critical both to his access to the community and to his aim of understanding why *moluwenes* made the choices they did with regard to sexual behavior.[13]

Researchers Nash and Bain defended their decision not to participate at the women's bathhouse events they studied on the grounds that one researcher was monogamous and that their "feminist ethics" prohibited them from doing so. Not surprisingly, though, their decision to wear street clothes and position themselves on the outskirts of the activity meant they felt "awkward" when play began. They worried about being perceived as inappropriately voyeuristic, inhibited, or judgmental by other attendees. Observers, after all, can themselves be observed. The organizers of the events, whom the researchers interviewed prior to attending the bathhouse events, made the researchers feel they were not being "honest" in their research if they did not participate.[14] This was not just because their decision was made ahead of time, but because they also were not "using the space in the ways [the organizers] had envisioned." When Nash and Bain broke etiquette in such a relatively small and tight-knit community, their fantasy of maintaining a "fly on the wall" researcher position was smashed by the "elephant in the room."

If anthropological and feminist ethics suggest attention to power differentials, what are the ethics of academic voyeurism, especially if it causes discomfort or confusion for others? When researchers decide ahead of time what they are willing to "see" and experience, might they become like tourists, disrespectful of local customs and oblivious to their own social impact? Do prior intentions *not* to engage sexually—or even erotically—in particular settings protect researchers against the vulnerability that participants expect and experience, and thus inhibit a researcher's ability to understand a field site? The researcher role, Nash and Bain admit, served as a "cover," providing psychological safety by offering little opportunity to "dwell on, or even discuss" insecurities about their attractiveness to other women.[15] Groes-Green acknowledges that his understanding of his informants grew when he personally experienced the "bodily momentary intensities that drive youngsters to play with death and danger, ecstasy and annihilation, orgies and frenzy."[16]

To their credit, these researchers raise these questions themselves in their published work. Researchers should never be required to participate in activities that violate their personal ethical or emotional commitments in the name of science. Well-trained researchers can conduct careful, thorough studies regardless of which methods they choose. In 2010, anthropologist Margot Weiss and sociologist Stacey Newmahr each published books on BDSM in the United States, based on research conducted during roughly the same time period. Weiss observed in a BDSM community without participating, while Newmahr became a BDSM player during her fieldwork. Their resulting ethnographies take different theoretical approaches: Weiss focuses more intently on BDSM as part of capitalist consumer culture while Newmahr spends more time exploring the creation of authentic "scenes." What each researcher observed, experienced, and concluded about BDSM was related to who she was and how she interacted with others at her field sites. Still, their descriptions of BDSM are factually similar, and both discerned the importance of authenticity for many contemporary BDSM practitioners. Weiss doesn't seem to have "missed" significant aspects of BDSM because of her nonparticipant status, although she contextualizes the scene more broadly in US culture than Newmahr does. Newmahr doesn't appear to have become too "close" to the community to analyze it effectively, although she homes in on the nuances of interaction and the phenomenology of BDSM play more than Weiss.

The point is that neither participation nor abstention from sexual activity is *inherently* unethical or problematic. Rather, such decisions are made by particular individuals in specific contexts and should be evaluated as such. Every research method has strengths and limitations and must be considered in relation to the questions being asked. Survey research may suffer from low response rates or from a community's dislike of being studied by outsiders. When limiting themselves to observation, researchers may not have access to back rooms, semiprivate exchanges, or less visible individuals. Participant-observers enjoy greater access but may feel conflicted over disseminating findings that portray a community negatively or find themselves stigmatized in the academic community. All researchers should reflect on the appropriateness of their methods to their questions and on power dynamics in the field, not just when contemplating sexual involvement with informants but at every stage of the process, from the choice of where to study to deciding what questions should be asked and of whom.

Notes

1. THE ELEMENTARY FORMS OF GROUP SEX

1. "Orgies, a Brief History," EIOBA, February 23, 2007, http://www.eioba.com/a/1ilc/orgies-a-brief-history.

2. Hugh Urban, *Magia Sexualis: Sex, Magic, and Liberation in Modern Western Esotericism* (Berkeley: University of California Press, 2006), 28.

3. Christopher C. Taylor, *Sacrifice as Terror: The Rwandan Genocide of 1994* (Oxford: Berg Press, 1999), 173.

4. Matthew Campbell, "French Teenagers Grab Free Love at Le Skins Orgy," *Sunday Times*, February 28, 2010, http://www.timesonline.co.uk/tol/news/world/europe/article7043885.ece.

5. "Teacher Gets Jail Time in Orgy Case," *Washington Times*, May 21, 2010, http:www.washingtontimes.com/news/2010/may/21/teacher-gets-jail-time-in-orgy-case/.

6. Leander Kahney, "Dogging Craze Has Brits in Heat," *Wired*, March 19, 2004, http://www.wired.com/culture/lifestyle/news/2004/03/62718.

7. Richard Byrne, "Setting the Boundaries: Tackling Public Sex Environments in Country Parks," in Proceedings of Royal Town Planning Institute Planning Research Conference (Oxford: Wadham College, University of Oxford, 2003).

8. Emmett Wilson, "Shame and the Other: Reflections on the Theme of Shame in French Psychoanalysis," in *The Many Faces of Shame*, ed. Donald Nathanson (New York: Guilford Press, 1987), 162–93.

9. Edward O. Laumann, John H. Gagnon, Robert T. Michael, and Stuart Michaels. *The Social Organization of Sexuality: Sexual Practices in the United States* (Chicago: University of Chicago Press, 1994).

10. A couple's addition of a third individual is perhaps less threatening of existing moral orders than an "orgy"; the couple, after all, are only trying to "spice up" their sex life and maintain their bond; the lone transgressor is still outnumbered.

11. Campbell, "French Teenagers Grab Free Love."

12. Lawrence G. Walters, "Obscenity Trial?" *New Statesman*, July 7, 2008, http://www.newstatesman.com/law-and-reform/2008/07/obscenity-community-google.

13. Thomas Gregor, *Anxious Pleasures: The Sexual Lives of an Amazonian People* (Chicago: University of Chicago Press, 1985).

14. David Kaiser and Lovisa Stannow, "The Way to Stop Prison Rape," *New York Review of Books*, March 25, 2010, http://www.nybooks.com/articles/archives/2010/mar/25/the-way-to-stop-prison-rape/?page=2.

15. I purposely do not use the term "participant observer" here, for I am here referring to experiences I had when I was not present in an official research capacity and did not anticipate writing a book on group sex. To me, the term "participant observation" should be reserved for a specific, purposeful method of data collection.

16. Eroticism can be conceptualized as the cultural elaboration of sexuality—a realm including the infinite variety of practices, institutions, rites, and representations "based upon constant invention, elaboration, taming and regulation of the sexual impulse." See M. Featherstone, ed., *Love and Eroticism* (Thousand Oaks, CA: Sage, 1999), 1. The term "erotics" is often used here to recognize that this cultural elaboration of sexuality interacts with individuals' unique bodies, histories, relationship patterns, and psychology.

17. *Why* humans seek relative privacy for sex remains speculative. Some scientists suggest that humans seek privacy because they are physically vulnerable while copulating. Yet humans are also physically vulnerable during experiences where others protect or guide them, such as childbirth, so this cannot be the only explanation. Other theories posit that a preference for related privacy was related to women's concealed estrus, protected against aggression caused by sexual jealousy, or was related to the evolution of social intelligence, which led to the development of a concept of self and the ability to make political calculations. See Ernestine Friedl, "Sex the Invisible," *American Anthropologist* 96, no. 4 (1994). Barrington Moore suggests that it may be related to aesthetic preferences or emotional needs because, like defecation and urination, copulation is a biological urge, arising in responses to internal and external stimuli, culminating in strong sensations, and "capable of arousing disgust." Moore also suggests that sexual passion can be "inherently threatening" to human societies. The use of gang rape as punishment and humiliation, he argues, indicates that "public sex can be especially exciting and that one of the sources of excitement may be the fusion with legitimate aggression." Norms of privacy may help "keep these explosive and socially dangerous impulses under control." This doesn't mean "human beings are potential sex maniacs," but that "erotic attractions can interfere with getting a job done." Barrington Moore Jr., *Privacy: Studies in Social and Cultural History* (Armonk, NY: M. E. Sharpe, 1984), 71.

18. Moore, *Privacy*, 70.

19. Moore, *Privacy*, 58.

20. Ibid., 78.

21. David Allyn, *Make Love, Not War: The Sexual Revolution: An Unfettered History* (Boston: Little, Brown, 2000), 206.

22. Moore, *Privacy*, 268.

23. "Orgies, a Brief History."

2. WHAT WE TALK ABOUT WHEN WE TALK ABOUT "ORGIES"

1. Alastair Blanshard, *Sex: Vice and Love from Antiquity to Modernity* (Malden, MA: Wiley-Blackwell, 2010), 50.

2. Janet Allured and Judith F. Gentry, *Louisiana Women: Their Lives and Times* (Athens: University of Georgia Press, 2009), 59.

3. *The Mystica*, s.v. "Laveau, Marie, (1794?–1881); (1827–1897)," by A. G. H., www.themystica.com/mystica/articles/l/laveau_marie.html.

4. Carolyn Morrow Long, *Spiritual Merchants: Religion, Magic, and Commerce* (Knoxville: University of Tennessee Press, 2001), 41.

5. Ibid., 42.

6. Allured and Gentry, *Louisiana Women*, 63.

7. Ibid.

8. Kimberly Daniels, "The Danger of Celebrating Halloween," *Charisma*, October 27, 2009, http://www.charismamag.com/index.php/prophetic-insight/23723-the-danger-of-celebrating-halloween?showall=1.

9. "Dennis Rodman Broadcasts Naughty Romp with 6 Women," Huffington Post, September 8, 2010, http://www.huffingtonpost.com/2010/09/08/dennis-rodman-broadcasts-_n_

708485.html; Hunter Davies, "Why I Didn't Tell the Whole Truth about the Beatles," *New Statesman*, October 25, 2012, http://www.newstatesman.com/culture/culture/2012/10/why-i-didnt-tell-whole-truth-about-beatles?page=1; Henry Samuel, "Dominique Strauss-Kahn: I Was Naive to Think I Could Get Away with Orgies," *Telegraph*, October 10, 2012, http://www.telegraph.co.uk/finance/dominique-strauss-kahn/9599236/Dominique-Strauss-Kahn-I-was-naive-to-think-I-could-get-away-with-orgies.html.

10.   Tommy Lee, Vince Neil, Mick Mars, Nikki Sixx, and Neil Strauss. *Mötley Crüe: The Dirt—Confessions of the World's Most Notorious Rock Band* (New York: HarperCollins, 2002), 146.

11.   Allan Hall, "Volkswagen Threw Orgies for MPs and Union Officials," *Mail Online*, May 31, 2007, http://www.dailymail.co.uk/news/article-458819/Volkswagen-threw-orgies-MPs-union-officials.html.

12.   Brian Ashcraft, "The DS Game, Japan Will Forgive. The Sexy Orgy, It Won't," *Kotaku* (blog), October 14, 2011, http://kotaku.com/5849764/the-ds-game-japan-will-forgive-the-sexy-orgy-it-wont.

13.   Hugh Urban, *Magia Sexualis: Sex, Magic, and Liberation in Modern Western Esotericism* (Berkeley: University of California Press, 2006), 26.

14.   Blanshard, *Sex*, 50.

15.   Judith Harris, *Pompeii Awakened: A Story of Rediscovery* (London: I. B. Tauris, 2007), 113.

16.   Ibid., 120.

17.   Mary Beard, "Frazer, Leach, and Virgil: The Popularity (and Unpopularity) of the Golden Bough," *Comparative Studies in Society and History* 34, no. 2 (1992): 220. *The Golden Bough* is also the source of many historical examples I ran across while researching this book, which is one reason I focus more on the contemporary meanings and practices of group sex instead of reporting cross-cultural historical rituals and practices if they cannot be substantiated.

18.   In the foreword to the abridged version of *The New Golden Bough*, Theodor Gaster admits that Frazer's sources were flawed. Still, he defends the project more generally, arguing that Frazer's ambitious attempt at devising a universal theory of human thought patterns fostered new understandings of culture; Sir James George Frazer, *The New Golden Bough*, ed. Theodor Gaster (New York: Criterion, 1959: xx. Such broadly comparative projects are rarely undertaken in recent decades by anthropologists and indeed would be impossible if one were to conduct only original fieldwork. I believe there is room in anthropology for multiple approaches to understanding—both specific local analyses of difference and the development of broader frameworks for understanding patterns across cultures—as long as comparative scholars maintain a reflexive and investigative stance toward their sources.

19.   Blanshard, *Sex*, 3. See also Tanya Corrin and Anna Moore, "New York, New Hedonists," *Observer*, July 20, 2002.

20.   Glen W. Bowersock, "The Vanishing Paradigm of the Fall of Rome," *Bulletin of the American Academy of Arts and Sciences* 49, no. 8 (1996): 31.

21.   Louise T. Higgins, Mo Zheng, Yali Liu, and Chun Hui Sun, "Attitudes to Marriage and Sexual Behaviors: A Survey of Gender and Culture Differences in China and United Kingdom," *Sex Roles* 46, no. 3/4 (2002):75–89.

22.   Urban, *Magia Sexualis*, 27.

23.   Ibid., 53.

24.   Blanshard, *Sex*, 58.

25.   Joseph Klaits, *Servants of Satan: The Age of the Witch Hunts* (Bloomington: Indiana University Press, 1987), 53.

26.   Ibid., 58.

27.   Helen Thomas, ed., *Dance in the City* (New York: St. Martin's, 1997), 185.

28.   Robert B. Edgerton, *Mau Mau: An African Crucible* (New York: Free Press, 1989), 112.

29.   "The Lowdown on Sex Parties," *Jet*, April 1, 1954, 56–58, available at http://www.flickr.com/photos/vieilles_annonces/1293887187/.

30. Robert C. Suggs, *Marquesan Sexual Behavior* (New York: Harcourt, Brace & World, 1966), 47.

31. Quoted in Craig MacAndrew and Robert B. Edgerton, *Drunken Comportment: A Social Explanation* (New York: Aldine, 1969), 95.

32. Bronislaw Malinowski, *The Sexual Life of Savages in North-Western Melanesia* (New York: Harcourt, Brace & World, 1929), 258.

33. Ben Zion Goldberg, *The Sacred Fire: The Story of Sex in Religion* (New Hyde Park, NY: University Books, 1930), 44.

34. Ibid., 5.

35. Ibid., 37, 45.

36. Ibid., 101.

37. Urban, *Magia Sexualis*, 22.

38. Mircea Eliade, *Patterns in Comparative Religion* (New York: Sheed & Ward, 1958), 357.

39. Ibid., 358.

40. Joseph Campbell with Bill Moyers, *The Power of Myth* (New York: Doubleday, 1988), 106–7.

41. Ibid., 108.

42. Suggs, *Marquesan Sexual Behavior,* 119.

43. Allured and Gentry, *Louisiana Women* , 62.

44. Long, *Spiritual Merchants*, 41.

45. Malinowski, *The Sexual Life of Savages*, 258.

46. Ibid., 275.

47. Neil Rennie, "The Point Venus 'Scene,'" in *Science and Exploration in the Pacific: European Voyages to the Southern Oceans in the Eighteenth Century*, ed. Margarette Lincoln (Woodbridge, Suffolk: Boydell & Brewer, 2002), 138.

48. Ibid., 242.

49. Nicholas Thomas, *Cook: The Extraordinary Sea Voyages of Captain James Cook* (New York: Bloomsbury Publishing, 2003), 156.

50. Alexander H. Bolyanatz, *Pacific Romanticism: Tahiti And The European Imagination* (Westport, CT: Praeger, 2004).

51. Thomas, *Cook*, 2003.

52. Ibid., 157.

53. Rennie, "The Point Venus 'Scene,'" 146.

54. Brian M. Fagan, *Clash of Cultures*, 2nd ed. (Lanham: Altamira Press, 1998), 147.

55. Rennie, "The Point Venus 'Scene,'" 249.

56. Burgo Partridge, *A History of Orgies* (1958; London: SevenOaks, 2005), 120.

57. Christopher Ryan and Cacilda Jethá, *Sex at Dawn: The Prehistoric Origins of Modern Sexuality* (New York: Harper, 2010), 129.

58. Kathryn Westcott, "At Last: An Explanation for 'Bunga Bunga,'" BBC News Europe, February 5, 2011, http://www.bbc.co.uk/news/world-europe-12325796.

59. Anna Louie Sussman, "The Berlusconi in Us All: Bunga Bunga's Real Meaning," *Atlantic*, April 6, 2011, http://www.theatlantic.com/international/archive/2011/04/the-berlusconi-in-us-all-bunga-bungas-real-meaning/236871/1/.

60. Lauren Frayer, "40 Lipsticked Virgins: Moammar Gadhafi's Best Bet for Survival," AOL News, May 23, 2011, http://www.aolnews.com/2011/03/23/moammar-40-lipsticked-virgins-gadhafis-best-bet-for-survival/.

61. David Steinberg, "Marco Vassi: My Aunt Nettie; *Where's Waldo?*" *Comes Naturally*, January 8, 1993, http://www.nearbycafe.com/loveandlust/steinberg/erotic/cn/cn3.html.

62. Marco Vassi, *The Stoned Apocalypse* (Sag Harbor, NY: Second Chance Press, 1993), 72.

63. Ibid., 70.

64. John Heidenry, *What Wild Ecstasy: The Rise and Fall of the Sexual Revolution* (New York: Simon & Schuster, 1997), 132.

65. Vassi, *Stoned Apocalypse*, 90, 96.

66. Ibid., 105.

67. Ibid., 108.

68. Ibid., 108–110.

69. This quote is often attributed to Sade, but without a source.

70. Aleister Crowley, John Symonds, and Kenneth Grant, *The Confessions of Aleister Crowley* (New York: Penguin, 1989).

71. Urban, *Magia Sexualis*.

72. Ibid.

73. Suggs, *Marquesan Sexual Behavior*, 117.

74. William Ellis, *Polynesian Researches, during a Residence of Nearly Six Years in the South Sea Islands; Including Descriptions of the Natural History and Scenery of the Islands, with Remarks on the History, Mythology, Traditions, Government, Arts, Manners, and Customs of the Inhabitants* (London: Fisher, Son, & Jackson, 1829), 1:25.

75. Myron A. Marty, *Daily Life in the United States, 1960–1990: Decades of Discord* (Westport, CT: Greenwood, 1997).

76. Jeff Nuttall, *Bomb Culture* (New York: Delacorte Press, 1968), 264.

77. "The Sexual Freedom Movement in the 1960s," $am $loan.com, http://www.anusha.com/sfl.htm.

78. Quoted in Nuttall, *Bomb Culture*, 213.

79. Urban, *Magia Sexualis*, 257.

80. Pat Califia, *Macho Sluts* (Boston: Alyson Books, 1994), 15.

81. MacAndrew and Edgerton, *Drunken Comportment*, 95.

82. Partridge, *A History of Orgies*, vii.

83. Dominic Pettman, *After the Orgy: Toward a Politics of Exhaustion* (Albany: SUNY Press, 2002), 49–51.

84. Urban, *Magia Sexualis*, 20.

85. Ibid., 258.

86. Richard Payne Knight, *The Symbolical Language of Ancient Art and Mythology: An Inquiry* (New York: J. W. Bouton, 1892), 49.

87. David Allyn, *Make Love, Not War: The Sexual Revolution: An Unfettered History* (Boston: Little, Brown, 2000), 210.

88. Groes-Green, 2012.

3. BECOMING AN ORGIAST

1. M. Marshall, "'Four Hundred Rabbits': An Anthropological View of Ethanol as a Disinhibitor," in *Alcohol and Disinhibition: Nature and Meaning of the Link*, ed. R. Room and G. Collins (research monograph no. 12; Rockville, MD: US Department of Health and Human Services, 1983), 200.

2. Craig MacAndrew and Robert B. Edgerton, *Drunken Comportment: A Social Explanation* (New York: Aldine, 1969).

3. Heterosexual swinging and BDSM are often referred to as "alternative sexual practices" or "alternative sexualities." This phrase unfortunately reinforces the idea that there is a corresponding "normal" or standard sexuality—monogamous, married, "vanilla," and so on. I retain the phrase on occasion here because it appears in both the academic and popular literature; "alternative sexualities" also signals that such practices are transgressive from a mainstream perspective (even if the ideal is unstable).

4. Here, "community" is defined as a group with shared means of communication (websites, online groups, national and local publications), leisure activities, beliefs, practices (including the development of skills, the production of knowledge, rituals, etc.), and ethics. Although debating the subtle distinctions between "communities" and "subcultures" could be done extensively, I generally use the same terminology as the authors I discuss.

5. Not all individuals who identify as part of these communities are involved in group sex or erotic activity.

6. The size of the US population involved in swinging is estimated at 1 to 2 percent of the overall total, although these figures are problematic. Studies have consistently found, however, that self-identified swingers tend to be white, middle and upper-middle class, above average in education and income, and in professional and managerial positions. Lifestylers may also be involved with other communities and/or sexual practices, such as polyamory or BDSM/kink. Whenever possible, I match the use of the term "swingers" or "lifestyle" to the texts or individuals being discussed. In my own work on the United States, I usually use swinging to refer to a practice and lifestyle as an identity.

7. Antoinette Kelly, "Swingers Groups in Ireland Are Growing at a Massive Rate," Irish Central, September 14, 2010, http://www.irishcentral.com/news/Swinging-in-Ireland-is-a-growing-at-a-massive-rate-102882449.html?showAll=y.

8. The term "girl-girl" is used in heterosexual pornography to discuss female same-sex activity and is widely used in discussions about types of lifestyle play.

9. Terry Gould, *The Lifestyle: A Look at the Erotic Rites of Swingers* (Toronto: Vintage Canada, 1999), 107.

10. As the complexity of practices, meanings, and local variations cannot be conveyed here, my discussion is primarily focused on two ethnographies of BDSM in the United States, *Playing on the Edge: Sadomasochism, Risk, and Intimacy* (Bloomington: Indiana University Press, 2010) by Staci Newmahr, a sociologist who participated in a heterosexual BDSM community while conducting her research, and *Techniques of Pleasure: BDSM and the Circuits of Sexuality* (Durham: Duke University Press, 2010) by Margot Weiss, an anthropologist who studied pansexual BDSM in San Francisco.

11. Russell Westhaver, "Party Boys: Identity, Community, and the Circuit" (PhD diss., Simon Fraser University, 2003).

12. Russell Westhaver, "Flaunting and Empowerment: Thinking about Circuit Parties, the Body and Power," *Journal of Contemporary Ethnography* 35, no. 6 (2006): 621.

13. Ibid., 612.

14. Martin S. Weinberg and Colin J. Williams, "Gay Baths and the Social Organization of Impersonal Sex," *Social Problems* 23 (1975): 124.

15. Maurice van Lieshout, "Leather Nights in the Woods: Locating Male Homosexuality and Sadomasochism in a Dutch Highway Rest Area," in *Queers in Space: Communities/Public Places/Sites of Resistance*, ed. Gordon Brent Ingram, Anne-Marie Bouthillette, and Yolanda Retter (Seattle: Bay Press, 1997), 347.

16. Ibid., 352.

17. Ibid., 353.

18. William Leap, "Sex in 'Private' Places: Gender, Erotics, and Detachment in Two Urban Locales," in *Public Sex, Gay Space*, ed. William L. Leap (New York: Columbia University Press, 1999), 136.

19. Ira Tattleman, "The Meaning at the Wall: Tracing the Gay Bathhouse," in *Queers in Space: Communities/Public Places/Sites of Resistance*, ed. Gordon Brent Ingram, Anne-Marie Bouthillette, and Yolanda Retter (Seattle: Bay Press, 1997), 400.

20. Weinberg and Williams, "Gay Baths," 130.

21. "What" explanation page, Darkness Falls Two, http://www.darknessfallstwo.org/.

22. Women have been less likely to utilize public places for sex, probably due at least in part to safety concerns.

23. John Grube, "'No More Shit': The Struggle for Democratic Gay Space in Toronto," in *Queers in Space: Communities/Public Places/Sites of Resistance*, ed. John M. Ingham, Anne-Marie Bouthillette, and Yolanda Retter (Seattle: Bay Press, 1997), 132–33.

24. "Guidelines," Club Bliss London, http://www.club-bliss-london.com/guide.htm.

25. Weinberg and Williams, "Gay Baths," 130.

26. Charles Moser,"S/M (Sadomasochistic) Interactions in Semi-Public Settings," *Journal of Homosexuality* 36, no. 2 (1998).

27. Richard Tewksbury, "Bathhouse Intercourse: Structural and Behavoral Aspects of an Erotic Oasis," *Deviant Behavior* 23 (2002): 104.

28. Weinberg and Williams, "Gay Baths," 130.

29. Corie Hammers, "An Examination of Lesbian/Queer Bathhouse Culture and the Social Organization of (Im)Personal Sex," *Journal of Contemporary Ethnography* 38, no. 3 (2009): 318.

30. Westhaver, "Flaunting and Empowerment," 619.

31. Westhaver, "Party Boys," 98.

32. Lieshout, "Leather Nights in the Woods," 347.

33. William Jankowiak and Laura Mixson, "'I Have His Heart, Swinging Is Just Sex': The Ritualization of Sex and the Rejuvenation of the Love Bond in an American Spouse Exchange Community," in *Intimacies: Love and Sex across Cultures*, ed. William R. Jankowiak (New York: Columbia University Press, 2008), 254.

4. DISGUST, SHAME, AND GUILT

1. Millet's book was translated into English as *The Sexual Life of Catherine M* in 2002.

2. Millet, Catherine. *The Sexual Life of Catherine M* (New York: Grove Press, 2003), 10.

3. Leslie Camhi, "Sex Obsession by the Numbers," *New York Times*, June 22, 2002, http://www.nytimes.com/2002/06/22/books/sex-obsession-by-the-numbers.html?pagewanted=all&src=pm.

4. "The Sexual Life of Catherine M—Is Just Not Sexy," *The Literary Kitty* (blog), September 21, 2010, http://literarykitty.wordpress.com/2010/09/21/the-sexual-life-of-catherine-m-is-just-not-sexy/.

5. Millet, *The Sexual Life of Catherine M*, 54.

6. Ibid., 36.

7. Ibid., 34.

8. Ibid., 14.

9. Ibid., 142.

10. Ibid.

11. Ibid., 197.

12. Ibid., 191.

13. Ibid., 180.

14. Ibid., 176.

15. Jessica Berens, "The Double Life of Catherine M," *Guardian*, May 19, 2002, http://www.guardian.co.uk/books/2002/may/19/biography.features.

16. Millet, *The Sexual Life of Catherine M*, 63.

17. Ibid., 23, 26.

18. Ibid., 175.

19. "Thai Zoo Hopes Porn Will Get Sluggish Pandas to Mate," *Fox News*, March 27, 2007, http://www.foxnews.com/story/0,2933,261569,00.html.

20. Clarissa Ward, "'Panda Porn' to Boost Male's Sex Drive," *ABC News*, February 15, 2010, http://abcnews.go.com/Nightline/AmazingAnimals/porn-boost-male-pandas-sex-drives/story?id=9718714.

21. Brian Handwerk, "Panda Porn to Boost Mating Efforts at Thai Zoo," *National Geographic News*, November 13, 2006, http://news.nationalgeographic.com/news/2006/11/061113-panda-mate.html.

22. Esther Perel, *Mating in Captivity: Unlocking Erotic Intelligence* (New York: Harper Perennial, 2007).

23. Rajesh Shrivana, "Zoo Keepers Go 'Blue' in the Face for a Chimp of the Old Block . . ." *Deccan Herald*, December 25, 2011, http://www.deccanherald.com/content/43307/zoo-keepers-go-blue-face.html.

24. Dennis Campbell, "Porn: The New Sex Education," *Joe Public Blog*, *Guardian*, March 30, 2009, http://www.guardian.co.uk/society/joepublic+education/sexeducation.

25. Alex Morris, "They Know What Boys Want," *New York Magazine*, January 30, 2011, http://nymag.com/news/features/70977/.

26. Nicola Abé, "Online Sex Education: Parents' Porn Fears Exaggerated, Experts Say," *Spiegel Online* , October 14, 2011, http://www.spiegel.de/international/zeitgeist/online-sex-education-parents-porn-fears-exaggerated-experts-say-a-790266-2.html.

27. Jessica Bennett, "Northwestern University's Live Sex Class," *Daily Beast* , March 2, 2011, http://www.thedailybeast.com/articles/2011/03/03/the-story-behind-northwestern-universitys-live-sex-class.html.

28. Joshua Rhett Miller, "Northwestern University Professor Defends Explicit Sex Toy Demonstration after Class," *Fox News* , March 3, 2011, http://www.foxnews.com/us/2011/03/03/northwestern-university-professor-defends-explicit-sex-toy-demonstration/?cmpid=cmty_%7BlinkBack%7D_Northwestern_University_Professor_Defends_Explicit_Sex_Toy_Demonstration_After_Class.

29. Stefano Esposito, "Church Nixed Helping Northwestern Students Because of Sex Toy Flap," *Herald-News* , 2011, http://heraldnews.suntimes.com/photos/galleries/4718726-417/church-nixed-helping-northwestern-students-because-of-sex-toy-flap.html.

30. Jacques Steinberg, "Extracurricular Sex Toy Lesson Draws Rebuke at Northwestern," *New York Times* , March 3, 2011, http://www.nytimes.com/2011/03/04/education/04northwestern.html?_r=2&.

31. While I retain these psychoanalytic insights, I am not committed to a Freudian view of "sexual instinct," his model of the unconscious, or a particular story of human development, such as the Oedipus complex. I draw on psychoanalysts from varying traditions, self psychology to object relations theory, and primarily from areas where their quibbles are irrelevant to my overall argument.

32. The academic literature on emotion fills volumes, taking up different aspects of emotional experience: how to define emotion and distinguish the concept from others, such as affect or feeling; immediate emotional reactions such as facial expressions, vocal utterances, or physiological responses; self-reported subjective emotional experiences or descriptions; how emotions are elicited or displayed in specific situations, contexts, and cultures; models of emotional experience; types of emotions; and so on. Some emotions, such as embarrassment or pride, can be observed in only some human (and occasionally animal) populations. Emotions can be conscious or unconscious, affecting us in multiple ways simultaneously. Many researchers believe that certain emotions can be considered biological, or universal, such as anger, disgust, fear, joy, sadness, and surprise, although they differ as to which emotions might be included and why. Some distinguish between primary and secondary emotions or between primary emotional states and "self-conscious emotional states."

33. David Matsumoto and Hyi Sung Hwang, "Culture and Emotion," *Journal of Cross-Cultural Psychology* 43, no. 1 (2012): 106.

34. Ibid., 94.

35. Diana Jean Schemo, "Sex Education with Just One Lesson: No Sex," *New York Times*, December 28, 2000, http://www.nytimes.com/2000/12/28/us/sex-education-with-just-one-lesson-no-sex.html?pagewanted=all&src=pm.

36. William Ian Miller, *The Anatomy of Disgust* (Cambridge, MA: Harvard University Press, 1997).

37. Ibid., 20.

38. Some film series in this genre, which I refer to as "consumption porn," are *Cocktails, Slap Happy, Gag Factor, Rough Sex*, and *Oral Consumption*.

39. Tim Dean, *Unlimited Intimacy: Reflections on the Subculture of Barebacking* (Chicago: University of Chicago Press, 2010), 136.

40. David Greenberg, *The Construction of Homosexuality*

41. Gilbert Herdt, *Sambia Sexual Culture: Essays from the Field* (Chicago: University of Chicago Press 1999), 18.

42. Deborah A. Elliston, "'Ritualized Homosexuality' in Melanesia and Beyond, *American Ethnologist* 22, no. 4 (1995): 862.

43. Ibid., 850.

44. Ibid., 858.

45. Ibid., 859.

46. Kelly, Raymond Case. 1993. Constructing inequality: the fabrication of a hierarchy of virtue among the Etoro. Ann Arbor: University of Michigan Press, p. 46 and Kelly Raymond Case. 1977. Etoro Social Structure: a study in Structural Contradiction. Ann Arbor: University of Michigan Press, p. 16.

47. Paul Gilbert, "Evolution, Social Roles, and the Differences in Shame and Guilt," *Social Research* 70, no. 4 (2003): 1215.

48. Richard Shweder, "Toward a Deep Cultural Psychology of Shame," *Social Research* 70, no. 4 (2003): 1115.

49. Michael Lewis, *Shame: The Exposed Self* (New York: Free Press, 1992), 195.

50. Ibid., 162.

51. Joseph D. Lichtenberg, *Sensuality and Sexuality across the Divide of Shame* (New York: Routledge, 2007), 144. Although Lichtenberg hopes that lovemaking between adults can be sensual, tender, and mutual, he also cautions that full arousal, excitement, and orgiastic release will require prohibitions and transgressions. Expressions of sexuality inevitably involve confrontation with a prohibitive barrier that, while it "may be more or less intense," "always involves a degree of ediginess and rebelliousness from infancy" (111).

52. Nicholas Thomas, *Cook: The Extraordinary Sea Voyages of Captain James Cook* (New York: Bloomsbury Publishing, 2003), 69.

53. Mario Perniola, "Between Clothing and Nudity," in *Fragments for a History of the Human Body*, ed. Michel Fehrer (New York: Zone, 1989), 237–65.

54. Alice Dreger, "Wanting Privacy versus Being Ashamed," *Fetishes I Don't Get: Thoughts on Life, Love, and Lust* (blog), *Psychology Today*, March 6, 2011, http://www.psychologytoday.com/blog/fetishes-i-dont-get/201103/wanting-privacy-versus-being-ashamed.

55. The phrase *in flagrante delicto* is occasionally used as a euphemism for being caught naked or having sex, though in very different contexts.

56. Gang rape, group rape, disciplining, streamlining, *lainap*, and waylaying are terms used to refer to forced sex in different contexts; unwanted sex can also occur with varying levels of coercion. In some situations, the individuals involved or those interpreting the events differ about whether "rape" is the appropriate term; when this is the case, I try to acknowledge the ambiguity across perspectives and use the same term as those who are closest to the experience. Thus, even though certain "ritual defloration" practices of young girls might be considered coercive or criminal in other contexts, I use the language found in the original source whenever possible.

57. Ed Yong, "Ballistic Penises and Corkscrew Vaginas—The Sexual Battles of Ducks," *Not Exactly Rocket Science* (blog), December 22, 2009, http://scienceblogs.com/notrocketscience/2009/12/22/ballistic-penises-and-corkscrew-vaginas-the-sexual-battles/.

58. Joanna Bourke, "Sexual Violence, Bodily Pain, and Trauma: A History," *Theory, Culture & Society* 29, no. 3 (2012): 32.

59. Darius Rejali, "Ordinary Betrayals: Conceptualizing Refugees Who Have Been Tortured in the Global Village," *Human Rights Review* 1, no. 4 (2000), available at http://academic.reed.edu/poli_sci/faculty/rejali/articles/HRRarticle.html.

60. Thomas Gregor, *Anxious Pleasures: The Sexual Lives of an Amazonian People* (Chicago: University of Chicago Press, 1985), 493.

61. Yolanda Murphy and Robert Francis Murphy, *Women of the Forest*, 2nd ed. (New York: Columbia University Press, 1985), 195.

62. Ibid.

63. Ibid., xlvii. The Murphys also discovered that assumptions of inferiority reversed once a woman was beyond her childbearing years; in the underlying cosmology of Mundurucu society, older women become "sociological males," suggesting a more complex power structure than one based only on gender. This is also from *Women of the Forest*, p. 18.

64. E. Adamson Hoebel, *The Cheyennes: Indians of the Great Plains* (New York: Holt, 1960), cited in Peggy R. Sanday, *Fraternity Gang Rape: Sex, Brotherhood, and Privilege on Campus* (New York: New York University Press, 1990), 100.

65. Kate Wood, "Contextualizing Group Rape in Post-apartheid South Africa," *Culture, Health, and Sexuality* 7, no. 4 (2005): 309.

66. Ibid., 310.

67. Phoebe Ferris-Rotman, "Prison Gang Rape of Mafia 'Poet' Prompts Government Response," *Pink News*, August 5, 2008, http://www.pinknews.co.uk/2008/08/05/prison-gang-rape-of-mafia-poet-prompts-government-response/.

68. Tali Woodward, "Life in Hell: In California Prisons, an Unconventional Gender Identity Can Be Like an Added Sentence," *San Francisco Bay Guardian*, March 15, 2006, http://www.sfbg.com/40/24/cover_life.html.

69. Jesse Ellison, "The Military's Secret Shame," *Newsweek*, April 3, 2011, http://www.newsweek.com/2011/04/03/the-military-s-secret-shame.html.

70. Marian T. A. Tankink, "The Silence of South-Sudanese Women: Social Risks in Talking about Experiences of Sexual Violence," *Culture, Health & Sexuality: An International Journal for Research, Intervention and Care* 15, no. 4 (2013): 400.

71. Ibid., 398.

72. Jay Pateakos, "Brothers Break Silence in Big Dan's Rape Case," *Herald News*, October 25, 2009, http://www.heraldnews.com/news/local_news/x665149028/After-26-years-brothers-break-silence.

73. Charles Winokoor, "Frank O'Boy Speaks out on Big Dan's Rape Case," *Taunton Daily Gazette*, May 28, 2009, http://www.tauntongazette.com/news/x313662945/Frank-O-Boy-speaks-out-on-Big-Dan-s-rape-case.

74. Ibid.

75. Paul Edward Parker, "Juries Hear Big Dan's Rape Case," *Bristol County Century* (*Providence Journal*), November 1, 1999, C1.

76. Winokoor, "Frank O'Boy."

77. James C. McKinley, "Vicious Assault Shakes Texas Town," *New York Times*, March 8, 2011.

78. David Edwards, "Republican Lawmaker Blames 11-Year-Old Victim of Alleged Gang Rape," *The Raw Story*, March 16, 2011, http://www.rawstory.com/rs/2011/03/16/republican-lawmaker-blames-11-year-old-victim-of-alleged-gang-rape/.

79. Cindy Horswell, "Defendant in Cleveland Gang Rape Case Gets Life Sentence," *Houston Chronicle*, November 28, 2012, http://www.chron.com/news/houston-texas/houston/article/Defendant-in-Cleveland-gang-rape-case-gets-life-4073766.php.

80. Miller, *Anatomy of Disgust*, 9.

81. Ibid., x.

82. "Photos of Gang Rape Go Viral on Facebook," *Globe and Mail*, September 16, 2010, http://www.theglobeandmail.com/news/national/british-columbia/photos-of-gang-rape-go-viral-on-facebook/article1710072/.

83. "Pitt Meadows, B.C. Gang Rape: Boy Who Posted Images of 16-Year-Old Victim Sentenced," Huffington Post, February 10, 2012, http://www.huffingtonpost.ca/2012/02/10/pitt-meadows-bc-gang-rape_n_1269269.html.

84. Kashmir Hill, "The Potential Financial Consequences of Sharing Gang-Rape Photos on Facebook," *Forbes*, September 17, 2010, http://blogs.forbes.com/kashmirhill/2010/09/17/the-potential-financial-consequences-of-sharing-gang-rape-photos-on-facebook/.

85. "Gang Rape 10,000," *Quantum Buddha's Blog* (blog), September 24, 2010, http://quantumbuddha.wordpress.com/2010/09/24/gang-rape-10000/, accessed November 2012. By February 2013, the blog entry had been deleted, although it can still be found at http://www.progressivebloggers.ca/2010/09/gang-rape-10000/.

86. "Gang Rape 8,000," *Quantum Buddha's Blog* (blog), September 2010, http://quantumbuddha.wordpress.com/2010/09/17/gang-rape-8000/, accessed November 2012. By February 2013, the blog entry had been deleted, although it can still be found at http://www.progressivebloggers.ca/2010/09/gang-rape-8000/.

87. Although discussed less in the media, and disputed by Bronwyn Curran, Mukhtaran Mai's brother Shaquoor was also reportedly sodomized by three Mastoi men just before her attack, as punishment for the supposed caste violations.

88. "Hudood Ordinances—The Crime and Punishment for Zina," Amnesty International in Asia & the Pacific, http://asiapacific.amnesty.org/apro/aproweb.nsf/pages/svaw_hudoo.

89. Bruce Loudon, "Pakistan Pack Rape as Reform Laws Stall," *Autstralian*, September 19, 2006, http://www.theaustralian.com.au/news/world/pakistan-pack-rape-as-reform-laws-stall/story-e6frg6so-1111112233324.

90. Bronwyn Curran, "Mukhtaran Mai: The Other Side of the Story," *News International*, April 30, 2011, http://www.thenews.com.pk/TodaysPrintDetail.aspx?ID=44406&Cat=9.

91. Caryn E. Neumann, *Sexual Crime: A Reference Handbook* (Santa Barbara: ABC-CLIO, 2009), 133.

92. "Outrage at Musharraf Rape Remarks," *BBC News*, September 16, 2005, http://news.bbc.co.uk/2/hi/south_asia/4251536.stm. Musharraf also claimed that he was misquoted: Glenn Kessler, "Musharraf Denies Rape Comments," *Washington Post*, September 19, 2005, http://www.washingtonpost.com/wp-dyn/content/article/2005/09/18/AR2005091800554.html.

93. Lynn G. Smith and James R. Smith, "Comarital Sex: The Incorporation of Extramarital Sex into the Marriage Relationship," in *Beyond Monogamy: Recent Studies of Sexual Alternatives in Marriage*, ed. James R. Smith and Lynn G. Smith (Baltimore: Johns Hopkins University Press, 1974), 133.

94. Curtis Bergstrand and Jennifer Blevins Sinski, *Swinging in America: Love, Sex, and Marriage in the 21st Century* (Santa Barbara: Praeger, 2010), 55.

95. Larsen, p. 5.

96. Larsen, p. 11.

97. Corie Hammers, "An Examination of Lesbian/Queer Bathhouse Culture and the Social Organization of (Im)Personal Sex," *Journal of Contemporary Ethnography* 38, no. 3 (2009): 325.

98. Ibid., 324.

99. Ibid., 325.

100. Ibid., 154.

101. Ibid., 156.

102. Ibid., 157.

103. Russell Westhaver, "Party Boys: Identity, Community, and the Circuit" (PhD diss., Simon Fraser University, 2003), 105.

104. Ibid., 619.

105. Russell Westhaver, "Flaunting and Empowerment: Thinking about Circuit Parties, the Body and Power," *Journal of Contemporary Ethnography* 35, no. 6 (2006): 617.

106. Ibid., 636.

107. Westhaver, "Party Boys," 112.

108. Westhaver, "Flaunting and Empowerment," 618.

109. Westhaver, "Party Boys," 270.

110. David McInnes, Jack Bradley, and Garrett Prestage, "The Discourse of Gay Men's Group Sex: The Importance of Masculinity," *Culture, Health & Sexuality: An International Journal for Research, Intervention and Care* 11, no. 6 (2009): 647.

111. Ibid., 651.

112. Erin Mantz, "Suburban Swingers: Beyond the Sex," *Today.com*, July 29, 2008, http://today.msnbc.msn.com/id/25851876/ns/today-relationships/t/suburban-swingers-beyond-sex/#.UNfESqX3AUs.

113. Harmon Leon, "A Night with the California Swingers Club," The Smoking Jacket, December 22, 2010, http://www.thesmokingjacket.com/humor/california-swingers-club.

114. Stephen Holden, review of *The Lifestyle: Group Sex in the Suburbs*, directed by David Schisgall, *New York Times*, March 16, 2000, http://movies.nytimes.com/movie/179829/The-Lifestyle/overview.

115. Ibid.

116. Unsigned review of *The Lifestyle: Group Sex in the Suburbs*, directed by David Schisgall, Nitrate Online, www.nitrateonline.com/1999/fsiff99-3.html#Lifestyle.

117. Phil Villarreal, review of *Sex with Strangers*, directed by Joe Gantz and Harry Gantz, *Arizona Daily Star*, August 30, 2002.

118. David Noh, review of *Sex with Strangers*, directed by Joe Gantz and Harry Gantz, *Film Journal International*, http://www.filmjournal.com/filmjournal/esearch/article_display.jsp?vnu_content_id=1000696179.

119. Jed Horne, review of *Sex with Strangers*, directed by Joe Gantz and Harry Gantz, *Tech Online Edition*, October 8, 2002, www-tech.mit.edu/V122/N46/Sex_with_strang.46a.html.

120. India Nicholas, "Swingers Go Wild for Bill Plympton," *Willamette Week* (staff blog), October 13, 2009, http://blogs.wweek.com/news/2009/10/13/swingers-go-wild-for-bill-plympton/.

121. Mantz, "Suburban Swingers."

122. Leon, "California Swingers Club."

123. Harmon Leon, *The American Dream: Walking in the Shoes of Carnies, Arms Dealers, Immigrant Dreamers, Pot Farmers, and Christian Believers* (New York: Nation Books, 2008).

124. Sanjiv Bhattacharya, "Meet the Mandingos," *Details*, 2007, http://www.details.com/sex-relationships/sex-and-other-releases/200703/meet-the-mandingos.

125. Carla Meyer, review of *Sex with Strangers*, directed by Joe Gantz and Harry Gantz, *SFGate*, February 22, 2002, www.sfgate.com/cgi-bin/article.cgi?f=/c/a/2002/02/22/DD77008.DTL.

126. Michael J. Mooney, "Swinging through South Florida's Underground Sex Clubs," *Broward Palm Beach New Times*, March 3, 2011, http://www.browardpalmbeach.com/content/printVersion/1375004/.

127. Ferrett Steinmetz, "Placing My First Swingers' Ad," *Ferrett* (blog), www.theferrett.com.

128. Unsigned review of *The Lifestyle*, Nitrate Online.

129. Miller, *Anatomy of Disgust*, 194.

130. Mooney, "South Florida's Underground Sex Clubs."

131. Larissa Nolan, "Collymore Revelation Lets 'Dogging' out of the Kennel," *Irish Independent*, March 7, 2004, http://www.independent.ie/irish-news/collymore-revelation-lets-dogging-out-of-the-kennel-26218546.html.

132. Stan Collymore, *Tackling My Demons* (London: CollinsWillow, 2004), 290.

133. Scott Barancik, "D.C. Swings! Couples Meet for Cocktails, Hors d'Oeuvres, and Blowjobs at a Washington Restaurant," *Washington City Paper*, December 15, 1995, http://www.washingtoncitypaper.com/articles/8031/dc-swings/.

134. "Crowning Cora," *Washington City Paper*, January 5, 1996, http://www.washingtoncitypaper.com/articles/9541/crowning-cora.

135. Terry Gould, *The Lifestyle: A Look at the Erotic Rites of Swingers* (Toronto: Vintage Canada, 1999).

CASE STUDY: THE "DARK ORGIES" OF THE MARIND-ANIM

1. Jan van Baal, with Father J. Verschueren, MSC, *Dema: Description and Analysis of Marind Culture* (The Hague: Martinus Nijhoff, 1966), 40.

2. Ibid., 540.

3. Bruce M. Knauft, *South Coast New Guinea Cultures: History, Comparison, Dialectic* (Cambridge: Cambridge University Press, 1993), 157, 162.

4. Baal, *Dema*, 709.

5. Ibid., 812.

6. Ibid., 549.

7. Ibid., 811.

8. Ibid., 162–63.

9. Ibid., 808.

10. Ibid., 821.

11. Ibid., 815.

12. Ibid., 816.

13. Ibid., 155.

14. Ibid., 165.

15. Ibid., 141.

16. Ibid., 171.

17. Ibid., 25.
18. Ibid., 819.
19. Ibid., 27.
20. Ibid., 492.
21. Jan van Baal, "The Dialectics of Sex in Marind-anim Culture," in *Ritualized Homosexuality in Melanesia* , ed. Gilbert H. Herdt (Berkeley: University of California Press, 1984), 128.
22. Jeroen A. Overweel, *The Marind in a Changing Environment: A Study on Social-Economic Change in Marind Society to Assist in the Formulation of a Long Term Strategy for the Foundation for Social, Economic and Environmental Development (YAPSEL)* (Irian Jaya, Indonesia: YAPSEL, 1993), 22.
23. Ibid., 28.
24. Ibid., 57.
25. Knauft, 165.
26. Lawrence Hammar, "The Dark Side to Donovanosis: Color, Climate, Race and Racism in American South Venereology," *Journal of Medical Humanities* 18, no. 1 (1997): 29–57.
27. Ibid., 33.

5. FROM THE COOLIDGE EFFECT TO COSMIC ECSTASY

1. Elaine Hatfield, *A New Look at Love* (Lanham: University Press of America, 2002), 75.
2. Joris M. Koene and Andries Ter Maat, "Coolidge Effect in Pond Snails: Male Motivation in a Simultaneous Hermaphrodite," *BMC Evolutionary Biology* 7 (2007): 212.
3. Hatfield, *A New Look at Love*, 75.
4. James G. Pfaus, "Revisiting the Concept of Sexual Motivation," *Annual Review of Sex Research* 10 (1999): 120.
5. Dietrich Klusmann, "Sexual Motivation and the Duration of Partnership," *Archives of Sexual Behavior* 31, no. 3 (2002): 275–87.
6. David Schnarch, *Passionate Marriage: Love, Sex, and Intimacy in Emotionally Committed Relationships* (New York: Henry Holt, 1997).
7. Garrett Prestage et al., *TOMS: Three or More Study* (Sydney, Australia: National Centre in HIV Epidemiology and Clinical Research, University of New South Wales, 2008), 23.
8. Russell Westhaver, "Flaunting and Empowerment: Thinking about Circuit Parties, the Body and Power," *Journal of Contemporary Ethnography* 35, no. 6 (2006): 630.
9. David McInnes, Jack Bradley, and Garrett Prestage, "The Discourse of Gay Men's Group Sex: The Importance of Masculinity," *Culture, Health & Sexuality: An International Journal for Research, Intervention and Care* 11, no. 6 (2009): 647.
10. Curtis Bergstrand, Nancy Schrepf, and Jennifer Williams-Sinski, "Civilization and Sexual Discontent: Monogamy and the Problem of Surplus Repression" (unpublished manuscript, December 1, 2003), Bellarmine University.
11. Curtis Bergstrand and Jennifer Blevins Sinski, *Swinging in America: Love, Sex, and Marriage in the 21st Century* (Santa Barbara: Praeger, 2010), 32.
12. Ibid., 75–76.
13. William Jankowiak and Laura Mixson, "'I Have His Heart, Swinging Is Just Sex': The Ritualization of Sex and the Rejuvenation of the Love Bond in an American Spouse Exchange Community," in *Intimacies: Love and Sex across Cultures*, ed. William R. Jankowiak (New York: Columbia University Press, 2008), 260. Also, NSSHB (2010) "Sexual Behavior in the United States: Results From a National Probability Sample of Men and Women Ages 14-94." www.kinseyinstitute.org/resources/faq.html#frequency.
14. Daniel Bergner, "What Do Women Want?" *New York Times Magazine*, January 22, 2009, http://www.nytimes.com/2009/01/25/magazine/25desire-t.html?pagewanted=all.
15. Men can feel aroused without erections, however, or experience penile response that does not match their psychological state.
16. Bergner, "What Do Women Want?"

17. Andy Campbell, "Horseshoe Crab Mating Ritual Is the Oldest Beach Orgy," *Weird News* (blog), Huffington Post, May 11, 2012, http://www.huffingtonpost.com/2012/05/11/horseshoe-crab-orgy_n_1509445.html.

18. Todd Shackelford and Aaron T. Goetz, "Psychological and Physiological Adaptations to Sperm Competition in Humans," *Review of General Psychology* 9, no. 3 (2005): 228–48.

19. Ibid.

20. Sarah J. Kilgallon and Leigh W Simmons, "Image Content Influences Men's Semen Quality," *Biology Letters* 1, no. 3 (2005): 253–55.

21. Ogi Ogas and Sai Gaddam, *A Billion Wicked Thoughts: What the World's Largest Experiment Reveals about Human Desire* (New York: Dutton, 2011).

22. David J. Ley, *Insatiable Wives:Women Who Stray and the Men Who Love Them* (Lanham: Rowman & Littlefield, 2009), xii.

23. Ibid., 51.

24. David J. Ley, "Is Kinky Sex Good for Your Marriage?" *Women Who Stray* (blog), *Psychology Today*, June 22, 2010, http://www.psychologytoday.com/blog/women-who-stray/201006/is-kinky-sex-good-your-marriage.

25. Ogas and Gaddam, *A Billion Wicked Thoughts*.

26. Ibid.

27. Ibid.

28. Dan Savage, "Husband Has No Interest in Hot Wife," *Savage Love*, *Creative Loafing Charlotte*, March 24, 2009, http://clclt.com/charlotte/husband-has-no-interest-in-hot-wife/Content?oid=2152344.

29. Terry Gould, *The Lifestyle: A Look at the Erotic Rites of Swingers* (Toronto: Vintage Canada, 1999), 214.

30. Ibid.

31. Bigg Texx, May 27, 2012 (3:03 a.m.), comment on *DoMyWife* (forum), http://www.domywife.com/forum/general-discussion/10884-hot-wife-swinging-polyamory-candaulism-compersion.html.

32. Mr. Fun, February 25, 2009 (9:32 a.m.), comment on "Rivals Spur Men to Produce Better Sperm," *Hot Wife Allie* (blog), http://www.hotwivesonline.com/2005/06/09/rivals-spur-men-to-produce-better-sperm/.

33. "Did You Ever Wonder Why You Just Needed to Fuck That Good Looking Guy?" *I Play & He Waits* (blog), http://iplayhewaits.blogspot.com/p/did-you-ever-wonder-why-you-just-needed.html?zx=f8645986ab54e251.

34. Quoted in Cuckoldress Roxanne, "The Science of Cuckolding," *A Cuckoldress World* (blog), December 20, 2004, http://www.xtcforums.com/main.php?page=cuckoldscientificexplanation.

35. Harvey Milkman and Stanley G. Sunderworth, *Craving for Ecstasy and Natural Highs: A Positive Approach to Mood Alteration* (Los Angeles: Sage, 2009), 153.

36. Donald Dutton and Arthur Aron, "Some Evidence for Heightened Sexual Attraction under Conditions of High Anxiety," *Journal of Personality and Social Psychology* 30, no. 4 (1974): 510–17.

37. Gary Lewandowski and Arthur Aron, "Distinguishing Arousal from Novelty and Challenge in Initial Romantic Attraction between Strangers," *Social Behavior and Personality* 32, no. 4 (2004): 361–72.

38. Jonathan W. Roberti, "A Review of Behavioral and Biological Correlates of Sensation Seeking," *Journal of Research in Personality* 38 (2004): 268; Marvin Zuckerman, "The Psychophysiology of Sensation Seeking," *Journal of Personality* 58, no. 1 (1990): 313–45.

39. Dan T. A. Eisenberg, Benjamin Campbell, James MacKillop, Meera Modi, David Dang, J. Koji Lum, and David S. Wilson, "Polymorphisms in the Dopamine D4 and D2 Receptor Genes and Reproductive and Sexual Behaviors," *Evolutionary Psychology* 5, no. 4 (2007): 696–715.

40. Roberti, "Correlates of Sensation Seeking," 269.

41. Ibid., 256.

42. Ibid., 262.

43. Ibid., 266.

44. G. Prestage et al., "Use of Illicit Drugs among Gay Men Living with HIV in Sydney," *AIDS* 21, Suppl. 1 (2007): S53.

45. Michael Hurley and Garrett Prestage, "Intensive Sex Partying Amongst Gay Men in Sydney," *Culture, Health & Sexuality: An International Journal for Research, Intervention and Care* 11, no. 6 (2009): 598.

46. Ibid., 601.

47. Jonathan Bollen and David McInnes, "Time, Relations and Learning in Gay Men's Experiences of Adventurous Sex," *Social Semiotics* 14, no. 1 (2004): 25.

48. John Tierney, "What's New? Exuberance for Novelty Has Benefits," *New York Times*, February 3, 2012, http://www.nytimes.com/2012/02/14/science/novelty-seeking-neophilia-can-be-a-predictor-of-well-being.html?_r=1&emc=eta1.

49. Abraham Maslow, *Toward a Psychology of Being* (New York: Van Nostrand, 1968), 73.

50. Ibid., 94.

51. Ibid., 105.

52. Ibid., 80.

53. I. M. Lewis, "Trance, Possession, Shamanism, and Sex," *Anthropology of Consciousness* 14, no. 1 (2003): 31.

54. Michel Maffesoli, *The Shadow of Dionysus: A Contribution to the Sociology of the Orgy*, trans. Cindy Linse and Mary Kristina Palmquist (Albany: SUNY Press, 1993), 64.

55. Harvey Whitehouse, "Terror," in *The Oxford Handbook of Religion and Emotion*, ed. John Corrigan (New York: Oxford).

56. Mark Thompson, ed., *Leatherfolk: Radical Sex, People, Politics, and Practice* (Boston: Alyson Publications, 1991), 285.

57. Ibid., 292.

58. Ibid., 289.

59. Kal Cobalt, "The Path of Pain: Spiritual BDSM," *Kal Cobalt's Blog* (blog), http://www.realitysandwich.com/path_pain_spiritual_bdsm.

60. Bill Brent, "Interview with Pat Califia by Bill Brent," *Black Sheets* 15 (1999), 30, cited in Patrick Moore, *Beyond Shame: Reclaiming the Abandoned History of Radical Sexuality* (Boston: Beacon Press, 2004), 57.

61. Mark Thompson, ed., *Leatherfolk : Radical Sex, People, Politics, and Practice* (Boston: Alyson Publications, 1991), 269, 287.

62. Gayle Rubin and Judith Butler, "Sexual Traffic," *Differences: A Journal of Feminist Cultural Studies* 6, no. 2/3 (1994): 78.

63. Alicia D. Horton, "Flesh Hook Pulling: Motivations and Meaning-Making from the 'Body Side' of Life," *Deviant Behavior* 34, no. 2 (2013): 120.

64. Hugh Urban, "The Beast with Two Backs: Aleister Crowley, Sex Magic and the Exhaustion of Modernity," *Journal of Alternative and Emergent Religions* 7, no. 3 (2004): 7.

65. Ibid., 24.

66. Ibid., 22.

67. Ibid., 105.

68. "Club Tantra," School of Tantra, http://www.schooloftantra.net/ClubTantra/ClubTantra2.htm.

69. Janet Kira Lessin, "Double Penetration: A Path to Enlightenment," Club Tantra, http://clubtantra.org/2012/11/04/double-penetration-a-path-to-enlightenment/.

70. Ibid.

71. "Compersion" is a term used by polyamorists to describe feelings of happiness upon seeing a partner experience joy, happiness, or pleasure, sexual or otherwise. Compersion is sometimes put forth as the opposite of jealousy; other times, it is conceptualized as a state that can be achieved through reflection.

72. Jack Morin, *The Erotic Mind: Unlocking the Inner Source of Sexual Passion and Fulfillment* (New York: HarperCollins, 1995), 22.

73. Ibid., 50.

74. Ibid., 107.

75. Ibid., 135.

76. Robert Greene, *The Art of Seduction* (New York: Penguin, 2001).

77. Morin, *The Erotic Mind*, 43.

78. "Is life exciting or dull?" GSS: 45.7 percent "exciting"; 54.4 percent "pretty routine or dull." Swingers: 75.9 percent "exciting"; 23.8 percent "pretty routine or dull." Bergstrand and Sinski, *Swinging in America*, 57.

79. Ibid., 52.

6. GAMES PEOPLE PLAY

1. I. M. Lewis, "Trance, Possession, Shamanism, and Sex," *Anthropology of Consciousness* 14, no. 1 (2003): 24.

2. Matt Wray, "Burning Man and the Rituals of Capitalism," *Bad Subjects* 21 (1995), http://bad.eserver.org/issues/1995/21/wray.html.

3. Tim Wayne, "Burning Man Review," *Tim Wayne* (blog), http://blog.hisnameistimmy.com/burning-man-our-review/12.

4. Larry Harvey, "Jiffy Lube 2001," Burning Man, http://www.burningman.com/blackrockcity_yearround/jrs/extras/jiffylube.html.

5. Jeremy Hockett, "Participant Observation and the Study of Self: Burning Man as Ethnographic Experience," In *After Burn: Reflections on Burning Man*, ed. Lee M Gilmore and Mark Van Proyen (Albuquerque: University of New Mexico Press, 2005), 69.

6. "Down n Dirty First Timers Guide to Burning Man," *Festival A Go-Go* (blog), April 28, 2010, http://festivalagogo.com/?p=412.

7. "Second Life Grid Survey—Economic Metrics," available at http://www.gridsurvey.com/economy.php.

8. Mike Wagner, "Sex in Second Life," *Information Week*, May 26, 2007, http://www.informationweek.com/news/199701944?cid=email.

9. Anshe Chung Studios, "Anshe Chung Becomes First Virtual World Millionaire," news release, November 26 2006, http://www.anshechung.com/include/press/press_release251106.html.

10. "State of Sex: Second Life," *MMOrgy* (blog), October 13, 2005, www.mmorgy.com/2005/10/state_of_sex_second_life_1.php.

11. User profile for Misty Crimsonlay, Smashwords, www.smashwords.com/profile/view/mistyc.

12. Misty Crimsonlay, *Second Life—Hot Orgies* (Amazon Digital Services, 2011), Kindle edition.

13. Tom Boellstorff, *Coming of Age in Second Life: An Anthropologist Explores the Virtually Human* (Princeton: Princeton University Press, 2008), 165.

14. "Revealed: The 'Other Woman' in Second Life Divorce . . . Who's Now Engaged to the Web Cheat She's Never Met," *Mail Online*, November 14, 2008, http://www.dailymail.co.uk/news/article-1085412/Revealed-The-woman-Second-Life-divorce--whos-engaged-web-cheat-shes-met.html.

15. Ashley John Craft, "Love 2.0: A Quantitative Exploration of Sex and Relationships in the Virtual World Second Life," *Archives of Sexual Behavior* 41, no. 4 (2012): 943.

16. Richard L. Gilbert, Monique A. Gonzalez, and Nora A. Murphy, "Sexuality in the 3D Internet and Its Relationship to Real-Life Sexuality," *Psychology & Sexuality* 2, no. 2 (2011): 119.

17. Craft, "Love 2.0," 946.

18. Gilbert, Gonzalez, and Murphy,"Sexuality in the 3D Internet," 118.

19. Craft, "Love 2.0," 944.

20. Male swinger, quoted in Curtis Bergstrand and Jennifer Blevins Sinski, *Swinging in America: Love, Sex, and Marriage in the 21st Century* (Santa Barbara: Praeger, 2010), 6.

21. Jonathan Bollen and David McInnes, "Time, Relations and Learning in Gay Men's Experiences of Adventurous Sex," *Social Semiotics* 14, no. 1 (2004): 21.

22. Jane Ward, "Dude-Sex: White Masculinities and 'Authentic' Heterosexuality among Dudes Who Have Sex with Dudes," *Sexualities* 11, no. 4 (2008): 420.

23. Bergstrand and Sinski, *Swinging in America*.

24. Ibid., 56.

25. Ibid., 36.

26. George C. O'Neill and Nena O'Neill, "Patterns in Group Sexual Activity," *Journal of Sex Research* 6, no. 2 (1970): 101–12; C. Symonds, "Pilot Study of the Peripheral Behavior of Sexual Mate Swappers" (master's thesis, University of California, Riverside, 1968).

27. "100 Signs You May Be a Swinger," *Kasidie*, http://www.kasidie.com/static/magazine/humor/100signs.html.

28. Rachel R. White, "Sex Parties," *Time Out New York*, September 28, 2011, http://www.timeout.com/newyork/clubs-nightlife/sex-parties.

29. Richard Martin, "Powerful Exchanges: Ritual and Subjectivity in Berlin's BDSM Scene" (PhD diss., Princeton University, 2011), 46.

30. Daniel H. Lende, Terri Leonard, Claire E. Sterk, and Kirk Elifson, "Functional Methamphetamine Use: The Insider's Perspective," *Addiction Research & Theory* 15, no. 5 (2007): 465–77.

31. Hans S. Crombag and Terry E. Robinson, "Drugs, Environment, Brain, and Behavior," *Current Directions in Psychological Science* 13, no. 3 (2004): 110.

32. Jonathan W. Roberti, "A Review of Behavioral and Biological Correlates of Sensation Seeking," *Journal of Research in Personality* 38 (2004): 270.

33. James Pfaus and John Pinel, "Alcohol Inhibits and Disinhibits Sexual Behavior in the Male Rat," *Psychobiology* 17, no. 2 (1989): 195–201.

34. James G. Pfaus et al., "Inhibitory and Disinhibitory Effects of Psychomotor Stimulants and Depressants on the Sexual Behavior of Male and Female Rats," *Hormones and Behavior* 58, no. 1 (2010): 163–76.

35. Ibid., 163.

36. Karla S. Frohmader et al., "Effects of Methamphetamine on Sexual Performance and Compulsive Sex Behavior in Male Rats," *Psychopharmacology* 212, no. 1 (2010): 93–104.

37. R. Cagiano et al., "Effects on Rat Sexual Behaviour of Acute MDMA (Ecstasy) Alone or in Combination with Loud Music," *European Review for Medical and Pharmacological Sciences* 12 (2008): 291.

38. Adam Isaiah Green and Perry N Halkitis, "Crystal Methamphetamine and Sexual Sociality in an Urban Gay Subculture: An Elective Affinity," *Culture, Health & Sexuality: An International Journal for Research, Intervention and Care* 8, no. 4 (2006): 329.

39. Ibid., 323–24.

40. Ibid., 329.

41. Ibid., 325.

42. Joseph J. Palamar et al., "A Qualitative Descriptive Study of Perceived Sexual Effects of Club Drug Use in Gay and Bisexual Men," *Psychology & Sexuality* ifirst (2012): 10, 12.

43. Garrett Prestage et al., *TOMS: Three or More Study* (Sydney, Australia: National Centre in HIV Epidemiology and Clinical Research, University of New South Wales, 2008), 23.

44. Pfaus et al., "Inhibitory and Disinhibitory Effects," 163–76.

45. Russell Westhaver, "Party Boys: Identity, Community, and the Circuit" (PhD diss., Simon Fraser University, 2003), 172.

46. Holly Williams, "Teen Spirit: The 'Skins' Sensation Sweeping France," *Indepdendent*, July 31, 2010, http://www.independent.co.uk/arts-entertainment/tv/features/teen-spirit-the-skins-sensation-sweeping-france-2037470.html.

47. Claudine Doury, "France, Skins Parties, 2010," VU' l'agence, www.agencevu.com.

48. The American version of *Skins*, which appeared on MTV in 2011, drew criticism as child pornography because the actors were under eighteen years old and the plotlines were heavily sexualized. The show was canceled after the first season, according to network representatives, because it "didn't connect with a US audience as much as we had hoped." Still, as a theme, Skins has emerged in the party scene.

49. Stewart Payne, "Police Arrest MySpace Party Girl," *Telegraph*, April 13, 2007, http://www.telegraph.co.uk/news/uknews/1548483/Police-arrest-MySpace-party-girl.html.

50. Nick Craven, "What Really Happened at the Myspace Party from Hell," *Mail Online*, April 21, 2007, http://www.dailymail.co.uk/femail/article-449819/What-REALLY-happened-Myspace-party-hell.html.

51. Ashley Steinberg, "Rebels without Cause," *Newsweek*, March 17, 2008, http://www.thedailybeast.com/newsweek/2008/03/17/rebels-without-cause.html.

52. "Kissing-Crazy 'Pokemon' Teens Shock Chilean Society," Agence France-Presse, August 19, 2008, http://afp.google.com/article/ALeqM5g8_oJjFpw4GepEhegk6MXX9DZ41A.

53. Alexei Barrionuevo, "In Tangle of Young Lips, a Sex Rebellion in Chile," *New York Times*, September 12, 2008, http://www.nytimes.com/2008/09/13/world/americas/13chile.html?_r=0.

54. Steinberg, "Rebels without Cause."

55. Andrea González Recabarren, "Tribus urbanas: Pokemones y peloláis . . . ¿Cuánto sabes de ellos?" *Universia*, January 16, 2008, http://noticias.universia.cl/vida-universitaria/noticia/2008/01/16/314616/tribus-urbanas-pokemones-pelolais-sabes.html.

56. Barrionuevo, "Sex Rebellion in Chile," 2008.

57. Seventy men were in attendance; many took multiple turns.

58. Soyon Im, "Sex: The Annabel Chong Story," *Seattle Weekly*, July 26, 2000, http://www.seattleweekly.com/2000-07-26/film/sex-the-annabel-chong-story/.

59. Amy Goodman, "Voice: An Interview with Annabel Chong," Nerve.com, June 22, 1999, http://www.nerve.com/dispatches/goodman/chong.

60. Ibid.

61. Chun (2000). www.asianweek.com/2000_05_04/ae_annabelchong.html.

62. Lawrence Van Gelder, review of *Sex: The Annabel Chong Story*, New York Times, February 11, 2000, http://partners.nytimes.com/library/film/021100sex-film-review.html.

63. Robin Askew, "Annabel Chong: *Sex: The Annabel Chong Story*," *Spike Magazine*, October 1, 2000, http://www.spikemagazine.com/1000annabelchong.php.

64. Ibid.

65. Goodman (1999). "Attitudes to Marriage."

66. Gayle Rubin, "Thinking Sex: Notes for a Radical Theory of the Politics of Sexuality," in *Pleasure and Danger: Exploring Female Sexuality*, ed. Carole S. Vance (Boston: Routledge and Kegan Paul, 1984), 267–319.

67. Annabel Chong's website, www.annabelchong.com (accessed September 2012). As of March 2013, the website was no longer operative.

7. FEAR AND BONDING IN LAS VEGAS (AND BEYOND)

1. Christopher Ryan and Cacilda Jethá, *Sex at Dawn: The Prehistoric Origins of Modern Sexuality* (New York: Harper, 2010), 93.

2. Whether ritual multipartner sex occurs in an actual group or sequentially is somewhat at issue in the literature, but I have included a discussion here because the Canela appear as one of the few documented examples of "group sex" in non-Western societies.

3. Ryan and Jethá, *Sex at Dawn*, 103 (emphasis in original).

4. Ibid., 93.

5. Ibid., 102.

6. Ibid., 48.

7. Ibid., 292.

8. Ibid., 180.

9. William H. Crocker, "Canela Marriage: Factors in Change," in *Marriage Practices in Lowland South America*, ed. Kenneth M. Kensinger (Urbana and Chicago: University of Illinois Press, 1984), available at http://anthropology.si.edu/canela/literature/marrriage.pdf. Also see *Mending Ways: The Canela Indians of Brazil* (1999; co-produced by National Human Studies Film Center, Smithsonian Institution), DVD.

10. (Crocker & Crocker p. 113)

11. William Lloyd Warner, *A Black Civilization: A Social Study of an Australian Tribe* (New York: Harper & Brothers, 1937), 311.

12. Ibid., 306.

13. Ibid., 308.

14. Ibid., 217.

15. Ibid., 307.

16. Ibid., 308.

17. Ibid., 233.

18. Joan Kimm, *A Fatal Conjunction: Two Laws, Two Cultures* (Sydney: Federation Press, 2004), 52.

19. Ryan and Jethá, *Sex at Dawn*, 185.

20. Bruce M. Knauft, *South Coast New Guinea Cultures: History, Comparison, Dialectic* (New York: Cambridge University Press, 1993), 157.

21. Ewen Callaway, "Loving Bonobos Have a Carnivorous Dark Side," *New Scientist*, October 13, 2008, http://www.newscientist.com/article/dn14926.

22. Ryan and Jethá, *Sex at Dawn*, 198.

23. While "bonding" hormones such as oxytocin may play roles in connections between some individuals involved in group sex, the term "bonding" is used here to talk about social processes rather than biological processes.

24. Cynthia McFadden, "Many Campus Assault Victims Stay Quiet, or Fail to Get Help," *Nightline*, September 6, 2010, http://abcnews.go.com/Nightline/college-campus-assaults-constant-threat/story?id=11410988#.UNvDWKX3Dq1.

25. "Family Sues College after Daughter's Suicide," WABC-TV *Eyewitness News*, July 11, 2008, http://abclocal.go.com/wabc/story?section=news/local&id=6259518.

26. McFadden, "Assault Victims Stay Quiet."

27. Gerald Eskenazi, "The Male Athlete and Sexual Assault," *New York Times on the Web*, June 3, 1990, http://www.nytimes.com/books/97/08/03/reviews/glenridge-athlete.html?_r=2.

28. Diana Scully and Joseph Marolla, "'Riding the Bull at Gilley's': Convicted Rapists Describe the Rewards of Rape," *Social Problems* 32, no. 3 (1985): 262.

29. Tracy Clark-Flory, "Yale Fraternity Pledges Chant about Rape," *Salon.com*, October 15, 2010, http://www.salon.com/life/broadsheet/2010/10/15/yale_fraternity_pledges_chant_about_rape/index.html.

30. Patricia Yancey Martin and Robert A. Hummer, "Fraternities and Rape on Campus," in *Race, Class, and Gender: An Anthology*, ed. Margaret Anderson and Patricia Hill Collins (Belmont, CA: Wadsworth, 1989), 162.

31. David Smith, "It Took Me 20 Years to Realise That I'd Done Something Wrong," *Guardian*, June 17, 2009, http://www.guardian.co.uk/world/2009/jun/17/rape-apology-south-africa.

32. Moni Basu and Nkepile Mabuse, "He Raped as a Teenager and Now Works to Stop Sexual Violence in South Africa," *CNN*, May 7, 2012, http://www.cnn.com/2012/05/05/world/africa/south-africa-rape.

33. Karen Franklin, "Enacting Masculinity: Antigay Violence and Group Rape as Participatory Theater," *Sexuality Research & Social Policy* 1, no. 2 (2004): 35.

34. Ibid.

35. Scully and Marolla, "'Riding the Bull at Gilley's,'" 260.

36. Peggy R. Sanday, *Fraternity Gang Rape: Sex, Brotherhood, and Privilege on Campus* (New York: New York University Press, 1990), 14.

37. Donald G. Dutton and Susan L. Painter, "Traumatic Bonding: The Development of Emotional Attachments in Battered Women and Other Relationships of Intermittent Abuse," *Victimology: An International Journal* 6, no. 1–4: 139–155. Quoted in Patrick J. Carnes, *The Betrayal Bond: Breaking Free of Exploitative Relationships* (Deerfield Beach, FL: Health Communications, 1997).

38. S. Mokwena, "The Era of the Jackrollers: Contextualizing the Rise of Youth Gangs in Soweto" (paper presented at the Centre for the Study of Violence and Reconciliation, Johannesburg, October 30, 1991).

39.   Janet Maia Wojcicki, "'She Drank His Money': Survival Sex and the Problem of Violence in Taverns in Gauteng Province, South Africa," *Medical Anthropology Quarterly* 16, no. 3 (2002): 270.

40.   Lloyd Vogelman and Sharon Lewis, "Gang Rape and the Culture of Violence in South Africa," *Der Überblick*, no. 2 (1993): 39–42.

41.   Mokwena, "The Era of the Jackrollers."

42.   Annie Kelly, "Raped and Killed for Being a Lesbian: South Africa Ignores 'Corrective' Attacks," *Guardian*, March 12, 2009, http://www.guardian.co.uk/world/2009/mar/12/eudy-simelane-corrective-rape-south-africa.

43.   Jonathan Clayton, "Where Sex Crime Is 'Just a Bit of a Game,'" *Times Online*, August 12, 2005, http://www.thetimes.co.uk/tto/news/uk/article1936778.ece.

44.   Rachel Jewkes and Naeema Abrahams, "The Epidemiology of Rape and Sexual Coercion in South Africa: An Overview," *Social Science & Medicine* 55 (2002): 1231–44.

45.   Kate Wood, "Contextualizing Group Rape in Post-apartheid South Africa," *Culture, Health, and Sexuality* 7, no. 4 (2005): 306.

46.   Heather Jones, "Rapex in South Africa," *Wilder Voice* 3, no. 5 (2008).

47.   Ben Hoyle, "'Jack Rolling' Link to Rape Gang," *Times Online*, August 12, 2005, http://www.thetimes.co.uk/tto/news/uk/article1936777.ece.

48.   Nancy Gibbs, Mary Cronin, and Melissa Ludtke, "Wilding in the Night," *Time*, May 8, 1989, http://www.time.com/time/magazine/article/0,9171,957631,00.html.

49.   Pamela Newkirk, *Within the Veil: Black Journalists, White Media* (New York: New York University Press, 2000), 28.

50.   Jamie Satterfield, "Slaying Victims Lost in the Furor," *Knoxnews.com*, May 27, 2007, http://www.knoxnews.com/news/2007/may/27/slaying-victims-lost-in-the-furor/.

51.   Marian T. A. Tankink, "The Silence of South-Sudanese Women: Social Risks in Talking about Experiences of Sexual Violence," *Culture, Health & Sexuality: An International Journal for Research, Intervention and Care* 15, no. 4 (2013): 391–403.

52.   Nicholas D. Kristof, "A Policy of Rape," *New York Times*, June 5, 2005.

53.   Amnesty International, "Sudan, Darfur Rape as a Weapon of War" (report, July 2004), available at http://www.amnesty.org/en/library/asset/AFR54/076/2004/en/f66115ea-d5b4-11dd-bb24-1fb85fe8fa05/afr540762004en.pdf.

54.   Daniel Jonah Goldhagen, *Worse Than War: Genocide, Eliminationism and the Ongoing Assault on Humanity* (New York: PublicAffairs, 2009), 456.

55.   Tankink, "Silence of South Sudanese Women," 395.

56.   Kristof, "A Policy of Rape."

57.   Adrian Croft, "Doctor, Gang-Raped in Sudan's Darfur, Wins Rights Award," *Reuters*, October   6,   2010,   http://www.reuters.com/article/2010/10/06/us-sudan-award-idUSTRE69552320101006 .

58.   National Center on Domestic and Sexual Violence, "Darfur: Gendered Violence and Rape as a Weapon of Genocide," available at http://www.ncdsv.org/images/DarfurGendered-ViolenceRapeWeapon.pdf.

59.   "History," Global Grassroots: Conscious Social Change for Women website, http://www.globalgrassroots.org/history.html.

60.   Katharine Houreld, "Women and Girls in Darfur Raped, Jailed, Fined," *The Age* (Australia), March 14, 2005, http://www.theage.com.au/news/World/Women-and-girls-in-Darfur-raped-jailed-fined/2005/03/13/1110649052906.html.

61.   Kristof, "A Policy of Rape."

62.   Jeffrey Gettleman, "A Taste of Hope Sends Refugees Back to Darfur," *New York Times*, February 26, 2012, http://www.nytimes.com/2012/02/27/world/africa/darfur-refugees-returning-home.html?ref=sudan&_r=0.

63.   Andrew Green, "Humanitarian Crisis Worsens as Fighting Escalates in Sudan," *Lancet* 381, no. 9863 (2013): 281, available at http://www.lancet.com/journals/lancet/article/PIIS0140-6736%2813%2960118-X/fulltext.

64.   Goldhagen, *Worse Than War*, 455.

65.   Claudia Card, "Rape as a Weapon of War," *Hypatia* 11, no. 4 (1996): 3.

66.   Goldhagen, *Worse Than War*, 453.

67. Card, "Rape as a Weapon of War."

68. "Bosniak" is the term used to refer to ethnic identity; the term "Bosnian" refers to all residents of Bosnia regardless of ethnicity or religion.

69. Goldhagen, *Worse Than War*, 460, 465.

70. Tankink, "Silence of South Sudanese Women," 392.

71. Emily Wax, "'We Want to Make a Light Baby,'" *Washington Post*, June 30, 2004.

72. Goldhagen, *Worse Than War*, 461.

73. Ibid., 463.

74. David McInnes, Jack Bradley, and Garrett Prestage, "The Discourse of Gay Men's Group Sex: The Importance of Masculinity," *Culture, Health & Sexuality: An International Journal for Research, Intervention and Care* 11, no. 6 (2009): 650.

75. Carol Jenkins, "The Homosexual Context of Heterosexual Practice in Papua New Guinea," in *Bisexualities and AIDS: International Perspectives*, ed. Peter Aggleton (London: Taylor & Francis, 1996), 188–203.

76. Gary W. Dowsett, "The Gay Plague Revisited: AIDS and Its Enduring Moral Panic," in *Moral Panics, Sex Panics: Fear and the Fight over Sexual Rights*, ed. Gilbert Herdt (New York: New York University Press, 2009), 130.

77. Kurt C. Organista, "HIV Prevention Models with Mexican Migrant Farmworkers," in *Practice Issues in HIV/AIDS Services: Empowerment-Based Models and Program Applications*, ed. Ronald J. Mancoske and James Donald Smith (Binghamton, NY: Haworth Press, 2004), 136.

78. "After Matthew Johns Affair, Why Sports Stars Like Group Sex," *Sunday Telegraph* (Australia), May 17, 2009, http://www.dailytelegraph.com.au/sport/sport-biography/after-matthew-johns-affair-why-sports-stars-like-group-sex/story-fn34og81-1225712999651.

79. Ryan and Jetha, *Sex at Dawn*, 93.

80. Amanda Hughes, "I Was a Football Groupie," *Guardian*, November 14, 2004, http://www.guardian.co.uk/football/2004/nov/15/newsstory.sport7.

81. Mark Vanlandingham and Nancy Grandjean, "Some Cultural Underpinnings of Male Sexual Behaviour Patterns in Thailand," in *Sexual Cultures and Migration in the Era of AIDS: Anthropological and Demographic Perspectives*, ed. Gilbert Herdt (Oxford: Clarendon Press, 1997), 136–37.

82. Matthew Gault-Williams, "Nat Young—From Collaroy to Hawai'i," *Legendary Surfers: A Definitive History of Surfing's Culture and Heroes* (blog), February 29, 2008, http://files.legendarysurfers.com/surf/legends/lsc215.html#nat_young_begins.

83. Patrick Doyle, "Exclusive: Former Stones, Dylan Superfan Pamela Des Barres on 'Greatest Groupies,'" *Rolling Stone*, December 15, 2010, http://www.rollingstone.com/music/news/exclusive-former-stones-dylan-superfan-pamela-debarres-on-greatest-groupies-20101215.

84. Hughes, "I Was a Football Groupie."

85. Lisa DePaulo and Kyla Jones, "The Days and Nights of an NBA Groupie," *GQ*, July 2006, http://www.gq.com/sports/profiles/200606/nba-men-women-groupies.

86. Katy Kelleher, "'Super Groupie' Kat Stacks Assaulted on Video," *Jezebel*, June 1, 2010, http://jezebel.com/5552387/super-groupie-kat-stacks-assaulted-on-video; Arati Patel, "Notorious Hip-Hop Groupie Kat Stacks Petitioning Obama Administration to Stop Her Deportation," *Hollywood Reporter*, August 23, 2012, http://www.hollywoodreporter.com/news/kat-stacks-hip-hop-groupie-deported-obama-petition-364907.

87. Jeff Baenen, "Culpepper, Three Other Vikings Charged in Boat-Party Scandal," *USA Today*, December 15, 2005, http://usatoday30.usatoday.com/sports/football/nfl/vikings/2005-12-15-boat-party-charges_x.htm#.

88. Michael Silver and George Dohrman, "Adrift on Lake Woebegone," *Sports Illustrated*, October 24, 2005, http://sportsillustrated.cnn.com/vault/article/magazine/MAG1113465/3/index.htm.

89. Jonathan Kaminsky, "Former Viking Fred Smoot Continues to Terrorize Neighborhood," *Citypages News*, October 1, 2008, http://www.citypages.com/2008-10-01/news/former-viking-fred-smoot-continues-to-terrorize-neighborhood/.

90. Silver and Dohrman, "Adrift on Lake Woebegone."

91. Terry Gould, *The Lifestyle: A Look at the Erotic Rites of Swingers* (Toronto: Vintage Canada, 1999).

92. Ibid., 30.

93. Christopher Ryan, "Not All Military Adultery Results in Scandal," *Psychology Today*, November 16, 2012, http://www.psychologytoday.com/em/111037.

94. Jen Miller, "I Did It for Science—Experiment: Key Party," *Nerve*, March 1, 2006, http://www.nerve.com/love-sex/i-did-it-for-science/i-did-it-for-science-key-party. Other preteen and teenage games I heard about while writing this book use dice, playing cards, straws, or blindfolds to select partners; these games aren't usually completely "random," however, but played at parties where the participants already know one another.

CASE STUDY: A LIFE FANTASTIC

1. Patrick Moore, *Beyond Shame: Reclaiming the Abandoned History of Radical Sexuality* (Boston: Beacon Press, 2004), xxiv.

2. George Chauncey, *Gay New York: Gender, Urban Culture, and the Making of the Gay Male World, 1890–1940* (New York: Basic Books, 1994), 356–58, 360.

3. Jeffrey Escoffier, *Bigger Than Life: The History of Gay Porn Cinema from Beefcake to Hardcore* (Philadelphia: Running Press, 2009), 91.

4. Ira Tattleman, "The Meaning at the Wall: Tracing the Gay Bathhouse," in *Queers in Space: Communities/Public Places/Sites of Resistance*, ed. Gordon Brent Ingram, Anne-Marie Bouthillette, and Yolanda Retter (Seattle: Bay Press, 1997), 403, 404.

5. Michael Bronski, *The Pleasure Principle: Sex, Backlash, and the Struggle for Gay Freedom* (New York: St. Martin's, 1998), xx.

6. Michael Pollack, "Homosexual Rituals and Safer Sex," *Journal of Homosexuality* 25, no. 3 (1993): 308.

7. Ibid., 312.

8. Mark Thompson, ed., *Leatherfolk: Radical Sex, People, Politics, and Practice* (Boston: Alyson Publications, 1991), 159.

9. R. H. Hopcke and M. Thompson, "S/M and the Psychology of Gay Male Initiation: An Archetypal Perspective," in *Leatherfolk: Radical Sex, People, Politics, and Practice*, ed. Mark Thompson (Boston: Alyson Publications, 1991), 72.

10. Tim Dean, *Unlimited Intimacy: Reflections on the Subculture of Barebacking* (Chicago: University of Chicago Press, 2010), 129. Dean is specifically referring to bareback gang bangs, although his comments refer to sexual witnessing more generally.

11. Gayle Rubin, "Thinking Sex: Notes for a Radical Theory of the Politics of Sexuality," in *Pleasure and Danger: Exploring Female Sexuality*, ed. Carole S. Vance (Boston: Routledge and Kegan Paul, 1984), 139.

12. Pat Califia, "San Francisco: Revisiting 'the City of Desire,'" in *Queers in Space: Communities/Public Places/Sites of Resistance*, ed. Gordon Brent Ingram, Anne-Marie Bouthillette, and Yolanda Retter (Seattle: Bay Press, 1997), 193.

13. Moore, *Beyond Shame*, 8, 9.

14. Martin P. Levine, *Gay Macho: The Life and Death of the Homosexual Clone* (New York: New York University Press, 1998), 92.

15. Moore, *Beyond Shame*, 49.

16. Ibid., 25.

17. Escoffier, *Bigger Than Life*, 149.

18. Levine, *Gay Macho*, 53.

19. Moore, *Beyond Shame*, 23.

20. Larry Kramer, *Faggots* (New York: Grove Press, 1978), 48.

21. Ibid., 86.

22. John Rechy, *The Sexual Outlaw: A Documentary* (New York: Grove Press, 1977), 285.

23. Ibid., 287.

24. Moore, *Beyond Shame*, 112.

25. Ibid., 13.

26. Ibid., 49.

27. Quoted in Dangerous Bedfellows [Eva Hoffman, Wayne Pendleton], *Policing Public Sex: Queer Politics and the Future of AIDS Activism* (Cambridge, MA: South End Press, 2008), 339.

28. Robert Reynolds and Gerard Sullivan, *Gay Men's Sexual Stories: Getting It!* (Binghamton, NY: Haworth SocialWork Practice Press, 2003), 67.

29. Ibid., 73.

30. Mains, Geoff. (1984). *Urban Aboriginals: A Celebration of Leathersexuality* (Daedalus Publishing).

31. Thompson, *Leatherfolk*, 301.

32. Comparing contemporary Western practices to tribal initiation rites is problematic in that we cannot assume that meanings translate across time and space. On the other hand, if a given practice—fisting or BDSM, for example—*feels* like an initiation rite or rite of passage to participants and is used for those purposes, a scholar can focus on that subjective experience.

33. Moore, *Beyond Shame*, 73.

34. Dangerous Bedfellows, *Policing Public Sex*, 351.

8. FROM REVOLUTIONARIES TO ROCK STARS (AND BACK AGAIN)

1. Pardis Mahdavi, *Passionate Uprisings: Iran's Sexual Revolution* (Stanford: Stanford University Press, 2009), 94.

2. Curtis Bergstrand and Jennifer Blevins Sinski, *Swinging in America: Love, Sex, and Marriage in the 21st Century* (Santa Barbara: Praeger, 2010), 57.

3. Mahdavi, *Passionate Uprisings*, 3.

4. Ibid., 97.

5. Ibid., 1.

6. Ibid., 146.

7. Ibid., 180.

8. Ibid., 91.

9. Ibid., 84.

10. Ibid., 66.

11. Ibid., 103.

12. Ibid., 22.

13. Ibid., 198.

14. Ibid., 101.

15. Ibid., 94.

16. Ibid., 307.

17. Brian Whitaker, *Unspeakable Love: Gay and Lesbian Life in the Middle East* (Berkeley: University of California Press, 2006).

18. Dennis Campbell,"Porn: The New Sex Education," *Joe Public Blog* (blog), *Guardian*, March 30, 2009, http://www.guardian.co.uk/society/joepublic+education/sexeducation.

19. Jean Baudrillard,"Paroxysm: The End of the Millennium or the Countdown," *Economy and Society* 26, no. 4 (November 1997): 22.

20. Ibid., 447–55.

21. This is a pseudonym.

22. Amira Polack,"Eric Stotz: Hollywood Fundraiser," *Business Today*, Fall 2009, http://www.businesstoday.org/magazine/its-always-christmas-washington/eric-stotz-hollywood-fundraiser.

23. "Kandy Masquerade Party" event announcement, Yahoo! Upcoming Events and Things to Do, http://upcoming.yahoo.com/event/1447379/GA/Holmby-Hills/Kandy-Masquerade-Party-at-the-Playboy-Mansion-Tickets-Available-HERE.

24. Steven Watts, *Mr Playboy: Hugh Hefner and the American Dream* (Hoboken, NJ: Wiley, 2008), 6.

25. Ibid., 209.

26. Barbara Isenberg, "Mr. Playboy: Hugh Hefner Tells How He Created an Identity in Order to Fulfill His Dreams," *Time Magazine*, October 2, 2005, http://www.time.com/time/magazine/article/0,9171,1112823,00.html#ixzz1yosR8m16.

27. Watts, *Mr Playboy*, 4, 104.

28. John Heidenry, *What Wild Ecstasy: The Rise and Fall of the Sexual Revolution* (New York: Simon & Schuster, 1997), 59.

29. Watts, *Mr Playboy*, 272.

30. Ibid., 281.

31. Heidenry, *What Wild Ecstasy*, 151.

32. Watts, *Mr Playboy*, 197.

33. Ibid., 282.

34. Izabella St. James, *Bunny Tales: Behind Closed Doors at the Playboy Mansion* (Philadelphia: Running Press, 2006), 60.

35. Ibid., 151.

36. Ibid., 154.

37. "Hugh Hefner Has Sex Twice a Week, Playmates Describe Orgies," Huffington Post, July 12, 2010, http://www.huffingtonpost.com/2010/07/12/hugh-hefner-i-have-sex-tw_n_643303.html.

38. Mike Larkin, "I've Still Got My Mojo! Hugh Hefner Bounces Back from Humiliating Bedroom Revelations with a Party at the Playboy Mansion," *Daily Mail*, August 9, 2011, http://www.dailymail.co.uk/tvshowbiz/article-2023796/Hugh-Hefner-puts-Crystal-Harris-bedroom-revelations-Playboy-party.html.

39. St. James, *Bunny Tales*, 176.

40. Grace Dent, "Has Hugh Hefner Finally Seen the Ghost of Playboy Future?" *Guardian*, March 1, 2012.

41. Lloyd Grove, "Getting a Rise out of Hef," *Daily Beast*, January 3, 2011, http://www.thedailybeast.com/articles/2011/01/04/hugh-hefner-newly-engaged-responds-to-complaints-from-ex-playboy-bunny.html.

42. Watts, *Mr Playboy*, 454.

43. Ibid.

44. Gerrie Lim, *Singapore Rebel: Searching for Annabel Chong* (Singapore: Monsoon Books, 2011).

45. Field notes, Las Vegas, 2004.

46. Mark Seal, "The Prince Who Blew through Billions," *Vanity Fair*, July 2011, http://www.vanityfair.com/society/features/2011/07/prince-jefri-201107.

47. Henry Samuel, "Dominique Strauss-Kahn Did Not Know He Was Sleeping with Prostitutes 'Because They Were All Naked,'" *Telegraph*, September 6, 2012.

48. Lydia Martin, "Lydia Has Lunch with Thomas Kramer," *Miami Herald*, November 13, 2011.

49. Hal K. Rothman, *Devil's Bargains: Tourism in the Twentieth-Century American West* (Lawrence: University Press of Kansas, 1998), xiii.

50. Terry Gould, *The Lifestyle: A Look at the Erotic Rites of Swingers* (Toronto: Vintage Canada, 1999).

51. Ibid., 33.

52. Gilbert Bartell, *Group Sex: A Scientist's Eyewitness Report on the American Way of Swinging* (New York: Peter H. Wyden, 1971), 125.

53. Ibid., 127.

54. Valerie Milano, "Playboy TV—'Sex Curious,'" *Hollywood Today*, February 8, 2011, http://www.hollywoodtoday.net/2011/02/08/playboy-tv-%E2%80%9Csex-curious%E2%80%9D/.

55. Stephen M. Silverman, "Prince Harry Party Girl Tells of the Naked Night: Report," *People*, September 1, 2012, http://www.people.com/people/package/article/0,,20395222_20626402,00.html.

56. "Prince Harry Nude Photos Boosting Las Vegas Tourism," Huffington Post, August 23, 2012, http://www.huffingtonpost.com/2012/08/23/prince-harry-nude-photos-boosting-las-vegas-tourism_n_1824848.html.

57. Rebecca Macatee, "Prince Harry's Naked Bonanza! Scandal Worth $23 Million Tourism Boost to Las Vegas," *E! Online*, October 10, 2012, http://www.eonline.com/news/353055/prince-harry-s-naked-bonanza-scandal-worth-23-million-tourism-boost-to-las-vegas; Rory Carroll, "Las Vegas Hails Prince Harry as a True Son of Sin City," *Guardian*, August 25, 2012, http://www.guardian.co.uk/uk/2012/aug/25/prince-harry-las-vegas-party.

58. Edward Wong, "18 Orgies Later, Chinese Swinger Gets Prison Bed," *New York Times*, May 20, 2010, http://www.nytimes.com/2010/05/21/world/asia/21china.html?_r=2&th&emc=th.

59. Malcolm Moore, "Chinese Professor Jailed for Three-and-a-Half Years for Swinging," *Telegraph*, May 20, 2010, http://www.telegraph.co.uk/news/worldnews/asia/china/7743547/Chinese-professor-jailed-for-three-and-a-half-years-for-swinging.html.

60. Excerpts from "Criminal Law of the People's Republic of China," All China Women's Federation, http://www.womenofchina.cn/html/node/75472-1.htm.

61. Ming Haoyue, "Is the 'Crime of Group Sex' Really Outdated?" *China Daily*, April 1, 2010, http://www.chinadaily.com.cn/cndy/2010-04/01/content_9672304.htm.

62. Austin Ramzy, "A Swinger's Case: China's Attitude toward Sex," *Time*, May 22, 2010, http://www.time.com/time/world/article/0,8599,1991029,00.html.

63. Julian Smisek, "Group Sex and the Cultural Revolution—A Translation," Danwei, May 23, 2010, http://www.danwei.org/sexuality/group_sex_and_the_cultural_rev.php.

64. Samantha Smithstein, "Marriage Like Water, 'Partner Swapping' Like Wine," *What the Wild Things Are* (blog), *Psychology Today*, May 20, 2010, http://www.psychologytoday.com/blog/what-the-wild-things-are/201005/marriage-water-partner-swapping-wine.

65. Ramzy, "A Swinger's Case."

66. Whitaker, *Unspeakable Love*.

67. Bartell, *Group Sex*, 45.

68. Annalee Newitz, "Swinging in the Suburbs," *Metro (Silicon Valley's Weekly Newspaper)*, 2000, 8.

69. Curtis Bergstrand, Nancy Schrepf, and Jennifer Williams-Sinski. "Civilization and Sexual Discontent: Monogamy and the Problem of Surplus Repression" (unpublished manuscript, Bellarmine University, 2003), 5.

70. Bergstrand and Blevins Sinski, *Swinging in America*, 97.

71. Julian Guthrie, "Partner Swapping Comes out of Closet . . .," *San Francisco Chronicle*, July 9, 2002, 2.

72. "Comments" section in Michael Bowen, "Swapping Stories," *Pacific Northwest Inlander*, November 17, 2010, http://www.inlander.com/spokane/article-15892-swapping-stories.html#dComments.

73. Mehdi Khalaji, "The Clerics vs. Modernity: Failure of the Islamic Republic's Soft Power," *Majalla*, June 2012, available at http://www.washingtoninstitute.org/policy-analysis/view/the-clerics-vs.-modernity-failure-of-the-islamic-republics-soft-power.

74. Kareem Fahim, "Slap to a Man's Pride Set Off Tumult in Tunisia," *New York Times*, January 21, 2011, http://www.nytimes.com/2011/01/22/world/africa/22sidi.html?pagewanted=1&_r=1&src=twrhp.

75. Carol Huang, "Facebook and Twitter Key to Arab Spring Uprisings: Report," *The National* (United Arab Emirates), June 6, 2011, http://www.thenational.ae/news/uae-news/facebook-and-twitter-key-to-arab-spring-uprisings-report.

76. Mohamed Fadel Fahmy, "Egyptian Blogger Aliaa Elmahdy: Why I Posed Naked," CNN, November 19, 2011, http://articles.cnn.com/2011-11-19/middleeast/world_meast_nude-blogger-aliaa-magda-elmahdy_1_egyptian-blogger-nude-photo-kareem-amer?_s=PM:MIDDLEEAST.

77. Alexander Bratersky, "Putin Jokes about Orgy, But Slams Pussy Riot," *Moscow Times*, September 7, 2012.

78. Carole Cadwalladr, "Pussy Riot: Will Vladimir Putin Regret Taking On Russia's Cool Women Punks?" *Observer*, July 28, 2012, http://www.guardian.co.uk/world/2012/jul/29/pussy-riot-protest-vladimir-putin-russia.

79. Miriam Elder, "Pussy Riot Member Freed as Two Bandmates Face Exile to Prison Camp," *Guardian*, October 10, 2012, http://www.guardian.co.uk/world/2012/oct/10/pussy-riot-member-free.

80. Lynn Berry, "Pussy Riot Band Members Should Be Freed, Says Russian Prime Minister Dmitry Medvedev," Huffington Post, September 12, 2012, http://www.huffingtonpost.com/2012/09/12/pussy-riot-dmitry-medvedev-should-be-freed_n_1877513.html.

81. "Dear General Public: Please Stop Sucking the Punk out of Pussy Riot, It's Crude and Disgusting," *Superchief*, September 1, 2012, http://superchief.tv/dear-general-public-please-stop-sucking-the-punk-out-of-pussy-riot-its-crude-and-disgusting/.

82. "Skins Secret Party," video uploaded by djbungle to YouTube, August 20, 2007, http://www.youtube.com/watch?v=MEvNY4IBKwQ.

83. Jon Landau, "The Rolling Stone Interviews: Paul Simon," Paul Simon.info, 1972, http://www.paul-simon.info/PHP/showarticle.php?id=13&kategorie=1.

84. Sheila Weller, "Suddenly That Summer," *Vanity Fair*, July 2012, http://www.vanityfair.com/culture/2012/07/lsd-drugs-summer-of-love-sixties.

85. Donald R. Sutherland, "The Religion of Gerrard Winstanley and Digger Communism," The Digger Archives, last updated January 31, 2013, http://www.diggers.org/diggers/religion_winstanley.htm.

86. Tim Dean, *Unlimited Intimacy: Reflections on the Subculture of Barebacking* (Chicago: University of Chicago Press, 2010), 5.

9. UPPING THE ANTE OR OVER THE EDGE?

1. Sarah Lyall. "Here's the Pub, Church and Field for Public Sex," *New York Times*, October 8, 2010.

2. Stan Collymore, *Tackling My Demons* (London: CollinsWillow, 2004), 307.

3. Ibid., 306.

4. Ibid., 289.

5. Ibid., 282.

6. Lyall, "Here's the Pub."

7. Collymore, *Tackling My Demons*, 315.

8. Rudiger M. Trimpop, *The Psychology of Risk Taking Behavior* (Amsterdam: North Holland, 1994), 296.

9. Annys Shin, "Engineering a Safer Burger: Technology Is Entrepreneur's Main Ingredient for Bacteria-Free Beef," *Washington Post*, June 12, 2008, http://www.washingtonpost.com/wp-dyn/content/article/2008/06/11/AR2008061103656_pf.html.

10. "2011 Estimates of Foodborne Illness: CDC 2011 Estimates: Findings," Centers for Disease Control and Prevention, available at http://www.cdc.gov/foodborneburden/2011-food-borne-estimates.html (last updated Ocrober 10, 2012).

11. Tom Laskaway, "'Pink Slime' Is the Tip of the Iceberg: Look What Else Is in Industrial Meat," *Grist: A Beacon in the Smog*, March 19, 2012, http://grist.org/factory-farms/pink-slime-is-the-tip-of-the-iceberg-look-what-else-is-in-industrial-meat/.

12. "Sexually Transmitted Diseases in the United States, 2008," Centers for Disease Control and Prevention, available at http://www.cdc.gov/std/stats08/trends.htm (last updated November 16, 2009).

13. In 2010, the most recent year with available data. "HIV/AIDS Statistics and Surveillance: Basic Statistics," Centers for Disease Control and Prevention, available at http://www.cdc.gov/hiv/topics/surveillance/basic.htm (last modified February 28, 2013).

14. Trimpop, *Risk Taking Behavior*, 271.

15. John Tulloch and Deborah Lupton, *Risk and Everyday Life* (London: Sage), 2003.

16. Trimpop, *Risk Taking Behavior*, 294.

17. Lee, Emma. (2012). "Girls Gone Wild: Female Sex Addiction on the Web," www.thefix.com/content/women-sex-addicts-and-internet8535?page=all.

18. Douglas Quenqua, "Recklessly Seeking Sex on Craigslist," *New York Times*, April 17, 2009, http://www.nytimes.com/2009/04/19/fashion/19craigslist.html?_r=1&pagewanted=all.

19. Catherine Hakim, *Erotic Capital: The Power of Attraction in the Boardroom and the Bedroom* (New York: Basic Books, 2011).

20. Henry Russell, *Craigslist Casual Encounters* (Los Angeles: Haha Publishing, 2010), 4.

21. Neva Chonin, "Sex and the City," *San Francisco Chronicle SF Gate*, September 17, 2006, http://www.sfgate.com/cgi-bin/article.cgi?file=/c/a/2006/09/17/PKG6BKQQA41.DTL.

22. "New Craigslist 'Group Sex' Bust," April 22, 2010, The Smoking Gun, http://www.thesmokinggun.com/documents/crime/new-craigslist-group-sex-bust.

23. "867-5309 Is Not Jenny," *Lakeland Ledger*, May 16, 1982, http://news.google.com/newspapers?id=PaVOAAAAIBAJ&sjid=PvsDAAAAIBAJ&pg=6320,11943.

24. Craigslist, Washington, DC, casual encounters, March 1, 2012.

25. David A. Moskowitz and Michael E. Roloff, "The Ultimate High: Sexual Addiction and the Bug Chasing Phenomenon," *Sexual Addiction & Compulsivity* 14, no. 1 (2007): 26.

26. International Institute for Trauma and Addiction Professionals website, www.sexhelp.com.

27. Yakima, WA Chapter 6.55 Sex Offenses, http://www.codepublishing.com/WA/Yakima/Yakima06/Yakima0655.html#6.55.020.

28. Keith Morrison, "Battling Sexual Addiction," *Dateline NBC*, February 24, 2004. http://www.msnbc.msn.com/id/4302347/ns/dateline_nbc/t/battling-sexual-addiction/#.T7RZ6464JlJ.

29. Janice M. Irvine, "Reinventing Perversion: Sex Addiction and Cultural Anxieties," *Journal of the History of Sexuality* 5, no. 3 (1995): 429–50.

30. Ibid., 442.

31. Ibid., 443.

32. Ibid., 446.

33. Ibid., 433.

34. John Heidenry, *What Wild Ecstasy: The Rise and Fall of the Sexual Revolution* (New York: Simon & Schuster, 1997), 151.

35. Lee et al., *Mötley Crüe*, 134.

36. A good psychologist would question someone who claimed sex was "boring," as such a statement begs to be unpacked as much as the statement that "sex is just fun." What each of these statements implies is that sex is—or is not—meeting the needs and fulfilling the desires that those particular individuals believe it should.

37. Straight pornography is usually still filmed without condoms. The industry instead relies on a system of STD testing where performers make their results public.

38. Serosorting is not considered safe by many physicians because of the risk of being "cross-infected" by different strains of HIV. Mark Honigsbaum, "West Side Story: A Tale of Unprotected Sex Which Could Be Link to New HIV Superbug," *Guardian*, March 25, 2005, http://www.guardian.co.uk/world/2005/mar/26/aids.usa.

39. The lifestyle, as discussed elsewhere, here refers to those individuals who identify as being in "the lifestyle" or make use of the websites, networks, events, conferences, etc. aimed at lifestylers. Swinging as a practice may occur more broadly, and nonmonogamy is, of course, an even broader category.

40. Comment in Busy Swingers Forum at Swing Life Style, http://www.swinglifestyle.com/forums/General_Discussions/3-Some/Female__Bareback_/thread-id_47405/viewarticle.cfm/maxrow_10/startrow_31/maxrow_10/startrow_11/maxrow_10/startrow_21/maxrow_10/startrow_31/maxrow_10/startrow_91/maxrow_10/startrow_121/maxrow_10/startrow_131/maxrow_10/startrow_141/maxrow_10/startrow_81/maxrow_10/startrow_91/maxrow_10/startrow_61/maxrow_10/startrow_51/maxrow_10/startrow_101 (accessed February 2013).

41. Tim Dean, *Unlimited Intimacy: Reflections on the Subculture of Barebacking* (Chicago: University of Chicago Press, 2010), 45.

42. Ibid., x.

43. Ibid., 2.

44. Peter Cassels, "Taking Aim at Barebacking Videos," Edge San Francisco, May 24, 2010, http://www.edgesanfrancisco.com/entertainment/culture///106024/taking_aim_at_barebacking_videos.

45. Marc Peyser, Elizabeth Roberts, and Frappa Stout, "A Deadly Dance," *Newsweek*, September 29, 1997, 77.

46. Garrett Prestage et al., *TOMS: Three or More Study* (Sydney, Australia: National Centre in HIV Epidemiology and Clinical Research, University of New South Wales, 2008), 38. Edits in the quotation are mine.

47. David McInnes, Jack Bradley, and Garrett Prestage, "The Discourse of Gay Men's Group Sex: The Importance of Masculinity," *Culture, Health & Sexuality: An International Journal for Research, Intervention and Care* 11, no. 6 (2009): 650.

48. Dean, *Unlimited Intimacy*, 45.

49. Michael Warner, "Why Gay Men Are Having Risky Sex," appendix to *What Do Gay Men Want? An Essay on Sex, Risk, and Subjectivity*, by David M. Halperin (Ann Arbor: University of Michigan Press, 2007).

50. Ibid.

51. Dean, *Unlimited Intimacy*, 39.

52. Ibid., 6.

53. Ibid., 128.

54. Ibid., 50.

55. Gregory A. Freeman, "Bug Chasers: The Men Who Long to Be HIV+," *Rolling Stone*, February 6, 2003, https://solargeneral.com/library/bug-chasers.pdf.

56. DeAnn K. Gauthier and Craig J. Forsyth. "Bareback Sex, Bug Chasers, and the Gift of Death," *Deviant Behavior* 20 (1998): 92.

57. Ibid., 85–100.

58. Dean, *Unlimited Intimacy*, 72; originally from www.ultimatebareback.com.

59. Ibid., 51.

60. Berg, Rigmor. (2008). "Barebacking Among MSM Internet Users," *Aids and Behavior* 12(5): 822-833.

61. Moskowitz and Roloff, "The Ultimate High," 21–40.

62. Colin Batrouney, "Gay Men and Sexual Adventurism: Where to from Here?" *Social Research Briefs* 15 (2009).

63. Margot D. Weiss, *Techniques of Pleasure: BDSM and the Circuits of Sexuality* (Durham: Duke University Press, 2010), 88.

64. "Recent Updates to Proposed Revisions for DSM-5," American Psychiatric Association, http://www.dsm5.org/Pages/RecentUpdates.aspx (accessed March 2013).

65. Thomas Weinberg, cited in Weiss, *Techniques of Pleasure*, 12.

66. Staci Newmahr, *Playing on the Edge: Sadomasochism, Risk, and Intimacy* (Bloomington: Indiana University Press, 2010), 76.

67. Ibid., 100.

68. Ibid., 95.

69. Stephen Lyng, "Edgework, Risk, and Uncertainty," in *Social Theories of Risk and Uncertainty: An Introduction*, edited by Jens O. Zinn (New York: Wiley-Blackwell, 2008), 107.

70. Ibid., 111.

71. Ibid., 120.

72. Jonathan Simon, "Taking Risks: Extreme Sports and the Embrace of Risk in Advanced Liberal Societies," in *Embracing Risk: The Changing Culture of Insurance and Responsibility*, edited by Tom Baker and Jonathan Simon (Chicago: University of Chicago Press, 2002), 193.

73. Newmahr, *Playing on the Edge*, 159.

74. Ibid., 163.

75. Weiss, *Techniques of Pleasure*, 62, 85.

76. Ibid., 85.

77. Newmahr, *Playing on the Edge*, 134–40.

78. Weiss, *Techniques of Pleasure*, 137.

79. Newmahr, *Playing on the Edge*, 149. Newmahr also points out that although some of the same effects are possible because of incompetence, such as losing consciousness, they are not considered edgeplay in such a context.

80. Weiss, *Techniques of Pleasure*, 89.

81. P. H. Connolly, "Psychological Functioning of Bondage/Domination/Sado-Masochism (BDSM) Practitioners," *Journal of Psychology and Human Sexuality* 81, no. 1 (2006): 79–120.

82. Richters, Juliet, Richard O. De Visser, Chris E. Rissel, Andrew E. Grulich, and Anthony M.A. Smith. "Demographic and Psychosocial Features of Participants in Bondage and Discipline, "Sadomasochism" or Dominance and Submission (Bdsm): Data from a National Survey." *The Journal of Sexual Medicine* 5, no. 7 (2008): 1660-68.
Juliet Richters, "Through a Hole in a Wall: Setting and Interaction in Sex-on-Premises Venues," *Sexualites* 10, no. 3 (2007): 275–97.

83. Newmahr, *Playing on the Edge*, 147.

84. Weiss, *Techniques of Pleasure*.

85. Ibid., 122.

86. Kayt Sukel, "50 Shades of Grey (Matter): How Science Is Defying BDSM Stereotypes," Huffington Post Women (blog), May 30, 2012, http://www.huffingtonpost.com/kaytsukel/bdsm_b_1554310.html.

10. WHAT ARE YOU DOING AFTER THE ORGY?

1. Leslie Camhi, "Sex Obsession by the Numbers," *New York Times*, June 22, 2002, http://www.nytimes.com/2002/06/22/books/sex-obsession-by-the-numbers.html?pagewanted=all&src=pm.

2. Christian Groes-Green, "Orgies of the Moment: Bataille's Anthropology of Transgression and the Defiance of Danger in Post-Socialist Mozambique," *Anthropological Theory* 10, no. 4 (2010): 394.

3. Ibid., 398.

4. Ibid., 397.

5. Ibid., 403.

6. Ibid., 400.

7. Marco Vassi, *The Stoned Apocalypse* (Sag Harbor, NY: Second Chance Press, 1993), 28.

8. Ibid., 139.

9. Ibid., 156.

10. Ibid., 137.

11. Ibid., 250.

12. David Steinberg, "Marco Vassi: My Aunt Nettie; *Where's Waldo?*" *Comes Naturally*, January 8, 1993, http://www.nearbycafe.com/loveandlust/steinberg/erotic/cn/cn3.html.

13. Mark Thompson, ed., *Leatherfolk: Radical Sex, People, Politics, and Practice* (Boston: Alyson Publications, 1991), 277.

14. David Allyn, *Make Love, Not War: The Sexual Revolution: An Unfettered History* (Boston: Little, Brown, 2000), 210.

APPENDIX A

1. Kate Kelland, "Disease Risk Higher for Swingers Than Prostitutes," Reuters, June 23, 2010, http://www.reuters.com/article/2010/06/23/us-sex-diseases-swingers-idUSTRE65M6NX20100623.

2. "Incidence, Prevalence, and Cost of Sexually Transmitted Infections in the United States," CDC Fact Sheet, February 13, 2013, http://www.cdc.gov/std/stats/STI-Estimates-Fact-Sheet-Feb-2013.pdf.

3. An HPV epidemiologist I consulted suggested that due to the limitations of existing studies, this is an underestimation.

4. "Genital Herpes," CDC Fact Sheet, www.cdc.gov/std/herpes/stdfact-herpes.htm (last updated February 11, 2013).

5. "Sexually Transmitted Infections," Be Well: Health Education Services, Georgetown University, http://be.georgetown.edu/48377.html.

6. Terri D. Conley et al., "Unfaithful Individuals Are Less Likely to Practice Safer Sex Than Openly Nonmonogamous Individuals," *Journal of Sexual Medicine* 9, no. 6 (2012): 1559–65.

APPENDIX B

1. Curtis Bergstrand and Jennifer Blevins Sinski, *Swinging in America: Love, Sex, and Marriage in the 21st Century* (Santa Barbara: Praeger, 2010), ix.

2. Laud Humphreys, *Tearoom Trade: Impersonal Sex in Public Places* (Chicago: Aldine, 1975), 28. While some critique Humphreys for his research overall, most social scientists recognize that his covert observations in tearooms did not have the potential to harm the men involved. The second part of his study, where he interviewed the men under false pretenses as part of another study, was far more controversial.

3. Richard Tewksbury, "Bathhouse Intercourse: Structural and Behavoral Aspects of an Erotic Oasis," *Deviant Behavior* 23 (2002): 75–112.

4. Alison L. Bain and Catherine J. Nash, "Undressing the Researcher: Feminism, Embodiment and Sexuality at a Queer Bathhouse Event," *Area* 38, no. 1 (2006): 99–106.

5. Maurice van Lieshout, "Leather Nights in the Woods: Locating Male Homosexuality and Sadomasochism in a Dutch Highway Rest Area," in *Queers in Space: Communities/Public Places/Sites of Resistance*, ed. Gordon Brent Ingram, Anne-Marie Bouthillette, and Yolanda Retter (Seattle: Bay Press, 1997), 345.

6. Tim Dean, *Unlimited Intimacy: Reflections on the Subculture of Barebacking* (Chicago: University of Chicago Press, 2010), 29–34.

7. Russell Westhaver, "Party Boys: Identity, Community, and the Circuit" (PhD diss., Simon Fraser University, 2003), 21.

8. Ralph Bolton, "Tricks, Friends, and Lovers: Erotic Encounters in the Field," in *Taboo: Sex, Identity, and Erotic Subjectivity in Anthropological Fieldwork*, ed. Don Kulick and Margaret Wilson (London: Routledge, 1995), 142.

9. Ibid., 148.

10. Ibid., 150.

11. Ibid., 151.

12. Christian Groes-Green, "Ambivalent Participation: Sex, Power, and the Anthropologist in Mozambique," *Medical Anthropology: Cross-Cultural Studies in Health and Illness* 31, no. 1 (2012): 49.

13. Ibid., 57.

14. Bain and Nash, "Undressing the Researcher," 104.

15. Ibid., 103.

16. Groes-Green, "Ambivalent Participation," 56.

Bibliography

Abé, Nicola. "Online Sex Education: Parents' Porn Fears Exaggerated, Experts Say." *Spiegel Online*, October 14, 2011. http://www.spiegel.de/international/zeitgeist/online-sex-education-parents-porn-fears-exaggerated-experts-say-a-790266-2.html.

Agence France-Presse. "Kissing-Crazy 'Pokemon' Teens Shock Chilean Society." August 19, 2008. http://afp.google.com/article/ALeqM5g8_oJjFpw4GepEhegk6MXX9DZ41A.

All China Women's Federation. Excerpts from "Criminal Law of the People's Republic of China." http://www.womenofchina.cn/html/node/75472-1.htm.

Allured, Janet, and Judith F. Gentry. *Louisiana Women: Their Lives and Times.* Athens: University of Georgia Press, 2009.

Allyn, David. *Make Love, Not War: The Sexual Revolution: An Unfettered History.* Boston: Little, Brown, 2000.

American Psychiatric Association. "Recent Updates to Proposed Revisions for DSM-5." http://www.dsm5.org/Pages/RecentUpdates.aspx. Accessed March 2013.

Amnesty International in Asia & the Pacific. "Hudood Ordinances—The Crime and Punishment for Zina." http://asiapacific.amnesty.org/apro/aproweb.nsf/pages/svaw_hudoo.

Andrew, Christopher M., and Vasili Mitrokhin. *The Sword and the Shield: The Mitrokhin Archive and the Secret History of the KGB.* New York: Basic Books, 1999.

Anshe Chung Studios. "Anshe Chung Becomes First Virtual World Millionaire." News release, November 26 2006. http://www.anshechung.com/include/press/press_release251106.html.

Ashcraft, Brian. "The DS Game, Japan Will Forgive. The Sexy Orgy, It Won't." *Kotaku* (blog), October 14, 2011. http://kotaku.com/5849764/the-ds-game-japan-will-forgive-the-sexy-orgy-it-wont.

Askew, Robin. "Annabel Chong: *Sex: The Annabel Chong Story.*" *Spike Magazine*, October 1, 2000. http://www.spikemagazine.com/1000annabelchong.php.

Baal, Jan van. "The Dialectics of Sex in Marind-anim Culture." In *Ritualized Homosexuality in Melanesia*, edited by Gilbert H. Herdt, 128–66. Berkeley: University of California Press, 1984.

Baal, Jan van, with J. Verschueren. *Dema: Description and Analysis of Marind Culture.* The Hague: Martinus Nijhoff, 1966.

Bain, Alison L., and Catherine J. Nash. "Undressing the Researcher: Feminism, Embodiment and Sexuality at a Queer Bathhouse Event." *Area* 38, no. 1 (2006): 99–106.

Barancik, Scott. "D.C. Swings! Couples Meet for Cocktails, Hors d'Oeuvres, and Blowjobs at a Washington Restaurant." *Washington City Paper*, December 15, 1995. http://www.washingtoncitypaper.com/articles/8031/dc-swings/.

Barrionuevo, Alexei."In Tangle of Young Lips, a Sex Rebellion in Chile." *New York Times*, September 12, 2008. http://www.nytimes.com/2008/09/13/world/americas/13chile.html?_r=0.

Bartell, Gilbert. *Group Sex: A Scientist's Eyewitness Report on the American Way of Swinging.* New York: Peter H. Wyden, 1971.

Batrouney, Colin. "Gay Men and Sexual Adventurism: Where to from Here?" *Social Research Briefs* 15 (2009).

Baudrillard, Jean. "Paroxysm: The End of the Millennium or the Countdown." *Economy and Society* 26, no. 4 (November 1997): 447–55.

———. *The Transparency of Evil: Essays on Extreme Phenomena.* London: Verso, 1993.

BBC News. "Outrage at Musharraf Rape Remarks." September 16, 2005. http://news.bbc.co.uk/2/hi/south_asia/4251536.stm.

Beard, Mary. "Frazer, Leach, and Virgil: The Popularity (and Unpopularity) of the Golden Bough." *Comparative Studies in Society and History* 34, no. 2 (1992): 203–24.

Bennett, Jessica. "Northwestern University's Live Sex Class." *Daily Beast*, March 2, 2011. http://www.thedailybeast.com/articles/2011/03/03/the-story-behind-northwestern-universi-tys-live-sex-class.html.

Berens, Jessica. "The Double Life of Catherine M." *Guardian*, May 19, 2002. http://www.guardian.co.uk/books/2002/may/19/biography.features.

Bergner, Daniel. "What Do Women Want?" *New York Times Magazine*, January 22, 2009. http://www.nytimes.com/2009/01/25/magazine/25desire-t.html?pagewanted=all.

Bergstrand, Curtis, Nancy Schrepf, and Jennifer Williams-Sinski. "Civilization and Sexual Discontent: Monogamy and the Problem of Surplus Repression." Unpublished manuscript, December 1, 2003, Bellarmine University.

Bergstrand, Curtis, and Jennifer Blevins Sinski. *Swinging in America: Love, Sex, and Marriage in the 21st Century.* Santa Barbara: Praeger, 2010.

Berry, Lynn. "Pussy Riot Band Members Should Be Freed, Says Russian Prime Minister Dmitry Medvedev." Huffington Post, September 12, 2012. http://www.huffingtonpost.com/2012/09/12/pussy-riot-dmitry-medvedev-should-be-freed_n_1877513.html.

Bhattacharya, Sanjiv. "Meet the Mandingos." *Details*, 2007. http://www.details.com/sex-rela-tionships/sex-and-other-releases/200703/meet-the-mandingos.

Blanchard, W. H. "The Group Process in Gang Rape." *Journal of Social Psychology* 49 (1959): 259-66.

Blanshard, Alastair. *Sex: Vice and Love from Antiquity to Modernity.* Malden, MA: Wiley-Blackwell, 2010.

Boellstorff, Tom. *Coming of Age in Second Life: An Anthropologist Explores the Virtually Human.* Princeton: Princeton University Press, 2008.

Bollen, Jonathan, and David McInnes. "Time, Relations and Learning in Gay Men's Experiences of Adventurous Sex." *Social Semiotics* 14, no. 1 (2004): 21–36.

Bolton, Ralph. "Tricks, Friends, and Lovers: Erotic Encounters in the Field." In *Taboo: Sex, Identity, and Erotic Subjectivity in Anthropological Fieldwork*, edited by Don Kulick and Margaret Wilson, 140–67. London: Routledge, 1995.

Bolyanatz, Alexander H. *Pacific Romanticism: Tahiti and the European Imagination.* Westport, CT: Praeger, 2004.

Bourke, Joanna. "Sexual Violence, Bodily Pain, and Trauma: A History." *Theory, Culture & Society* 29, no. 3 (2012): 25–51.

Bowersock, Glen W. "The Vanishing Paradigm of the Fall of Rome." *Bulletin of the American Academy of Arts and Sciences* 49, no. 8 (1996): 29–43.

Bratersky, Alexander. "Putin Jokes about Orgy, But Slams Pussy Riot." *Moscow Times*, September 7, 2012.

Bronski, Michael. *The Pleasure Principle: Sex, Backlash, and the Struggle for Gay Freedom.* New York: St. Martin's, 1998.

Byrne, Richard. "Setting the Boundaries: Tackling Public Sex Environments in Country Parks." In *Proceedings of Royal Town Planning Institute Planning Research Conference.* Oxford: Wadham College, University of Oxford, 2003.

Cadwalladr, Carole. "Pussy Riot: Will Vladimir Putin Regret Taking On Russia's Cool Women Punks?" *Observer*, July 28, 2012. http://www.guardian.co.uk/world/2012/jul/29/pussy-riot-protest-vladimir-putin-russia.

Cagiano, R., I. Bera, R. Sabatini, P. Flace, D. Vermesan, H. Vermesan, S. I. Dragulescu, L. Bottalico, and L. Santacroce. "Effects on Rat Sexual Behaviour of Acute MDMA (Ecstasy) Alone or in Combination with Loud Music." *European Review for Medical and Pharmacological Sciences* 12 (2008): 285–92.

Califia, Pat. *Macho Sluts*. Boston: Alyson Books, 1994.

———. "San Francisco: Revisiting 'the City of Desire.'" In *Queers in Space: Communities/Public Places/Sites of Resistance*, edited by Gordon Brent Ingram, Anne-Marie Bouthillette, and Yolanda Retter, 177–96. Seattle: Bay Press, 1997.

Camhi, Leslie. "Sex Obsession by the Numbers." *New York Times*, June 22, 2002. http://www.nytimes.com/2002/06/22/books/sex-obsession-by-the-numbers.html?pagewanted=all&src=pm.

Campbell, Andy. "Horseshoe Crab Mating Ritual Is the Oldest Beach Orgy." *Weird News* (blog), Huffington Post, May 11, 2012. http://www.huffingtonpost.com/2012/05/11/horseshoe-crab-orgy_n_1509445.html.

Campbell, Dennis. "Porn: The New Sex Education." *Joe Public Blog*, *Guardian*, March 30, 2009. http://www.guardian.co.uk/society/joepublic+education/sexeducation.

Campbell, Joseph, with Bill Moyers. *The Power of Myth*. New York: Doubleday, 1988.

Campbell, Matthew. "French Teenagers Grab Free Love at Le Skins Orgy." *Sunday Times*, February 28, 2011. http://www.timesonline.co.uk/tol/news/world/europe/article7043885.ece.

———. "French Led Astray by Louche Skins Parties." *Australian*, March 1, 2010. http://www.theaustralian.com.au/news/world/french-led-astray-by-louche-skins-parties/story-e6frg6so-1225835329894?sv=33a43ffd8309d2578b95a23b3f454d5a.

Card, Claudia. "Rape as a Weapon of War." *Hypatia* 11, no. 4 (1996): 5–18.

Carmichael, Mary. "His Cheating Brain." *Newsweek*, March 11, 2008. http://www.thedailybeast.com/newsweek/2008/03/12/his-cheating-brain.html.

Carnes, Patrick J. *The Betrayal Bond: Breaking Free of Exploitative Relationships*. Deerfield Beach, FL: Health Communications, 1997.

Carroll, Rory. "Las Vegas Hails Prince Harry as a True Son of Sin City." *Guardian*, August 25, 2012. http://www.guardian.co.uk/uk/2012/aug/25/prince-harry-las-vegas-party.

Cassels, Peter. "Taking Aim at Barebacking Videos." Edge San Francisco, May 24, 2010. http://www.edgesanfrancisco.com/entertainment/culture///106024/taking_aim_at_barebacking_videos.

Centers for Disease Control and Prevention. "2011 Estimates of Foodborne Illness: CDC 2011 Estimates: Findings." Available at http://www.cdc.gov/foodborneburden/2011-foodborne-estimates.html. Last updated Ocrober 10, 2012.

———. "Genital Herpes." CDC Fact Sheet. www.cdc.gov/std/herpes/stdfact-herpes.htm. Last updated February 11, 2013.

———. "HIV/AIDS Statistics and Surveillance: Basic Statistics." Available at http://www.cdc.gov/hiv/topics/surveillance/basic.htm. Last modified February 28, 2013.

———. "Incidence, Prevalence, and Cost of Sexually Transmitted Infections in the United States." CDC Fact Sheet, February 13, 2013. http://www.cdc.gov/std/stats/STI-Estimates-Fact-Sheet-Feb-2013.pdf.

———. "Sexually Transmitted Diseases in the United States, 2008." Available at http://www.cdc.gov/std/stats08/trends.htm. Last updated November 16, 2009.

Chauncey, George. *Gay New York: Gender, Urban Culture, and the Making of the Gay Male World, 1890–1940*. New York: Basic Books, 1994.

Chonin, Neva. "Sex and the City." *San Francisco Chronicle SF Gate*, September 17, 2006. http://www.sfgate.com/cgi-bin/article.cgi?file=/c/a/2006/09/17/PKG6BKQQA41.DTL.

Chun, Kimberly. "Sex: The Annabel Chong Story." *Asian Week*, May 4, 2000. http://asianweek.com/2000_05_04/ae_annabelchong.html.

Clark-Flory, Tracy. "Yale Fraternity Pledges Chant about Rape." *Salon.com*, October 15, 2010. http://www.salon.com/life/broadsheet/2010/10/15/yale_fraternity_pledges_chant_about_rape/index.html.

Club Bliss London. "Guidelines." http://www.club-bliss-london.com/guide.htm.

Cobalt, Kal."The Path of Pain: Spiritual BDSM." *Kal Cobalt's Blog* (blog). http://www.realitysandwich.com/path_pain_spiritual_bdsm.

Collymore, Stan. *Tackling My Demons*. London: CollinsWillow, 2004.

Conley, Terri D., Amy C. Moors, Ali Ziegler, and Constantina Karathanasis. "Unfaithful Individuals Are Less Likely to Practice Safer Sex Than Openly Nonmonogamous Individuals." *Journal of Sexual Medicine* 9, no. 6 (2012): 1559–65.

Connolly, P. H. "Psychological Functioning of Bondage/Domination/Sado-Masochism (BDSM) Practitioners." *Journal of Psychology and Human Sexuality* 81, no. 1 (2006): 79–120.

Corrin, Tanya, and Anna Moore. "New York, New Hedonists." *Observer*, July 20, 2002.

Craft, Ashley John. "Love 2.0: A Quantitative Exploration of Sex and Relationships in the Virtual World Second Life." *Archives of Sexual Behavior* 41, no. 4 (2012): 939–47.

Craven, Nick. "What Really Happened at the Myspace Party from Hell." *Mail Online*, April 21, 2007. http://www.dailymail.co.uk/femail/article-449819/What-REALLY-happened-Myspace-party-hell.html.

Crimsonlay, Misty. *Second Life—Hot Orgies*. Amazon Digital Services, 2011. Kindle edition.

Crocker, William H. "Canela Marriage: Factors in Change." In *Marriage Practices in Lowland South America*, ed. Kenneth M. Kensinger (Urbana and Chicago: University of Illinois Press, 1984). Available at http://anthropology.si.edu/canela/literature/marrriage.pdf.

Croft, Adrian. "Doctor, Gang-Raped in Sudan's Darfur, Wins Rights Award." *Reuters*, October 6, 2010. http://www.reuters.com/article/2010/10/06/us-sudan-award-idUSTRE69552320101006.

Crombag, Hans S., and Terry E. Robinson. "Drugs, Environment, Brain, and Behavior." *Current Directions in Psychological Science* 13, no. 3 (2004): 107–11.

Crowley, Aleister, John Symonds, and Kenneth Grant. *The Confessions of Aleister Crowley*. New York: Penguin, 1989.

Cuckoldress Roxanne. "The Science of Cuckolding." *A Cuckoldress World* (blog), December 20, 2004. http://www.xtcforums.com/main.php?page=cuckoldscientificexplanation.

Curran, Bronwyn. "Mukhtaran Mai: The Other Side of the Story." *News International*, April 30, 2011. http://www.thenews.com.pk/TodaysPrintDetail.aspx?ID=44406&Cat=9.

Dangerous Bedfellows [Eva Hoffman, Wayne Pendleton]. *Policing Public Sex: Queer Politics and the Future of AIDS Activism*. Cambridge, MA: South End Press, 1996.

Daniels, Kimberly. "The Danger of Celebrating Halloween." *Charisma*, October 27, 2009. http://www.charismamag.com/index.php/prophetic-insight/23723-the-danger-of-celebrating-halloween?showall=1.

Darkness Falls Two. "What" explanation page. http://www.darknessfallstwo.org/.

Davies, Hunter. "Why I Didn't Tell the Whole Truth about the Beatles." *New Statesman*, October 25, 2012. http://www.newstatesman.com/culture/culture/2012/10/why-i-didnt-tell-whole-truth-about-beatles?page=1.

Dean, Tim. *Unlimited Intimacy: Reflections on the Subculture of Barebacking*. Chicago: University of Chicago Press, 2010.

Dent, Grace. "Has Hugh Hefner Finally Seen the Ghost of Playboy Future?" *Guardian*, March 1, 2012.

Doury, Claudine. "France, Skins Parties, 2010." VU' l'agence, www.agencevu.com.

Dowsett, Gary W. "The Gay Plague Revisited: AIDS and Its Enduring Moral Panic." In *Moral Panics, Sex Panics: Fear and the Fight over Sexual Rights*, ed. Gilbert Herdt, 130–156. New York: New York University Press, 2009.

Dreger, Alice. "Wanting Privacy versus Being Ashamed." *Fetishes I Don't Get: Thoughts on Life, Love, and Lust* (blog), *Psychology Today*, March 6, 2011. http://www.psychologytoday.com/blog/fetishes-i-dont-get/201103/wanting-privacy-versus-being-ashamed.

Dutton, Donald, and Arthur Aron. "Some Evidence for Heightened Sexual Attraction under Conditions of High Anxiety." *Journal of Personality and Social Psychology* 30, no. 4 (1974): 510–17.

Edgerton, Robert B. *Mau Mau: An African Crucible*. New York: Free Press, 1989.

Edwards, David. "Republican Lawmaker Blames 11-Year-Old Victim of Alleged Gang Rape." *Raw Story*, March 16, 2011. http://www.rawstory.com/rs/2011/03/16/republican-lawmaker-blames-11-year-old-victim-of-alleged-gang-rape/.

EIOBA. "Orgies, a Brief History." http://www.eioba.com/a70752/orgies_a_brief_history.

Eisenberg, Dan T. A., Benjamin Campbell, James MacKillop, Meera Modi, David Dang, J. Koji Lum, and David S. Wilson. "Polymorphisms in the Dopamine D4 and D2 Receptor Genes and Reproductive and Sexual Behaviors." *Evolutionary Psychology* 5, no. 4 (2007): 696–715.

Elder, Miriam. "Pussy Riot Member Freed as Two Bandmates Face Exile to Prison Camp." *Guardian*, October 10, 2012. http://www.guardian.co.uk/world/2012/oct/10/pussy-riot-member-free.

Eliade, Mircea. *Patterns in Comparative Religion*. New York: Sheed & Ward, 1958.

Ellis, William. *Polynesian Researches, during a Residence of Nearly Six Years in the South Sea Islands; Including Descriptions of the Natural History and Scenery of the Islands, with Remarks on the History, Mythology, Traditions, Government, Arts, Manners, and Customs of the Inhabitants*. Vol. 1. London: Fisher, Son, & Jackson, 1829.

Ellison, Jesse. "The Military's Secret Shame." *Newsweek*, April 3, 2011. http://www.newsweek.com/2011/04/03/the-military-s-secret-shame.html.

Elliston, Deborah A. "'Ritualized Homosexuality' in Melanesia and Beyond. *American Ethnologist* 22, no. 4 (1995): 848–67.

Escoffier, Jeffrey. *Bigger Than Life: The History of Gay Porn Cinema from Beefcake to Hardcore*. Philadelphia: Running Press, 2009.

Eskenazi, Gerald. "The Male Athlete and Sexual Assault." *New York Times*, June 3, 1990. http://www.nytimes.com/books/97/08/03/reviews/glenridge-athlete.html?_r=2.

Esposito, Stefano. "Church Nixed Helping Northwestern Students Because of Sex Toy Flap." *Herald-News*, 2011. http://heraldnews.suntimes.com/photos/galleries/4718726-417/church-nixed-helping-northwestern-students-because-of-sex-toy-flap.html.

Fagan, Brian M. *Clash of Cultures*. 2nd ed. Lanham: Altamira Press, 1998.

Fahim, Kareem. "Slap to a Man's Pride Set Off Tumult in Tunisia." *New York Times*, January 21, 2011. http://www.nytimes.com/2011/01/22/world/africa/22sidi.html?pagewanted=1&_r=1&src=twrhp.

Fahmy, Mohamed Fadel. "Egyptian Blogger Aliaa Elmahdy: Why I Posed Naked." CNN, November 19, 2011. http://articles.cnn.com/2011-11-19/middleeast/world_meast_nude-blogger-aliaa-magda-elmahdy_1_egyptian-blogger-nude-photo-kareem-amer?_s=PM:MIDDLEEAST.

Featherstone, M., ed. *Love and Eroticism*. Thousand Oaks, CA: Sage, 1999.

Ferris-Rotman, Phoebe. "Prison Gang Rape of Mafia 'Poet' Prompts Government Response." *Pink News*, August 5, 2008. http://www.pinknews.co.uk/2008/08/05/prison-gang-rape-of-mafia-poet-prompts-government-response/.

Festival A Go-Go (blog). "Down n Dirty First Timers Guide to Burning Man." April 28, 2010. http://festivalagogo.com/?p=412.

Fox News. "Thai Zoo Hopes Porn Will Get Sluggish Pandas to Mate." March 27, 2007. http://www.foxnews.com/story/0,2933,261569,00.html.

Franklin, Karen. "Enacting Masculinity: Antigay Violence and Group Rape as Participatory Theater." *Sexuality Research & Social Policy* 1, no. 2 (2004): 25–40.

Frayer, Lauren. "40 Lipsticked Virgins: Moammar Gadhafi's Best Bet for Survival." AOL News, May 23, 2011. http://www.aolnews.com/2011/03/23/moammar-40-lipsticked-virgins-gadhafis-best-bet-for-survival/.

Frazer, Sir James George. *Aftermath: A Supplement to the Golden Bough*. London: MacMillan, 1955.

———. *The New Golden Bough*. Edited, with notes and foreword, by Theodor Gaster. New York: Criterion, 1959.

Freeman, Gregory A. "Bug Chasers: The Men Who Long to Be HIV+." *Rolling Stone*, February 6, 2003. https://solargeneral.com/library/bug-chasers.pdf.

Freud, Sigmund. *Three Essays on the Theory of Sexuality*. Edited by James Strachey. New York: Basic Books, 1962.

Friedl, Ernestine. "Sex the Invisible." *American Anthropologist* 96, no. 4 (1994): 833–44.

Frohmader, Karla S., Katherine L. Bateman, Michael N. Lehman, and Lique M. Coolen. "Effects of Methamphetamine on Sexual Performance and Compulsive Sex Behavior in Male Rats." *Psychopharmacology* 212, no. 1 (2010): 93–104.

Gauthier, DeAnn K., and Craig J. Forsyth. "Bareback Sex, Bug Chasers, and the Gift of Death." *Deviant Behavior* 20 (1998): 85–100.

Gelder, Lawrence Van. Review of *Sex: The Annabel Chong Story*. *New York Times*, February 11, 2000. http://partners.nytimes.com/library/film/021100sex-film-review.html.

Georgetown University Health Education Services. "Sexually Transmitted Infections." http://be.georgetown.edu/48377.html.

Gibbs, Nancy, Mary Cronin, and Melissa Ludtke. "Wilding in the Night." *Time*, May 8, 1989. http://www.time.com/time/magazine/article/0,9171,957631,00.html.

Gilbert, Paul. "Evolution, Social Roles, and the Differences in Shame and Guilt." *Social Research* 70, no. 4 (2003): 1205–29.

Gilbert, Richard L., Monique A. Gonzalez, and Nora A. Murphy. "Sexuality in the 3D Internet and Its Relationship to Real-Life Sexuality." *Psychology & Sexuality* 2, no. 2 (2011): 107–22.

Globe and Mail. "Photos of Gang Rape Go Viral on Facebook." September 16, 2010. http://www.theglobeandmail.com/news/national/british-columbia/photos-of-gang-rape-go-viral-on-facebook/article1710072/.

Goldberg, Ben Zion. *The Sacred Fire: The Story of Sex in Religion*. New Hyde Park, NY: University Books, 1930.

Goldhagen, Daniel Jonah. *Worse Than War: Genocide, Eliminationism and the Ongoing Assault on Humanity*. New York: PublicAffairs, 2009.

Goodman, Amy. "Voice: An Interview with Annabel Chong." Nerve.com, June 22, 1999. http://www.nerve.com/dispatches/goodman/chong.

Gould, Terry. *The Lifestyle: A Look at the Erotic Rites of Swingers*. Toronto: Vintage Canada, 1999.

Green, Adam Isaiah, and Perry N Halkitis. "Crystal Methamphetamine and Sexual Sociality in an Urban Gay Subculture: An Elective Affinity." *Culture, Health & Sexuality: An International Journal for Research, Intervention and Care* 8, no. 4 (2006): 317–33.

Green, Andrew. "Humanitarian Crisis Worsens as Fighting Escalates in Sudan." *Lancet* 381, no. 9863 (2013): 281, available at http://www.lancet.com/journals/lancet/article/PIIS0140-6736%2813%2960118-X/fulltext.

Greenberg, David. *The Construction of Homosexuality*. Chicago: University of Chicago Press, 1990.

Greene, Robert. *The Art of Seduction*. New York: Penguin, 2001.

Gregor, Thomas. *Anxious Pleasures: The Sexual Lives of an Amazonian People*. Chicago: University of Chicago Press, 1987.

Groes-Green, Christian. "Ambivalent Participation: Sex, Power, and the Anthropologist in Mozambique." *Medical Anthropology: Cross-Cultural Studies in Health and Illness* 31, no. 1 (2012): 44–60.

———. "Orgies of the Moment: Bataille's Anthropology of Transgression and the Defiance of Danger in Post-Socialist Mozambique." *Anthropological Theory* 10, no. 4 (2010): 385–407.

Grove, Lloyd. "Getting a Rise out of Hef." *Daily Beast*, January 3, 2011. http://www.thedailybeast.com/articles/2011/01/04/hugh-hefner-newly-engaged-responds-to-complaints-from-ex-playboy-bunny.html.

Grube, John. "'No More Shit': The Struggle for Democratic Gay Space in Toronto." In *Queers in Space: Communities/Public Places/Sites of Resistance*, edited by John M. Ingham, Anne-Marie Bouthillette, and Yolanda Retter, 127–46. Seattle: Bay Press, 1997.

Guthrie, Julian. "Partner Swapping Comes out of Closet . . ." *San Francisco Chronicle*, July 9, 2002.

Hakim, Catherine. *Erotic Capital: The Power of Attraction in the Boardroom and the Bedroom*. New York: Basic Books, 2011.

Hall, Allan. "Volkswagen Threw Orgies for MPs and Union Officials." *Mail Online*, May 31, 2007. http://www.dailymail.co.uk/news/article-458819/Volkswagen-threw-orgies-MPs-union-officials.html.

Hammar, Lawrence. "The Dark Side to Donovanosis: Color, Climate, Race and Racism in American South Venereology." *Journal of Medical Humanities* 18, no. 1 (1997): 29–57.

Hammers, Corie. "Bodies That Speak and the Promises of Queer: Looking to Two Lesbian/Queer Bathhouses For a Third Way." *Journal of Gender Studies* 17, no. 2 (June 2008): 147-164.

Hammers, Corie. "An Examination of Lesbian/Queer Bathhouse Culture and the Social Organization of (Im)Personal Sex." *Journal of Contemporary Ethnography* 38, no. 3 (2009): 308-55.

Handwerk, Brian. "Panda Porn to Boost Mating Efforts at Thai Zoo." *National Geographic News*, November 13, 2006. http://news.nationalgeographic.com/news/2006/11/061113-panda-mate.html.

Harris, Judith. *Pompeii Awakened: A Story of Rediscovery*. London: I. B. Tauris, 2007.

Harvey, Larry. "Jiffy Lube 2001." Burning Man. http://www.burningman.com/blackrock-city_yearround/jrs/extras/jiffylube.html.

Hatfield, Elaine. *A New Look at Love*. Lanham: University Press of America, 2002.

Heidenry, John. *What Wild Ecstasy: The Rise and Fall of the Sexual Revolution*. New York: Simon & Schuster, 1997.

Herdt, Gilbert. *Sambia Sexual Culture: Essays from the Field*. Chicago: University of Chicago Press 1999.

Higgins, Louise T., Mo Zheng, Yali Liu, and Chun Hui Sun. "Attitudes to Marriage and Sexual Behaviors: A Survey of Gender and Culture Differences in China and United Kingdom." *Sex Roles* 46, no. 3/4 (2002): 75–89.

Hill, Kashmir. "The Potential Financial Consequences of Sharing Gang-Rape Photos on Facebook." *Forbes*, September 17, 2010. http://blogs.forbes.com/kashmirhill/2010/09/17/the-potential-financial-consequences-of-sharing-gang-rape-photos-on-facebook/.

Hockett, Jeremy. "Participant Observation and the Study of Self: Burning Man as Ethnographic Experience." In *After Burn: Reflections on Burning Man*, edited by Lee M Gilmore and Mark Van Proyen. Albuquerque: University of New Mexico Press, 2005.

Holden, Stephen. Review of *The Lifestyle: Group Sex in the Suburbs*, directed by David Schisgall. *New York Times*, March 16, 2000. http://movies.nytimes.com/movie/179829/The-Lifestyle/overview.

Honigsbaum, Mark. "West Side Story: A Tale of Unprotected Sex Which Could Be Link to New HIV Superbug." *Guardian*, March 25, 2005. http://www.guardian.co.uk/world/2005/mar/26/aids.usa.

Hopcke, R. H., and M. Thompson. "S/M and the Psychology of Gay Male Initiation: An Archetypal Perspective." In *Leatherfolk: Radical Sex, People, Politics, and Practice*, edited by Mark Thompson, 65–76. Boston: Alyson Publications, 1991.

Horne, Jed. Review of *Sex with Strangers*, directed by Joe Gantz and Harry Gantz. *Tech Online Edition*, October 8, 2002. www-tech.mit.edu/V122/N46/Sex_with_strang.46a.html.

Horswell, Cindy. "Defendant in Cleveland Gang Rape Case Gets Life Sentence." *Houston Chronicle*, November 28, 2012. http://www.chron.com/news/houston-texas/houston/article/Defendant-in-Cleveland-gang-rape-case-gets-life-4073766.php.

Horton, Alicia D. "Flesh Hook Pulling: Motivations and Meaning-Making from the 'Body Side' of Life." *Deviant Behavior* 34, no. 2 (2013): 115–34.

Houreld, Katharine. "Women and Girls in Darfur Raped, Jailed, Fined." *Age* (Australia), March 14, 2005. http://www.theage.com.au/news/World/Women-and-girls-in-Darfur-raped-jailed-fined/2005/03/13/1110649052906.html.

Hoyle, Ben. "'Jack Rolling' Link to Rape Gang." *Times Online*, August 12, 2005. http://www.thetimes.co.uk/tto/news/uk/article1936777.ece.

Huang, Carol."Facebook and Twitter Key to Arab Spring Uprisings: Report." *National* (United Arab Emirates), June 6, 2011. http://www.thenational.ae/news/uae-news/facebook-and-twitter-key-to-arab-spring-uprisings-report.

Huffington Post. "Dennis Rodman Broadcasts Naughty Romp with 6 Women." September 8, 2010. http://www.huffingtonpost.com/2010/09/08/dennis-rodman-broadcasts-_n_708485.html.

———. "Hugh Hefner Has Sex Twice a Week, Playmates Describe Orgies." July 12, 2010. http://www.huffingtonpost.com/2010/07/12/hugh-hefner-i-have-sex-tw_n_643303.html.

———. "Pitt Meadows, B.C. Gang Rape: Boy Who Posted Images of 16-Year-Old Victim Sentenced." February 10, 2012. http://www.huffingtonpost.ca/2012/02/10/pitt-meadows-bc-gang-rape_n_1269269.html.

———. "Prince Harry Nude Photos Boosting Las Vegas Tourism." Huffington Post, August 23, 2012. http://www.huffingtonpost.com/2012/08/23/prince-harry-nude-photos-boosting-las-vegas-tourism_n_1824848.html.

Humphreys, Laud. *Tearoom Trade: Impersonal Sex in Public Places.* Chicago: Aldine, 1975.

Hurley, Michael, and Garrett Prestage. "Intensive Sex Partying Amongst Gay Men in Sydney." *Culture, Health & Sexuality: An International Journal for Research, Intervention and Care* 11, no. 6 (2009): 597–610.

Im, Soyon. "Sex: The Annabel Chong Story." *Seattle Weekly*, July 26, 2000. http://www.seattleweekly.com/2000-07-26/film/sex-the-annabel-chong-story/.

I Play & He Waits (blog). "Did You Ever Wonder Why You Just Needed to Fuck That Good Looking Guy?" http://iplayhewaits.blogspot.com/p/did-you-ever-wonder-why-you-just-needed.html?zx=f8645986ab54e251.

Irvine, Janice M. "Reinventing Perversion: Sex Addiction and Cultural Anxieties." *Journal of the History of Sexuality* 5, no. 3 (1995): 429–50.

Isenberg, Barbara. "Mr. Playboy: Hugh Hefner Tells How He Created an Identity in Order to Fulfill His Dreams." *Time*, October 2, 2005. http://www.time.com/time/magazine/article/0,9171,1112823,00.html#ixzz1yosR8m16.

Jankowiak, William, and Laura Mixson. "'I Have His Heart, Swinging Is Just Sex': The Ritualization of Sex and the Rejuvenation of the Love Bond in an American Spouse Exchange Community." In *Intimacies: Love and Sex across Cultures*, edited by William R. Jankowiak, 245–266. New York: Columbia University Press, 2008.

Jenkins, Carol. "The Homosexual Context of Heterosexual Practice in Papua New Guinea." In *Bisexualities and AIDS: International Perspectives*, edited by Peter Aggleton, 188–203. London: Taylor & Francis, 1996.

Jet. "The Lowdown on Sex Parties." April 1, 1954, 56–58. Available at http://www.flickr.com/photos/vieilles_annonces/1293887187/.

Jewkes, Rachel, and Naeema Abrahams. "The Epidemiology of Rape and Sexual Coercion in South Africa: An Overview." *Social Science & Medicine* 55 (2002): 1231–44.

Jones, Heather. "Rapex in South Africa." *Wilder Voice* 3, no. 5 (2008).

Kahney, Leander. "Dogging Craze Has Brits in Heat." *Wired*, March 19, 2004. http://www.wired.com/culture/lifestyle/news/2004/03/62718.

Kaiser, David, and Lovisa Stannow. "The Way to Stop Prison Rape." *New York Review of Books*, March 25, 2010. http://www.nybooks.com/articles/archives/2010/mar/25/the-way-to-stop-prison-rape/?page=2.

Kasidie. "100 Signs You May Be a Swinger." http://www.kasidie.com/static/magazine/humor/100signs.html.

Kelland, Kate. "Disease Risk Higher for Swingers Than Prostitutes." Reuters, June 23, 2010. http://www.reuters.com/article/2010/06/23/us-sex-diseases-swingers-idUSTRE65M6NX20100623.

Kelly, Antoinette. "Swingers Groups in Ireland Are Growing at a Massive Rate." Irish Central, September 14, 2010. http://www.irishcentral.com/news/Swinging-in-Ireland-is-a-growing-at-a-massive-rate-102882449.html?showAll=y.

Kessler, Glenn. "Musharraf Denies Rape Comments." *Washington Post*, September 19, 2005, http://www.washingtonpost.com/wp-dyn/content/article/2005/09/18/AR2005091800554.html.

Kessler, Pamela. *Undercover Washington: Where Famous Spies Lived, Worked and Loved.* Herndon, VA: Capitol Books, 2005.

Khalaji, Mehdi. "The Clerics vs. Modernity: Failure of the Islamic Republic's Soft Power." *Majalla*, June 2012. Available at http://www.washingtoninstitute.org/policy-analysis/view/the-clerics-vs.-modernity-failure-of-the-islamic-republics-soft-power.

Kilgallon, Sarah J., and Leigh W. Simmons. "Image Content Influences Men's Semen Quality." *Biology Letters* 1, no. 3 (2005): 253–55.

Kimm, Joan. *A Fatal Conjunction: Two Laws, Two Cultures.* Sydney: Federation Press, 2004.

Klaits, Joseph. *Servants of Satan: The Age of the Witch Hunts.* Bloomington: Indiana University Press, 1987.

Klusmann, Dietrich. "Sexual Motivation and the Duration of Partnership." *Archives of Sexual Behavior* 31, no. 3 (2002): 275–87.

Knauft, Bruce M. *South Coast New Guinea Cultures: History, Comparison, Dialectic.* Cambridge: Cambridge University Press, 1993.

Knight, Richard Payne. *The Symbolical Language of Ancient Art and Mythology: An Inquiry.* New York: J. W. Bouton, 1892.

Koene, Joris M, and Andries Ter Maat. "Coolidge Effect in Pond Snails: Male Motivation in a Simultaneous Hermaphrodite." *BMC Evolutionary Biology* 7 (2007): 212.

Kramer, Larry. *Faggots.* New York: Grove Press, 1978.

Kristof, Nicholas D. "A Policy of Rape." *New York Times*, June 5, 2005.

Lakeland Ledger. "867-5309 Is Not Jenny." May 16, 1982, http://news.google.com/newspapers?id=PaVOAAAAIBAJ&sjid=PvsDAAAAIBAJ&pg=6320,11943.

Landau, Jon. "The Rolling Stone Interviews: Paul Simon." Paul Simon.info, 1972. http://www.paul-simon.info/PHP/showarticle.php?id=13&kategorie=1.

Larkin, Mike. "I've Still Got My Mojo! Hugh Hefner Bounces Back from Humiliating Bedroom Revelations with a Party at the Playboy Mansion." *Daily Mail*, August 9, 2011. http://www.dailymail.co.uk/tvshowbiz/article-2023796/Hugh-Hefner-puts-Crystal-Harris-bedroom-revelations-Playboy-party.html.

Larsen, Josefine (2010) "The social vagina: labia elongation and social capital among women in Rwanda", Culture, Health & Sexuality, First published on: 27 July 2010 (iFirst); p. 1-14.

Laskaway, Tom. "'Pink Slime' Is the Tip of the Iceberg: Look What Else Is in Industrial Meat." *Grist: A Beacon in the Smog*, March 19, 2012. http://grist.org/factory-farms/pink-slime-is-the-tip-of-the-iceberg-look-what-else-is-in-industrial-meat/.

Laumann, Edward O., John H. Gagnon, Robert T. Michael, and Stuart Michaels. *The Social Organization of Sexuality: Sexual Practices in the United States.* Chicago: University of Chicago Press, 1994.

Leap, William L. "Sex in 'Private' Places: Gender, Erotics, and Detachment in Two Urban Locales." In *Public Sex, Gay Space*, edited by William L. Leap, 115–39. New York: Columbia University Press, 1999.

———. *Public Sex, Gay Space.* New York: Columbia University Press, 1999.

Lee, Tommy, Vince Neil, Mick Mars, Nikki Sixx, and Neil Strauss. *Mötley Crüe: The Dirt—Confessions of the World's Most Notorious Rock Band.* New York: HarperCollins, 2002.

Lende, Daniel H., Terri Leonard, Claire E. Sterk, and Kirk Elifson. "Functional Methamphetamine Use: The Insider's Perspective." *Addiction Research & Theory* 15, no. 5 (2007): 465–77.

Leon, Harmon. *The American Dream: Walking in the Shoes of Carnies, Arms Dealers, Immigrant Dreamers, Pot Farmers, and Christian Believers.* New York: Nation Books, 2008.

———. "A Night with the California Swingers Club." The Smoking Jacket, December 22, 2010. http://www.thesmokingjacket.com/humor/california-swingers-club.

Lessin, Janet Kira. "Double Penetration: A Path to Enlightenment." Club Tantra. http://clubtantra.org/2012/11/04/double-penetration-a-path-to-enlightenment/.

Levine, Martin P. *Gay Macho: The Life and Death of the Homosexual Clone.* New York: New York University Press, 1998.

Lewandowski, Gary, and Arthur Aron. "Distinguishing Arousal from Novelty and Challenge in Initial Romantic Attraction between Strangers." *Social Behavior and Personality* 32, no. 4 (2004): 361–72.

Lewis, I. M. "Trance, Possession, Shamanism, and Sex." *Anthropology of Consciousness* 14, no. 1 (2003): 20–39.

Lewis, Michael. *Shame: The Exposed Self.* New York: Free Press, 1992.

Ley, David J. *Insatiable Wives: Women Who Stray and the Men Who Love Them.* Lanham: Rowman & Littlefield, 2009.

———. "Is Kinky Sex Good for Your Marriage?" *Women Who Stray* (blog), *Psychology Today*, June 22, 2010. http://www.psychologytoday.com/blog/women-who-stray/201006/is-kinky-sex-good-your-marriage.

Lichtenberg, Joseph D. *Sensuality and Sexuality across the Divide of Shame.* New York: Routledge, 2007.

Lieshout, Maurice van. "Leather Nights in the Woods: Locating Male Homosexuality and Sadomasochism in a Dutch Highway Rest Area." In *Queers in Space: Communities/Public Places/Sites of Resistance*, edited by Gordon Brent Ingram, Anne-Marie Bouthillette, and Yolanda Retter, 339–57. Seattle: Bay Press, 1997.

Lim, Gerrie. *Singapore Rebel: Searching for Annabel Chong.* Singapore: Monsoon Books, 2011.

Long, Carolyn Morrow. *Spiritual Merchants: Religion, Magic, and Commerce.* Knoxville: University of Tennessee Press, 2001.

Loudon, Bruce. "Pakistan Pack Rape as Reform Laws Stall." *Autstralian*, September 19, 2006. http://www.theaustralian.com.au/news/world/pakistan-pack-rape-as-reform-laws-stall/story-e6frg6so-1111112233324.

Lyall, Sarah. "Here's the Pub, Church and Field for Public Sex." *New York Times*, October 7, 2010. http://www.nytimes.com/2010/10/08/world/europe/08puttenham.html?_r=3&page-wanted=print.

Lyng, Stephen. "Edgework, Risk, and Uncertainty." In *Social Theories of Risk and Uncertainty: An Introduction*, edited by Jens O. Zinn, 106–37. New York: Wiley-Blackwell, 2008.

MacAndrew, Craig, and Robert B. Edgerton. *Drunken Comportment: A Social Explanation.* New York: Aldine, 1969.

Macatee, Rebecca. "Prince Harry's Naked Bonanza! Scandal Worth $23 Million Tourism Boost to Las Vegas." *E! Online*, October 10, 2012. http://www.eonline.com/news/353055/prince-harry-s-naked-bonanza-scandal-worth-23-million-tourism-boost-to-las-vegas.

Maffesoli, Michel. *The Shadow of Dionysus: A Contribution to the Sociology of the Orgy.* Translated by Cindy Linse and Mary Kristina Palmquist. Albany: SUNY Press, 1993.

Mahdavi, Pardis. *Passionate Uprisings: Iran's Sexual Revolution.* Stanford: Stanford University Press, 2009.

Mail Online. "Revealed: The 'Other Woman' in Second Life Divorce . . . Who's Now Engaged to the Web Cheat She's Never Met." November 14, 2008. http://www.dailymail.co.uk/news/article-1085412/Revealed-The-woman-Second-Life-divorce--whos-engaged-web-cheat-shes-met.html.

Mains, Geoff. (1984). *Urban Aboriginals: A Celebration of Leathersexuality* (Daedalus Publishing).

Maines, Rachel. *The Technology of Orgasm: "Hysteria," the Vibrator, and Women's Sexual Satisfaction.* Baltimore: Johns Hopkins University Press, 1999.

Malinowski, Bronislaw. *The Sexual Life of Savages in North-Western Melanesia.* New York: Harcourt, Brace & World, 1929.

Mantz, Erin. "Suburban Swingers: Beyond the Sex." *Today.com*, July 29, 2008. http://to-day.msnbc.msn.com/id/25851876/ns/today-relationships/t/suburban-swingers-beyond-sex/#.UNfESqX3AUs.

Marshall, M. "'Four Hundred Rabbits': An Anthropological View of Ethanol as a Disinhibitor." In *Alcohol and Disinhibition: Nature and Meaning of the Link*, edited by R. Room and G. Collins, 186–204. Research monograph no. 12. Rockville, MD: US Department of Health and Human Services, 1983.

Martin, Lydia. "Lydia Has Lunch with Thomas Kramer." *Miami Herald*, November 13, 2011.

Martin, Patricia Yancey, and Robert A. Hummer. "Fraternities and Rape on Campus." In *Race, Class, and Gender: An Anthology*, edited by Margaret Anderson and Patricia Hill Collins. Belmont, CA: Wadsworth, 1989, 413–29.

Martin, Richard. "Powerful Exchanges: Ritual and Subjectivity in Berlin's BDSM Scene." PhD diss., Princeton University, 2011.

Marty, Myron A. *Daily Life in the United States, 1960–1990: Decades of Discord.* Westport, CT: Greenwood, 1997.

Maslow, Abraham. *Toward a Psychology of Being.* New York: Van Nostrand, 1968.

Matsumoto, David, and Hyi Sung Hwang. "Culture and Emotion." *Journal of Cross-Cultural Psychology* 43, no. 1 (2012): 91–118.

McInnes, David, Jack Bradley, and Garrett Prestage. "The Discourse of Gay Men's Group Sex: The Importance of Masculinity." *Culture, Health & Sexuality: An International Journal for Research, Intervention and Care* 11, no. 6 (2009): 641–54.

McKinley, James C. "Vicious Assault Shakes Texas Town." *New York Times*, March 8, 2011.

Meyer, Carla. Review of *Sex with Strangers*, directed by Joe Gantz and Harry Gantz. *SFGate*, February 22, 2002. www.sfgate.com/cgi-bin/article.cgi?f=/c/a/2002/02/22/DD77008.DTL.

Milano, Valerie. "Playboy TV—'Sex Curious.'" *Hollywood Today*, February 8, 2011. http://www.hollywoodtoday.net/2011/02/08/playboy-tv-%E2%80%9Csex-curious%E2%80%9D/.

Milkman, Harvey, and Stanley G. Sunderworth. *Craving for Ecstasy and Natural Highs: A Positive Approach to Mood Alteration.* Los Angeles: Sage, 2009.

Miller, Joshua Rhett. "Northwestern University Professor Defends Explicit Sex Toy Demonstration after Class." *Fox News*, March 3, 2011. http://www.foxnews.com/us/2011/03/03/northwestern-university-professor-defends-explicit-sex-toy-demonstration/?cmpid=cmty_%7BlinkBack%7D_Northwestern_University_Professor_Defends_Explicit_Sex_Toy_Demonstration_After_Class.

Miller, William Ian. *The Anatomy of Disgust.* Cambridge, MA: Harvard University Press, 1997.

Millet, Catherine. *The Sexual Life of Catherine M.* New York: Grove Press, 2003.

Ming Haoyue. "Is the 'Crime of Group Sex' Really Outdated?" *China Daily*, April 1, 2010. http://www.chinadaily.com.cn/cndy/2010-04/01/content_9672304.htm.

MMOrgy (blog). "State of Sex: Second Life." October 13, 2005. www.mmorgy.com/2005/10/state_of_sex_second_life_1.php.

Mokwena, S. "The Era of the Jackrollers: Contextualizing the Rise of Youth Gangs in Soweto." Paper presented at the Centre for the Study of Violence and Reconciliation, Johannesburg, October 30, 1991.

Mooney, Michael J. "Swinging through South Florida's Underground Sex Clubs." *Broward Palm Beach New Times*, March 3, 2011. http://www.browardpalmbeach.com/content/printVersion/1375004/.

Moore, Barrington Jr. *Privacy: Studies in Social and Cultural History.* Armonk, NY: M. E. Sharpe, 1984.

Moore, Malcolm. "Chinese Professor Jailed for Three-and-a-Half Years for Swinging." *Telegraph*, May 20, 2010. http://www.telegraph.co.uk/news/worldnews/asia/china/7743547/Chinese-professor-jailed-for-three-and-a-half-years-for-swinging.html.

Moore, Patrick. *Beyond Shame: Reclaiming the Abandoned History of Radical Sexuality.* Boston: Beacon Press, 2004.

Morin, Jack. *The Erotic Mind: Unlocking the Inner Source of Sexual Passion and Fulfillment.* New York: HarperCollins, 1995.

Morris, Alex. "They Know What Boys Want." *New York Magazine*, January 30, 2011. http://nymag.com/news/features/70977/.

———. "The Cuddle Puddle of Stuyvesant High School." *New York* Magazine, 2006. http://nymag.com/news/features/15589/.

Morrison, Keith. "Battling Sexual Addiction." *Dateline NBC*, February 24, 2004. http://www.msnbc.msn.com/id/4302347/ns/dateline_nbc/t/battling-sexual-addiction/#.T7RZ6464JlJ.

Moser, Charles. "S/M (Sadomasochistic) Interactions in Semi-Public Settings." *Journal of Homosexuality* 36, no. 2 (1998): 19–29.

Moskowitz, David A., and Michael E. Roloff. "The Ultimate High: Sexual Addiction and the Bug Chasing Phenomenon." *Sexual Addiction & Compulsivity* 14, no. 1 (2007): 21–40.

Murphy, Robert, and Leonard Kasdan. *The Structure of Parallel Cousin Marriage*. Indianapolis: Bobbs-Merrill, 1959.

Murphy, Yolanda, and Robert Francis Murphy. *Women of the Forest*. 2nd ed. New York: Columbia University Press, 1985.

Neumann, Caryn E. *Sexual Crime: A Reference Handbook*. Santa Barbara: ABC-CLIO, 2009.

Newitz, Annalee. "Swinging in the Suburbs." *Metro (Silicon Valley's Weekly Newspaper)*, 2000, 1–19.

Newkirk, Pamela. *Within the Veil: Black Journalists, White Media*. New York: New York University Press, 2000.

Newmahr, Staci. *Playing on the Edge: Sadomasochism, Risk, and Intimacy*. Bloomington: Indiana University Press, 2010.

Nicholas, India. "Swingers Go Wild for Bill Plympton." *Willamette Week* (staff blog), October 13, 2009. http://blogs.wweek.com/news/2009/10/13/swingers-go-wild-for-bill-plympton/.

Nitrate Online. Unsigned review of *The Lifestyle: Group Sex in the Suburbs*, directed by David Schisgall. www.nitrateonline.com/1999/fsiff99-3.html#Lifestyle.

Noh, David. Review of *Sex with Strangers*, directed by Joe Gantz and Harry Gantz. *Film Journal International*. http://www.filmjournal.com/filmjournal/esearch/article_display.jsp?vnu_content_id=1000696179.

Nolan, Larissa. "Collymore Revelation Lets 'Dogging' out of the Kennel." *Irish Independent*, March 7, 2004. http://www.independent.ie/irish-news/collymore-revelation-lets-dogging-out-of-the-kennel-26218546.html.

Nuttall, Jeff. *Bomb Culture*. New York: Delacorte Press, 1968.

Ogas, Ogi, and Sai Gaddam. *A Billion Wicked Thoughts: What the World's Largest Experiment Reveals about Human Desire*. New York: Dutton, 2011.

O'Neill, George C., and Nena O'Neill. "Patterns in Group Sexual Activity." *Journal of Sex Research* 6, no. 2 (1970): 101–12.

Organista, Kurt C. "HIV Prevention Models with Mexican Migrant Farmworkers." In *Practice Issues in HIV/AIDS Services: Empowerment-Based Models and Program Applications*, edited by Ronald J. Mancoske and James Donald Smith, 127–60. Binghamton, NY: Haworth Press, 2004.

Overweel, Jeroen A. *The Marind in a Changing Environment: A Study on Social-Economic Change in Marind Society to Assist in the Formulation of a Long Term Strategy for the Foundation for Social, Economic and Environmental Development (YAPSEL)*. Irian Jaya, Indonesia: YAPSEL, 1993.

Palamar, Joseph J., Mathew V. Kiang, Erik D. Storholm, and Perry N. Halkitis. "A Qualitative Descriptive Study of Perceived Sexual Effects of Club Drug Use in Gay and Bisexual Men." *Psychology & Sexuality ifirst* (2012): 1–18.

Parker, Paul Edward. "Juries Hear Big Dan's Rape Case." *Bristol County Century* (*Providence Journal*), November 1, 1999, C1.

Partridge, Burgo. *A History of Orgies*. London: SevenOaks, 2005. First published 1958.

Pateakos, Jay. "Brothers Break Silence in Big Dan's Rape Case." *Herald News*, October 25. 2009, http://www.heraldnews.com/news/local_news/x665149028/After-26-years-brothers-break-silence.

Payne, Stewart. "Police Arrest MySpace Party Girl." *Telegraph*, April 13, 2007. http://www.telegraph.co.uk/news/uknews/1548483/Police-arrest-MySpace-party-girl.html.

Perel, Esther. *Mating in Captivity: Unlocking Erotic Intelligence*. New York: Harper Perennial, 2007.

Perniola, Mario. "Between Clothing and Nudity." In *Fragments for a History of the Human Body*, edited by Michel Fehrer, 237–65. New York: Zone, 1989.

Pettman, Dominic. *After the Orgy: Toward a Politics of Exhaustion*. Albany: SUNY Press, 2002.

Peyser, Marc, Elizabeth Roberts, and Frappa Stout. "A Deadly Dance." *Newsweek*, September 29, 1997, 76–77.

Pfaus, James. "Revisiting the Concept of Sexual Motivation." *Annual Review of Sex Research* 10 (1999): 120.

Pfaus, James G., Mark F. Wilkins, Nina DiPietro, Michael Benibgui, Rachel Toledano, Anna Rowe, and Melissa Castro Couch. "Inhibitory and Disinhibitory Effects of Psychomotor Stimulants and Depressants on the Sexual Behavior of Male and Female Rats." *Hormones and Behavior* 58, no. 1 (2010): 163–76.

Pfaus, James, and John Pinel. "Alcohol Inhibits and Disinhibits Sexual Behavior in the Male Rat." *Psychobiology* 17, no. 2 (1989): 195–201.

Polack, Amira. "Eric Stotz: Hollywood Fundraiser." *Business Today*, Fall 2009. http://www.businesstoday.org/magazine/its-always-christmas-washington/eric-stotz-hollywood-fundraiser.

Pollack, Michael. "Homosexual Rituals and Safer Sex." *Journal of Homosexuality* 25, no. 3 (1993): 307–18.

Prestage, G., A. S. Fogarty, P. Rawstorne, J. Grierson, I. Zablotska, A. Grulich, and S. C. Kippax, "Use of Illicit Drugs among Gay Men Living with HIV in Sydney." *AIDS* 21, Suppl. 1 (2007): S49–55.

Prestage, Garrett, Jeff Hudson, Jack Bradley, Ian Down, Rob Sutherland, Nick Corrigan, Brad Gray, Baden Chalmers, Colin Batrouney, Paul Martin, David McInnes, Jeffrey Grierson, and Andrew Grulich. *TOMS: Three or More Study.* Sydney, Australia: National Centre in HIV Epidemiology and Clinical Research, University of New South Wales, 2008.

Quantum Buddha's Blog (blog). "Gang Rape 10,000." September 24, 2010. http://quantumbuddha.wordpress.com/2010/09/24/gang-rape-10000/. Accessed November 2012. By February 2013, the blog entry had been deleted, although it can still be found at http://www.progressivebloggers.ca/2010/09/gang-rape-10000/.

———. "Gang Rape 8,000." September 2010. http://quantumbuddha.wordpress.com/2010/09/17/gang-rape-8000/. Accessed November 2012. By February 2013, the blog entry had been deleted, although it can still be found at http://www.progressivebloggers.ca/2010/09/gang-rape-8000/.

Quenqua, Douglas. "Recklessly Seeking Sex on Craigslist." *New York Times*, April 17, 2009. http://www.nytimes.com/2009/04/19/fashion/19craigslist.html?_r=1&pagewanted=all.

Ramzy, Austin. "A Swinger's Case: China's Attitude toward Sex." *Time*, May 22, 2010. http://www.time.com/time/world/article/0,8599,1991029,00.html.

Recabarren, Andrea González. "Tribus urbanas: Pokemones y peloláis . . . ¿Cuánto sabes de ellos?" *Universia*, January 16, 2008. http://noticias.universia.cl/vida-universitaria/noticia/2008/01/16/314616/tribus-urbanas-pokemones-pelolais-sabes.html.

Rechy, John. *The Sexual Outlaw: A Documentary.* New York: Grove Press, 1977.

Rejali, Darius. "Ordinary Betrayals: Conceptualizing Refugees Who Have Been Tortured in the Global Village." *Human Rights Review* 1, no. 4 (2000): 8–25. Available at http://academic.reed.edu/poli_sci/faculty/rejali/articles/HRRarticle.html.

Rennie, Neil. "The Point Venus 'Scene.'" In *Science and Exploration in the Pacific: European Voyages to the Southern Oceans in the Eighteenth Century*, edited by Margarette Lincoln, 135–48. Woodbridge, Suffolk: Boydell & Brewer, 2002.

Reynolds, Robert, and Gerard Sullivan. *Gay Men's Sexual Stories: Getting It!* Binghamton, NY: Haworth SocialWork Practice Press, 2003.

Richters, Juliet. "Through a Hole in a Wall: Setting and Interaction in Sex-on-Premises Venues." *Sexualites* 10, no. 3 (2007): 275–97.

Roberti, Jonathan W. "A Review of Behavioral and Biological Correlates of Sensation Seeking." *Journal of Research in Personality* 38 (2004): 256–79.

Rothman, Hal K. *Devil's Bargains: Tourism in the Twentieth-Century American West.* Lawrence: University Press of Kansas, 1998.

Rubin, Gayle. "Thinking Sex: Notes for a Radical Theory of the Politics of Sexuality." In *Pleasure and Danger: Exploring Female Sexuality*, edited by Carole S. Vance, 267–319. Boston: Routledge and Kegan Paul, 1984.

Rubin, Gayle, and Judith Butler. "Sexual Traffic." *Differences: A Journal of Feminist Cultural Studies* 6, no. 2/3 (1994): 62–99.

Russell, Henry. *Craigslist Casual Encounters.* Los Angeles: Haha Publishing, 2010.

Ryan, Christopher, and Cacilda Jethá. *Sex at Dawn: The Prehistoric Origins of Modern Sexuality.* New York: Harper, 2010.

$am $loan.com. "The Sexual Freedom Movement in the 1960s." http://www.anusha.com/ sfl.htm.

Samuel, Henry. "Dominique Strauss-Kahn Did Not Know He Was Sleeping with Prostitutes 'Because They Were All Naked.'" *Telegraph*, September 6, 2012.

Samuel, Henry. "Dominique Strauss-Kahn: I Was Naive to Think I Could Get Away with Orgies." *Telegraph*, October 10, 2012. http://www.telegraph.co.uk/finance/dominique-strauss-kahn/9599236/Domi   nique-Strauss-Kahn-I-was-naive-to-think-I-could-get-away-with-orgies.html.

Sanday, Peggy R. *Fraternity Gang Rape: Sex, Brotherhood, and Privilege on Campus*. New York: New York University Press, 1990.

Satterfield, Jamie. "Slaying Victims Lost in the Furor." *Knoxnews.com*, May 27, 2007. http:// www.knoxnews.com/news/2007/may/27/slaying-victims-lost-in-the-furor/.

Savage, Dan. "Husband Has No Interest in Hot Wife." *Savage Love, Creative Loafing Charlotte*, March 24, 2009. http://clclt.com/charlotte/husband-has-no-interest-in-hot-wife/Content?oid=2152344.

Schemo, Diana Jean. "Sex Education with Just One Lesson: No Sex." *New York Times*, December 28, 2000. http://www.nytimes.com/2000/12/28/us/sex-education-with-just-one-lesson-no-sex.html?pagewanted=all&src=pm.

Scheper-Hughes, Nancy. *Death without Weeping: The Violence of Everyday Life in Brazil*. Berkeley: University of California Press, 1992.

Schnarch, David. *Passionate Marriage: Love, Sex, and Intimacy in Emotionally Committed Relationships*. New York: Henry Holt, 1997.

Scully, Diana, and Joseph Marolla. "'Riding the Bull at Gilley's': Convicted Rapists Describe the Rewards of Rape." *Social Problems* 32, no. 3 (1985): 251–62.

Seal, Mark. "The Prince Who Blew through Billions." *Vanity Fair*, July 2011. http:// www.vanityfair.com/society/features/2011/07/prince-jefri-201107.

Shackelford, Todd, and Aaron T. Goetz. "Psychological and Physiological Adaptations to Sperm Competition in Humans." *Review of General Psychology* 9, no. 3 (2005): 228-48.

Shin, Annys. "Engineering a Safer Burger: Technology Is Entrepreneur's Main Ingredient for Bacteria-Free Beef." *Washington Post*, June 12, 2008. http://www.washingtonpost.com/wp-dyn/content/article/2008/06/11/AR2008061103656_pf.html.

Shrivana, Rajesh. "Zoo Keepers Go 'Blue' in the Face for a Chimp off the Old Block . . ." *Deccan Herald*, December 25, 2011. http://www.deccanherald.com/content/43307/zoo-keepers-go-blue-face.html.

Shweder, Richard. "Toward a Deep Cultural Psychology of Shame." *Social Research* 70, no. 4 (2003): 1109–29.

Silver, Michael, and George Dohrman. "Adrift on Lake Woebegone." *Sports Illustrated*, October 24, 2005. http://sportsillustrated.cnn.com/vault/article/magazine/MAG1113465/3/index.htm.

Silverman, Stephen M. "Prince Harry Party Girl Tells of the Naked Night: Report." *People*, September   1,   2012.   http://www.people.com/people/package/article/0,,20395222_ 20626402,00.html.

Simon, Jonathan. "Taking Risks: Extreme Sports and the Embrace of Risk in Advanced Liberal Societies." In *Embracing Risk: The Changing Culture of Insurance and Responsibility*, edited by Tom Baker and Jonathan Simon, 177–208. Chicago: University of Chicago Press, 2002.

Smisek, Julian. "Group Sex and the Cultural Revolution—A Translation." Danwei, May 23, 2010. http://www.danwei.org/sexuality/group_sex_and_the_cultural_rev.php.

Smith, Lynn G., and James R. Smith. "Comarital Sex: The Incorporation of Extramarital Sex into the Marriage Relationship." In *Beyond Monogamy: Recent Studies of Sexual Alternatives in Marriage*, edited by James R. Smith and Lynn G. Smith, 84–102. Baltimore: Johns Hopkins University Press, 1974.

Smithstein, Samantha. "Marriage Like Water, 'Partner Swapping' Like Wine." *What the Wild Things Are* (blog), *Psychology Today*, May 20, 2010. http://www.psychologytoday.com/ blog/what-the-wild-things-are/201005/marriage-water-partner-swapping-wine.

Smoking Gun. "New Craigslist 'Group Sex' Bust." April 22, 2010. http://www.thesmokinggun.com/documents/crime/new-craigslist-group-sex-bust.

St. James, Izabella. *Bunny Tales: Behind Closed Doors at the Playboy Mansion*. Philadelphia: Running Press, 2006.

Steinberg, Ashley. "Rebels without Cause." *Newsweek*, March 17, 2008. http://www.thedailybeast.com/newsweek/2008/03/17/rebels-without-cause.html.

Steinberg, David. "Marco Vassi: My Aunt Nettie; *Where's Waldo?*" *Comes Naturally*, January 8, 1993. http://www.nearbycafe.com/loveandlust/steinberg/erotic/cn/cn3.html.

Steinberg, Jacques. "Extracurricular Sex Toy Lesson Draws Rebuke at Northwestern." *New York Times*, March 3, 2011. http://www.nytimes.com/2011/03/04/education/04northwestern.html?_r=2&.

Steinmetz, Ferrett. "Placing My First Swingers' Ad." *Ferrett* (blog), www.theferrett.com.

Suggs, Robert C. *The Hidden Worlds of Polynesia*. New York: New American Library, 1962.

———. *Marquesan Sexual Behavior*. New York: Harcourt, Brace & World, 1966.

Sukel, Kayt. "50 Shades of Grey (Matter): How Science Is Defying BDSM Stereotypes." Huffington Post, *Women* (blog), May 30, 2012. http://www.huffingtonpost.com/kayt-sukel/bdsm_b_1554310.html.

Superchief. "Dear General Public: Please Stop Sucking the Punk out of Pussy Riot, It's Crude and Disgusting." September 1, 2012. http://superchief.tv/dear-general-public-please-stop-sucking-the-punk-out-of-pussy-riot-its-crude-and-disgusting/.

Sussman, Anna Louie Sussman. "The Berlusconi in Us All: Bunga Bunga's Real Meaning." *Atlantic*, April 6, 2011. http://www.theatlantic.com/international/archive/2011/04/the-berlusconi-in-us-all-bunga-bungas-real-meaning/236871/1/.

Sutherland, Donald R. "The Religion of Gerrard Winstanley and Digger Communism." The Digger Archives, last updated January 31, 2013. http://www.diggers.org/diggers/religion_winstanley.htm.

Symonds, C. "Pilot Study of the Peripheral Behavior of Sexual Mate Swappers." Master's thesis, University of California, Riverside, 1968.

Tankink, Marian T. A. "The Silence of South-Sudanese Women: Social Risks in Talking about Experiences of Sexual Violence." *Culture, Health & Sexuality: An International Journal for Research, Intervention and Care* 15, no. 4 (2013): 391–403.

Tattleman, Ira. "The Meaning at the Wall: Tracing the Gay Bathhouse." In *Queers in Space: Communities/Public Places/Sites of Resistance*, edited by Gordon Brent Ingram, Anne-Marie Bouthillette, and Yolanda Retter, 391–406. Seattle: Bay Press, 1997.

Taylor, Christopher C. *Sacrifice as Terror: The Rwandan Genocide of 1994*. Oxford: Berg Press, 1999.

Tewksbury, Richard. "Bathhouse Intercourse: Structural and Behavoral Aspects of an Erotic Oasis." *Deviant Behavior* 23 (2002): 75–112.

Thomas, Helen, ed. *Dance in the City*. New York: St. Martin's, 1997.

Thomas, Nicholas. *Cook: The Extraordinary Sea Voyages of Captain James Cook*. New York: Bloomsbury Publishing, 2003.

Thompson, Mark, ed. *Leatherfolk: Radical Sex, People, Politics, and Practice*. Boston: Alyson Publications, 1991.

Tierney, John. "What's New? Exuberance for Novelty Has Benefits." *New York Times*, February 3, 2012. http://www.nytimes.com/2012/02/14/science/novelty-seeking-neophilia-can-be-a-predictor-of-well-being.html?_r=1&emc=eta1.

Trimpop, Rudiger M. *The Psychology of Risk Taking Behavior*. Amsterdam: North Holland, 1994.

Tulloch, John, and Deborah Lupton. *Risk and Everyday Life*. London: Sage, 2003.

Urban, Hugh. "The Beast with Two Backs: Aleister Crowley, Sex Magic and the Exhaustion of Modernity." *Journal of Alternative and Emergent Religions* 7, no. 3 (2004): 7–25.

———. *Magia Sexualis: Sex, Magic, and Liberation in Modern Western Esotericism*. Berkeley: University of California Press, 2006.

Vanlandingham, Mark, and Nancy Grandjean. "Some Cultural Underpinnings of Male Sexual Behaviour Patterns in Thailand." In *Sexual Cultures and Migration in the Era of AIDS:*

Anthropological and Demographic Perspectives, edited by Gilbert Herdt, 127–42. Oxford: Clarendon Press.

Vassi, Marco. *The Stoned Apocalypse*. Sag Harbor, NY: Second Chance Press, 1993.

Villarreal, Phil. Review of *Sex with Strangers*, directed by Joe Gantz and Harry Gantz. *Arizona Daily Star*, August 30, 2002.

Vogelman, Lloyd, and Sharon Lewis. "Gang Rape and the Culture of Violence in South Africa." *Der Überblick*, no. 2 (1993): 39–42.

Wagner, Mike. "Sex in Second Life." *Information Week*, May 26, 2007. http://www.informationweek.com/news/199701944?cid=email.

Walters, Lawrence G. "Obscenity Trial?" *New Statesman*, July 7, 2008. http://www.newstatesman.com/law-and-reform/2008/07/obscenity-community-google.

Ward, Clarissa. "'Panda Porn' to Boost Male's Sex Drive." *ABC News*, February 15, 2010. http://abcnews.go.com/Nightline/AmazingAnimals/porn-boost-male-pandas-sex-drives/story?id=9718714.

Ward, Jane. "Dude-Sex: White Masculinities and 'Authentic' Heterosexuality among Dudes Who Have Sex with Dudes." *Sexualities* 11, no. 4 (2008): 414–34.

Warner, Michael. "Why Gay Men Are Having Risky Sex." Appendix to *What Do Gay Men Want? An Essay on Sex, Risk, and Subjectivity*, by David M. Halperin. Ann Arbor: University of Michigan Press, 2007.

Warner, William Lloyd. *A Black Civilization: A Social Study of an Australian Tribe*. New York: Harper & Brothers, 1937.

Warner, William Lloyd. "Morphology and Functions of the Australian Murngin Type of Kinship." *American Anthropologist* 32, no. 2 (1930): 207–56.

Washington City Paper. "Crowning Cora." January 5, 1996. http://www.washingtoncitypaper.com/articles/9541/crowning-cora.

Washington Times. "Teacher Gets Jail Time in Orgy Case." May 21, 2010. http:www.washingtontimes.com/news/2010/may/21/teacher-gets-jail-time-in-orgy-case/.

Watts, Steven. *Mr Playboy: Hugh Hefner and the American Dream*. Hoboken, NJ: Wiley, 2008.

Wax, Emily. "'We Want to Make a Light Baby.'" *Washington Post*, June 30, 2004.

Wayne, Tim."Burning Man Review." *Tim Wayne* (blog). http://blog.hisnameistimmy.com/burning-man-our-review/12.

Weinberg, Martin S., and Colin J. Williams. "Gay Baths and the Social Organization of Impersonal Sex." *Social Problems* 23 (1975): 124–36.

Weiss, Margot D. *Techniques of Pleasure: BDSM and the Circuits of Sexuality*. Durham: Duke University Press, 2010.

Weller, Sheila. "Suddenly That Summer." *Vanity Fair*, July 2012. http://www.vanityfair.com/culture/2012/07/lsd-drugs-summer-of-love-sixties.

Westcott, Kathryn. "At Last: An Explanation for 'Bunga Bunga.'" *BBC News Europe*, February 5, 2011. http://www.bbc.co.uk/news/world-europe-12325796.

Westhaver, Russell. "Coming out of Your Skin: Circuit Parties, Pleasure, and the Subject." *Sexualites* 8, no. 3 (2005): 347-74.

Westhaver, Russell. "Flaunting and Empowerment: Thinking about Circuit Parties, the Body and Power." *Journal of Contemporary Ethnography* 35, no. 6 (2006): 611–44.

———. "Party Boys: Identity, Community, and the Circuit." PhD diss., Simon Fraser University, 2003.

Whitaker, Brian. *Unspeakable Love: Gay and Lesbian Life in the Middle East*. Berkeley: University of California Press, 2006.

White, Rachel R. "Sex Parties." *Time Out New York*, September 28, 2011. http://www.timeout.com/newyork/clubs-nightlife/sex-parties.

Whitehouse, Harvey. "Terror." In *The Oxford Handbook of Religion and Emotion*, edited by John Corrigan, 259–75. New York: Oxford University Press, 2008.

Williams, Holly. "Teen Spirit: The 'Skins' Sensation Sweeping France." *Independent*, July 31, 2010. http://www.independent.co.uk/arts-entertainment/tv/features/teen-spirit-the-skins-sensation-sweeping-france-2037470.html.

Wilson, Emmett. "Shame and the Other: Reflections on the Theme of Shame in French Psycho-analysis." In *The Many Faces of Shame*, edited by Donald Nathanson, 162–93. New York: Guilford Press, 1987.

Winokoor, Charles. "Frank O'Boy Speaks out on Big Dan's Rape Case." *Taunton Daily Gazette*, May 28, 2009. http://www.tauntongazette.com/news/x313662945/Frank-O-Boy-speaks-out-on-Big-Dan-s-rape-case.

Wojcicki, Janet Maia. "'She Drank His Money': Survival Sex and the Problem of Violence in Taverns in Gauteng Province, South Africa." *Medical Anthropology Quarterly* 16, no. 3 (2002): 267–93.

Wong, Edward. "18 Orgies Later, Chinese Swinger Gets Prison Bed." *New York Times*, May 20, 2010. http://www.nytimes.com/2010/05/21/world/asia/21china.html?_r=2&th&emc=th.

Wood, Kate. "Contextualizing Group Rape in Post-apartheid South Africa." *Culture, Health, and Sexuality* 7, no. 4 (2005): 303–17.

Woodward, Tali. "Life in Hell: In California Prisons, an Unconventional Gender Identity Can Be Like an Added Sentence." *San Francisco Bay Guardian*, March 15, 2006. http://www.sfbg.com/40/24/cover_life.html.

Wray, Matt. "Burning Man and the Rituals of Capitalism." *Bad Subjects* 21 (1995). http://bad.eserver.org/issues/1995/21/wray.html.

Yong, Ed. "Ballistic Penises and Corkscrew Vaginas—The Sexual Battles of Ducks." *Not Exactly Rocket Science* (blog), December 22, 2009. http://scienceblogs.com/notrocketscience/2009/12/22/ballistic-penises-and-corkscrew-vaginas-the-sexual-battles/.

Zuckerman, Marvin. "The Psychophysiology of Sensation Seeking." *Journal of Personality* 58, no. 1 (1990): 313–45.

Index